50% OFF
Online CRRN Prep Course!

By Mometrix

Dear Customer,

We consider it an honor and a privilege that you chose our CRRN Study Guide. As a way of showing our appreciation and to help us better serve you, we are offering **50% off our online CRRN Prep Course**. Many CRRN courses are needlessly expensive and don't deliver enough value. With our course, you get access to the best CRRN prep material, and **you only pay half price**.

We have structured our online course to perfectly complement your printed study guide. The CRRN Prep Course contains **in-depth lessons** that cover all the most important topics, **50+ video reviews** that explain difficult concepts, over **500 practice questions** to ensure you feel prepared, and more than **650 digital flashcards**, so you can study while you're on the go.

Online CRRN Prep Course

Topics Included:

- Nursing Models and Theories
    - Evidence-Based Practice
    - Nursing Process
- Functional Health Problems
    - Neurological Functions
    - Sensory Function
- The Function of the Rehabilitation Team and Transitions of Care
    - Collaboration
    - Community Reintegration or Transition to the Next Level Care
- Legislative, Economic, Ethical, and Legal Issues
    - Integration of Legislation and Regulations in Care Management
    - Cost-Effective Patient-Centered Care

Course Features:

- CRRN Study Guide
    - Get content that complements our best-selling study guide.
- Full-Length Practice Tests
    - With over 500 practice questions, you can test yourself again and again.
- Mobile Friendly
    - If you need to study on the go, the course is easily accessible from your mobile device.
- CRRN Flashcards
    - Our course includes a flashcard mode with over 650 content cards to help you study.

To receive this discount, visit us at <u>mometrix.com/university/crrn</u> or simply scan this QR code with your smartphone. At the checkout page, enter the discount code: **crrn50off**

If you have any questions or concerns, please contact us at <u>support@mometrix.com</u>.

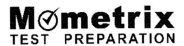

FREE Study Skills Videos/DVD Offer

Dear Customer,

Thank you for your purchase from Mometrix! We consider it an honor and a privilege that you have purchased our product and we want to ensure your satisfaction.

As part of our ongoing effort to meet the needs of test takers, we have developed a set of Study Skills Videos that we would like to give you for <u>FREE</u>. These videos cover our *best practices* for getting ready for your exam, from how to use our study materials to how to best prepare for the day of the test.

All that we ask is that you email us with feedback that would describe your experience so far with our product. Good, bad, or indifferent, we want to know what you think!

To get your FREE Study Skills Videos, you can use the **QR code** below, or send us an **email** at studyvideos@mometrix.com with *FREE VIDEOS* in the subject line and the following information in the body of the email:

- The name of the product you purchased.
- Your product rating on a scale of 1-5, with 5 being the highest rating.
- Your feedback. It can be long, short, or anything in between. We just want to know your impressions and experience so far with our product. (Good feedback might include how our study material met your needs and ways we might be able to make it even better. You could highlight features that you found helpful or features that you think we should add.)

If you have any questions or concerns, please don't hesitate to contact me directly.

Thanks again!

Sincerely,

Jay Willis
Vice President
jay.willis@mometrix.com
1-800-673-8175

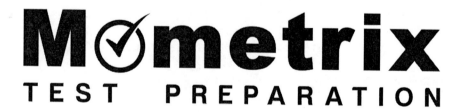

CRRN
Exam
Secrets

Study Guide
Your Key to Exam Success

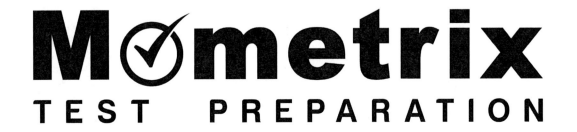

Written and edited by the Mometrix Nursing Certification Test Team

Printed in the United States of America

This paper meets the requirements of ANSI/NISO Z39.48-1992 (Permanence of Paper).

Mometrix offers volume discount pricing to institutions. For more information or a price quote, please contact our sales department at sales@mometrix.com or 888-248-1219.

Mometrix Media LLC is not affiliated with or endorsed by any official testing organization. All organizational and test names are trademarks of their respective owners.

Paperback
ISBN 13: 978-1-60971-533-5
ISBN 10: 1-60971-533-0

Ebook
ISBN 13: 978-1-62120-297-4
ISBN 10: 1-62120-297-6

DEAR FUTURE EXAM SUCCESS STORY

First of all, **THANK YOU** for purchasing Mometrix study materials!

Second, congratulations! You are one of the few determined test-takers who are committed to doing whatever it takes to excel on your exam. **You have come to the right place.** We developed these study materials with one goal in mind: to deliver you the information you need in a format that's concise and easy to use.

In addition to optimizing your guide for the content of the test, we've outlined our recommended steps for breaking down the preparation process into small, attainable goals so you can make sure you stay on track.

We've also analyzed the entire test-taking process, identifying the most common pitfalls and showing how you can overcome them and be ready for any curveball the test throws you.

Standardized testing is one of the biggest obstacles on your road to success, which only increases the importance of doing well in the high-pressure, high-stakes environment of test day. Your results on this test could have a significant impact on your future, and this guide provides the information and practical advice to help you achieve your full potential on test day.

Your success is our success

We would love to hear from you! If you would like to share the story of your exam success or if you have any questions or comments in regard to our products, please contact us at **800-673-8175** or **support@mometrix.com**.

Thanks again for your business and we wish you continued success!

Sincerely,
The Mometrix Test Preparation Team

> **Need more help? Check out our flashcards at:**
> **http://mometrixflashcards.com/CRRN**

TABLE OF CONTENTS

INTRODUCTION _____ 1
   REVIEW VIDEO DIRECTORY _____ 1

SECRET KEY #1 – PLAN BIG, STUDY SMALL _____ 2

SECRET KEY #2 – MAKE YOUR STUDYING COUNT _____ 3

SECRET KEY #3 – PRACTICE THE RIGHT WAY _____ 4

SECRET KEY #4 – PACE YOURSELF _____ 6

SECRET KEY #5 – HAVE A PLAN FOR GUESSING _____ 7

TEST-TAKING STRATEGIES _____ 10

NURSING MODELS AND THEORIES _____ 15
   EVIDENCE-BASED PRACTICE _____ 15
   NURSING THEORIES AND MODELS SIGNIFICANT TO REHABILITATION _____ 18
   NURSING PROCESS _____ 23
   RELATED THEORIES AND MODELS _____ 24
   REHABILITATION STANDARDS AND SCOPE OF PRACTICE _____ 30
   TECHNOLOGY _____ 33

FUNCTIONAL HEALTH PATTERNS _____ 34
   RESTORATION AND PRESERVATION OF HEALTH AND WELLBEING _____ 34
   OPTIMAL PSYCHOSOCIAL PATTERNS AND HOLISTIC WELLBEING _____ 47
   COPING AND STRESS MANAGEMENT SKILLS _____ 56
   MUSCULOSKELETAL FUNCTIONAL ABILITY _____ 68
   RESPIRATORY FUNCTIONAL ABILITY _____ 91
   CARDIOVASCULAR FUNCTIONAL ABILITY _____ 99
   NEUROLOGICAL FUNCTION _____ 107
   SENSORY FUNCTION _____ 139
   SAFETY CONCERNS _____ 145
   ABILITY TO COMMUNICATE EFFECTIVELY _____ 150
   OPTIMAL NUTRITION AND HYDRATION _____ 157
   ELIMINATION PATTERNS _____ 179
   SLEEP AND REST PATTERNS _____ 196

THE FUNCTION OF THE REHABILITATION TEAM AND TRANSITIONS OF CARE ____ 200
   COLLABORATION _____ 200
   COMMUNITY REINTEGRATION OR TRANSITION TO THE NEXT LEVEL OF CARE _____ 203

LEGISLATIVE, ECONOMIC, ETHICAL, AND LEGAL ISSUES _____ 208
   INTEGRATION OF LEGISLATION AND REGULATIONS IN CARE MANAGEMENT _____ 208
   COST-EFFECTIVE PATIENT-CENTERED CARE _____ 214
   ETHICAL CONSIDERATIONS AND LEGAL OBLIGATIONS THAT AFFECT PRACTICE ____ 216
   PROMOTING A SAFE ENVIRONMENT _____ 221
   QUALITY IMPROVEMENT PROCESSES _____ 223

CRRN PRACTICE TEST #1 _____ 226

ANSWER KEY AND EXPLANATIONS FOR TEST#1 _____ 253

CRRN PRACTICE TEST #2 _____ 274

HOW TO OVERCOME TEST ANXIETY _____ 275

ADDITIONAL BONUS MATERIAL _____ 281

Introduction

Thank you for purchasing this resource! You have made the choice to prepare yourself for a test that could have a huge impact on your future, and this guide is designed to help you be fully ready for test day. Obviously, it's important to have a solid understanding of the test material, but you also need to be prepared for the unique environment and stressors of the test, so that you can perform to the best of your abilities.

For this purpose, the first section that appears in this guide is the **Secret Keys**. We've devoted countless hours to meticulously researching what works and what doesn't, and we've boiled down our findings to the five most impactful steps you can take to improve your performance on the test. We start at the beginning with study planning and move through the preparation process, all the way to the testing strategies that will help you get the most out of what you know when you're finally sitting in front of the test.

We recommend that you start preparing for your test as far in advance as possible. However, if you've bought this guide as a last-minute study resource and only have a few days before your test, we recommend that you skip over the first two Secret Keys since they address a long-term study plan.

If you struggle with **test anxiety**, we strongly encourage you to check out our recommendations for how you can overcome it. Test anxiety is a formidable foe, but it can be beaten, and we want to make sure you have the tools you need to defeat it.

Review Video Directory

As you work your way through this guide, you will see numerous review video links interspersed with the written content. If you would like to access all of these review videos in one place, click on the video directory link found on the bonus page: **mometrix.com/bonus948/crrn**

Secret Key #1 – Plan Big, Study Small

There's a lot riding on your performance. If you want to ace this test, you're going to need to keep your skills sharp and the material fresh in your mind. You need a plan that lets you review everything you need to know while still fitting in your schedule. We'll break this strategy down into three categories.

Information Organization

Start with the information you already have: the official test outline. From this, you can make a complete list of all the concepts you need to cover before the test. Organize these concepts into groups that can be studied together, and create a list of any related vocabulary you need to learn so you can brush up on any difficult terms. You'll want to keep this vocabulary list handy once you actually start studying since you may need to add to it along the way.

Time Management

Once you have your set of study concepts, decide how to spread them out over the time you have left before the test. Break your study plan into small, clear goals so you have a manageable task for each day and know exactly what you're doing. Then just focus on one small step at a time. When you manage your time this way, you don't need to spend hours at a time studying. Studying a small block of content for a short period each day helps you retain information better and avoid stressing over how much you have left to do. You can relax knowing that you have a plan to cover everything in time. In order for this strategy to be effective though, you have to start studying early and stick to your schedule. Avoid the exhaustion and futility that comes from last-minute cramming!

Study Environment

The environment you study in has a big impact on your learning. Studying in a coffee shop, while probably more enjoyable, is not likely to be as fruitful as studying in a quiet room. It's important to keep distractions to a minimum. You're only planning to study for a short block of time, so make the most of it. Don't pause to check your phone or get up to find a snack. It's also important to **avoid multitasking**. Research has consistently shown that multitasking will make your studying dramatically less effective. Your study area should also be comfortable and well-lit so you don't have the distraction of straining your eyes or sitting on an uncomfortable chair.

 The time of day you study is also important. You want to be rested and alert. Don't wait until just before bedtime. Study when you'll be most likely to comprehend and remember. Even better, if you know what time of day your test will be, set that time aside for study. That way your brain will be used to working on that subject at that specific time and you'll have a better chance of recalling information.

Finally, it can be helpful to team up with others who are studying for the same test. Your actual studying should be done in as isolated an environment as possible, but the work of organizing the information and setting up the study plan can be divided up. In between study sessions, you can discuss with your teammates the concepts that you're all studying and quiz each other on the details. Just be sure that your teammates are as serious about the test as you are. If you find that your study time is being replaced with social time, you might need to find a new team.

Secret Key #2 – Make Your Studying Count

You're devoting a lot of time and effort to preparing for this test, so you want to be absolutely certain it will pay off. This means doing more than just reading the content and hoping you can remember it on test day. It's important to make every minute of study count. There are two main areas you can focus on to make your studying count.

Retention

It doesn't matter how much time you study if you can't remember the material. You need to make sure you are retaining the concepts. To check your retention of the information you're learning, try recalling it at later times with minimal prompting. Try carrying around flashcards and glance at one or two from time to time or ask a friend who's also studying for the test to quiz you.

To enhance your retention, look for ways to put the information into practice so that you can apply it rather than simply recalling it. If you're using the information in practical ways, it will be much easier to remember. Similarly, it helps to solidify a concept in your mind if you're not only reading it to yourself but also explaining it to someone else. Ask a friend to let you teach them about a concept you're a little shaky on (or speak aloud to an imaginary audience if necessary). As you try to summarize, define, give examples, and answer your friend's questions, you'll understand the concepts better and they will stay with you longer. Finally, step back for a big picture view and ask yourself how each piece of information fits with the whole subject. When you link the different concepts together and see them working together as a whole, it's easier to remember the individual components.

Finally, practice showing your work on any multi-step problems, even if you're just studying. Writing out each step you take to solve a problem will help solidify the process in your mind, and you'll be more likely to remember it during the test.

Modality

Modality simply refers to the means or method by which you study. Choosing a study modality that fits your own individual learning style is crucial. No two people learn best in exactly the same way, so it's important to know your strengths and use them to your advantage.

For example, if you learn best by visualization, focus on visualizing a concept in your mind and draw an image or a diagram. Try color-coding your notes, illustrating them, or creating symbols that will trigger your mind to recall a learned concept. If you learn best by hearing or discussing information, find a study partner who learns the same way or read aloud to yourself. Think about how to put the information in your own words. Imagine that you are giving a lecture on the topic and record yourself so you can listen to it later.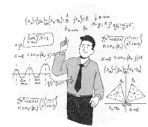

For any learning style, flashcards can be helpful. Organize the information so you can take advantage of spare moments to review. Underline key words or phrases. Use different colors for different categories. Mnemonic devices (such as creating a short list in which every item starts with the same letter) can also help with retention. Find what works best for you and use it to store the information in your mind most effectively and easily.

Secret Key #3 – Practice the Right Way

Your success on test day depends not only on how many hours you put into preparing, but also on whether you prepared the right way. It's good to check along the way to see if your studying is paying off. One of the most effective ways to do this is by taking practice tests to evaluate your progress. Practice tests are useful because they show exactly where you need to improve. Every time you take a practice test, pay special attention to these three groups of questions:

- The questions you got wrong
- The questions you had to guess on, even if you guessed right
- The questions you found difficult or slow to work through

This will show you exactly what your weak areas are, and where you need to devote more study time. Ask yourself why each of these questions gave you trouble. Was it because you didn't understand the material? Was it because you didn't remember the vocabulary? Do you need more repetitions on this type of question to build speed and confidence? Dig into those questions and figure out how you can strengthen your weak areas as you go back to review the material.

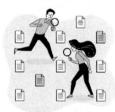

Additionally, many practice tests have a section explaining the answer choices. It can be tempting to read the explanation and think that you now have a good understanding of the concept. However, an explanation likely only covers part of the question's broader context. Even if the explanation makes perfect sense, **go back and investigate** every concept related to the question until you're positive you have a thorough understanding.

As you go along, keep in mind that the practice test is just that: practice. Memorizing these questions and answers will not be very helpful on the actual test because it is unlikely to have any of the same exact questions. If you only know the right answers to the sample questions, you won't be prepared for the real thing. **Study the concepts** until you understand them fully, and then you'll be able to answer any question that shows up on the test.

It's important to wait on the practice tests until you're ready. If you take a test on your first day of study, you may be overwhelmed by the amount of material covered and how much you need to learn. Work up to it gradually.

On test day, you'll need to be prepared for answering questions, managing your time, and using the test-taking strategies you've learned. It's a lot to balance, like a mental marathon that will have a big impact on your future. Like training for a marathon, you'll need to start slowly and work your way up. When test day arrives, you'll be ready.

Start with the strategies you've read in the first two Secret Keys—plan your course and study in the way that works best for you. If you have time, consider using multiple study resources to get different approaches to the same concepts. It can be helpful to see difficult concepts from more than one angle. Then find a good source for practice tests. Many times, the test website will suggest potential study resources or provide sample tests.

Practice Test Strategy

If you're able to find at least three practice tests, we recommend this strategy:

UNTIMED AND OPEN-BOOK PRACTICE

Take the first test with no time constraints and with your notes and study guide handy. Take your time and focus on applying the strategies you've learned.

TIMED AND OPEN-BOOK PRACTICE

Take the second practice test open-book as well, but set a timer and practice pacing yourself to finish in time.

TIMED AND CLOSED-BOOK PRACTICE

Take any other practice tests as if it were test day. Set a timer and put away your study materials. Sit at a table or desk in a quiet room, imagine yourself at the testing center, and answer questions as quickly and accurately as possible.

Keep repeating timed and closed-book tests on a regular basis until you run out of practice tests or it's time for the actual test. Your mind will be ready for the schedule and stress of test day, and you'll be able to focus on recalling the material you've learned.

Secret Key #4 – Pace Yourself

Once you're fully prepared for the material on the test, your biggest challenge on test day will be managing your time. Just knowing that the clock is ticking can make you panic even if you have plenty of time left. Work on pacing yourself so you can build confidence against the time constraints of the exam. Pacing is a difficult skill to master, especially in a high-pressure environment, so **practice is vital**.

Set time expectations for your pace based on how much time is available. For example, if a section has 60 questions and the time limit is 30 minutes, you know you have to average 30 seconds or less per question in order to answer them all. Although 30 seconds is the hard limit, set 25 seconds per question as your goal, so you reserve extra time to spend on harder questions. When you budget extra time for the harder questions, you no longer have any reason to stress when those questions take longer to answer.

Don't let this time expectation distract you from working through the test at a calm, steady pace, but keep it in mind so you don't spend too much time on any one question. Recognize that taking extra time on one question you don't understand may keep you from answering two that you do understand later in the test. If your time limit for a question is up and you're still not sure of the answer, mark it and move on, and come back to it later if the time and the test format allow. If the testing format doesn't allow you to return to earlier questions, just make an educated guess; then put it out of your mind and move on.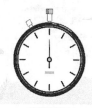

On the easier questions, be careful not to rush. It may seem wise to hurry through them so you have more time for the challenging ones, but it's not worth missing one if you know the concept and just didn't take the time to read the question fully. Work efficiently but make sure you understand the question and have looked at all of the answer choices, since more than one may seem right at first.

Even if you're paying attention to the time, you may find yourself a little behind at some point. You should speed up to get back on track, but do so wisely. Don't panic; just take a few seconds less on each question until you're caught up. Don't guess without thinking, but do look through the answer choices and eliminate any you know are wrong. If you can get down to two choices, it is often worthwhile to guess from those. Once you've chosen an answer, move on and don't dwell on any that you skipped or had to hurry through. If a question was taking too long, chances are it was one of the harder ones, so you weren't as likely to get it right anyway.

On the other hand, if you find yourself getting ahead of schedule, it may be beneficial to slow down a little. The more quickly you work, the more likely you are to make a careless mistake that will affect your score. You've budgeted time for each question, so don't be afraid to spend that time. Practice an efficient but careful pace to get the most out of the time you have.

Secret Key #5 – Have a Plan for Guessing

When you're taking the test, you may find yourself stuck on a question. Some of the answer choices seem better than others, but you don't see the one answer choice that is obviously correct. What do you do?

The scenario described above is very common, yet most test takers have not effectively prepared for it. Developing and practicing a plan for guessing may be one of the single most effective uses of your time as you get ready for the exam.

In developing your plan for guessing, there are three questions to address:

- When should you start the guessing process?
- How should you narrow down the choices?
- Which answer should you choose?

When to Start the Guessing Process

Unless your plan for guessing is to select C every time (which, despite its merits, is not what we recommend), you need to leave yourself enough time to apply your answer elimination strategies. Since you have a limited amount of time for each question, that means that if you're going to give yourself the best shot at guessing correctly, you have to decide quickly whether or not you will guess.

Of course, the best-case scenario is that you don't have to guess at all, so first, see if you can answer the question based on your knowledge of the subject and basic reasoning skills. Focus on the key words in the question and try to jog your memory of related topics. Give yourself a chance to bring the knowledge to mind, but once you realize that you don't have (or you can't access) the knowledge you need to answer the question, it's time to start the guessing process.

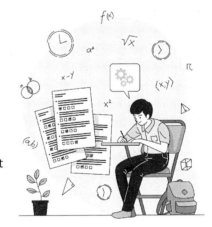

It's almost always better to start the guessing process too early than too late. It only takes a few seconds to remember something and answer the question from knowledge. Carefully eliminating wrong answer choices takes longer. Plus, going through the process of eliminating answer choices can actually help jog your memory.

Summary: Start the guessing process as soon as you decide that you can't answer the question based on your knowledge.

How to Narrow Down the Choices

The next chapter in this book (**Test-Taking Strategies**) includes a wide range of strategies for how to approach questions and how to look for answer choices to eliminate. You will definitely want to read those carefully, practice them, and figure out which ones work best for you. Here though, we're going to address a mindset rather than a particular strategy.

Your odds of guessing an answer correctly depend on how many options you are choosing from.

Number of options left	5	4	3	2	1
Odds of guessing correctly	20%	25%	33%	50%	100%

You can see from this chart just how valuable it is to be able to eliminate incorrect answers and make an educated guess, but there are two things that many test takers do that cause them to miss out on the benefits of guessing:

- Accidentally eliminating the correct answer
- Selecting an answer based on an impression

We'll look at the first one here, and the second one in the next section.

To avoid accidentally eliminating the correct answer, we recommend a thought exercise called **the $5 challenge**. In this challenge, you only eliminate an answer choice from contention if you are willing to bet $5 on it being wrong. Why $5? Five dollars is a small but not insignificant amount of money. It's an amount you could afford to lose but wouldn't want to throw away. And while losing $5 once might not hurt too much, doing

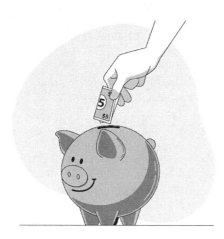

it twenty times will set you back $100. In the same way, each small decision you make—eliminating a choice here, guessing on a question there—won't by itself impact your score very much, but when you put them all together, they can make a big difference. By holding each answer choice elimination decision to a higher standard, you can reduce the risk of accidentally eliminating the correct answer.

The $5 challenge can also be applied in a positive sense: If you are willing to bet $5 that an answer choice *is* correct, go ahead and mark it as correct.

Summary: Only eliminate an answer choice if you are willing to bet $5 that it is wrong.

Which Answer to Choose

You're taking the test. You've run into a hard question and decided you'll have to guess. You've eliminated all the answer choices you're willing to bet $5 on. Now you have to pick an answer. Why do we even need to talk about this? Why can't you just pick whichever one you feel like when the time comes?

The answer to these questions is that if you don't come into the test with a plan, you'll rely on your impression to select an answer choice, and if you do that, you risk falling into a trap. The test writers know that everyone who takes their test will be guessing on some of the questions, so they intentionally write wrong answer choices to seem plausible. You still have to pick an answer though, and if the wrong answer choices are designed to look right, how can you ever be sure that you're not falling for their trap? The best solution we've found to this dilemma is to take the decision out of your hands entirely. Here is the process we recommend:

Once you've eliminated any choices that you are confident (willing to bet $5) are wrong, select the first remaining choice as your answer.

Whether you choose to select the first remaining choice, the second, or the last, the important thing is that you use some preselected standard. Using this approach guarantees that you will not be enticed into selecting an answer choice that looks right, because you are not basing your decision on how the answer choices look.

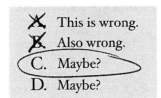

This is not meant to make you question your knowledge. Instead, it is to help you recognize the difference between your knowledge and your impressions. There's a huge difference between thinking an answer is right because of what you know, and thinking an answer is right because it looks or sounds like it should be right.

Summary: To ensure that your selection is appropriately random, make a predetermined selection from among all answer choices you have not eliminated.

Test-Taking Strategies

This section contains a list of test-taking strategies that you may find helpful as you work through the test. By taking what you know and applying logical thought, you can maximize your chances of answering any question correctly!

It is very important to realize that every question is different and every person is different: no single strategy will work on every question, and no single strategy will work for every person. That's why we've included all of them here, so you can try them out and determine which ones work best for different types of questions and which ones work best for you.

Question Strategies

☑ READ CAREFULLY

Read the question and the answer choices carefully. Don't miss the question because you misread the terms. You have plenty of time to read each question thoroughly and make sure you understand what is being asked. Yet a happy medium must be attained, so don't waste too much time. You must read carefully and efficiently.

☑ CONTEXTUAL CLUES

Look for contextual clues. If the question includes a word you are not familiar with, look at the immediate context for some indication of what the word might mean. Contextual clues can often give you all the information you need to decipher the meaning of an unfamiliar word. Even if you can't determine the meaning, you may be able to narrow down the possibilities enough to make a solid guess at the answer to the question.

☑ PREFIXES

If you're having trouble with a word in the question or answer choices, try dissecting it. Take advantage of every clue that the word might include. Prefixes can be a huge help. Usually, they allow you to determine a basic meaning. *Pre-* means before, *post-* means after, *pro-* is positive, *de-* is negative. From prefixes, you can get an idea of the general meaning of the word and try to put it into context.

☑ HEDGE WORDS

Watch out for critical hedge words, such as *likely, may, can, sometimes, often, almost, mostly, usually, generally, rarely,* and *sometimes.* Question writers insert these hedge phrases to cover every possibility. Often an answer choice will be wrong simply because it leaves no room for exception. Be on guard for answer choices that have definitive words such as *exactly* and *always.*

☑ SWITCHBACK WORDS

Stay alert for *switchbacks.* These are the words and phrases frequently used to alert you to shifts in thought. The most common switchback words are *but, although,* and *however.* Others include *nevertheless, on the other hand, even though, while, in spite of, despite,* and *regardless of.* Switchback words are important to catch because they can change the direction of the question or an answer choice.

☑ FACE VALUE

When in doubt, use common sense. Accept the situation in the problem at face value. Don't read too much into it. These problems will not require you to make wild assumptions. If you have to go beyond creativity and warp time or space in order to have an answer choice fit the question, then you should move on and consider the other answer choices. These are normal problems rooted in reality. The applicable relationship or explanation may not be readily apparent, but it is there for you to figure out. Use your common sense to interpret anything that isn't clear.

10

Answer Choice Strategies

☑ ANSWER SELECTION

The most thorough way to pick an answer choice is to identify and eliminate wrong answers until only one is left, then confirm it is the correct answer. Sometimes an answer choice may immediately seem right, but be careful. The test writers will usually put more than one reasonable answer choice on each question, so take a second to read all of them and make sure that the other choices are not equally obvious. As long as you have time left, it is better to read every answer choice than to pick the first one that looks right without checking the others.

☑ ANSWER CHOICE FAMILIES

An answer choice family consists of two (in rare cases, three) answer choices that are very similar in construction and cannot all be true at the same time. If you see two answer choices that are direct opposites or parallels, one of them is usually the correct answer. For instance, if one answer choice says that quantity x increases and another either says that quantity x decreases (opposite) or says that quantity y increases (parallel), then those answer choices would fall into the same family. An answer choice that doesn't match the construction of the answer choice family is more likely to be incorrect. Most questions will not have answer choice families, but when they do appear, you should be prepared to recognize them.

☑ ELIMINATE ANSWERS

Eliminate answer choices as soon as you realize they are wrong, but make sure you consider all possibilities. If you are eliminating answer choices and realize that the last one you are left with is also wrong, don't panic. Start over and consider each choice again. There may be something you missed the first time that you will realize on the second pass.

☑ AVOID FACT TRAPS

Don't be distracted by an answer choice that is factually true but doesn't answer the question. You are looking for the choice that answers the question. Stay focused on what the question is asking for so you don't accidentally pick an answer that is true but incorrect. Always go back to the question and make sure the answer choice you've selected actually answers the question and is not merely a true statement.

☑ EXTREME STATEMENTS

In general, you should avoid answers that put forth extreme actions as standard practice or proclaim controversial ideas as established fact. An answer choice that states the "process should be used in certain situations, if…" is much more likely to be correct than one that states the "process should be discontinued completely." The first is a calm rational statement and doesn't even make a definitive, uncompromising stance, using a hedge word *if* to provide wiggle room, whereas the second choice is far more extreme.

☑ BENCHMARK

As you read through the answer choices and you come across one that seems to answer the question well, mentally select that answer choice. This is not your final answer, but it's the one that will help you evaluate the other answer choices. The one that you selected is your benchmark or standard for judging each of the other answer choices. Every other answer choice must be compared to your benchmark. That choice is correct until proven otherwise by another answer choice beating it. If you find a better answer, then that one becomes your new benchmark. Once you've decided that no other choice answers the question as well as your benchmark, you have your final answer.

⊘ PREDICT THE ANSWER

Before you even start looking at the answer choices, it is often best to try to predict the answer. When you come up with the answer on your own, it is easier to avoid distractions and traps because you will know exactly what to look for. The right answer choice is unlikely to be word-for-word what you came up with, but it should be a close match. Even if you are confident that you have the right answer, you should still take the time to read each option before moving on.

General Strategies

⊘ TOUGH QUESTIONS

If you are stumped on a problem or it appears too hard or too difficult, don't waste time. Move on! Remember though, if you can quickly check for obviously incorrect answer choices, your chances of guessing correctly are greatly improved. Before you completely give up, at least try to knock out a couple of possible answers. Eliminate what you can and then guess at the remaining answer choices before moving on.

⊘ CHECK YOUR WORK

Since you will probably not know every term listed and the answer to every question, it is important that you get credit for the ones that you do know. Don't miss any questions through careless mistakes. If at all possible, try to take a second to look back over your answer selection and make sure you've selected the correct answer choice and haven't made a costly careless mistake (such as marking an answer choice that you didn't mean to mark). This quick double check should more than pay for itself in caught mistakes for the time it costs.

⊘ PACE YOURSELF

It's easy to be overwhelmed when you're looking at a page full of questions; your mind is confused and full of random thoughts, and the clock is ticking down faster than you would like. Calm down and maintain the pace that you have set for yourself. Especially as you get down to the last few minutes of the test, don't let the small numbers on the clock make you panic. As long as you are on track by monitoring your pace, you are guaranteed to have time for each question.

⊘ DON'T RUSH

It is very easy to make errors when you are in a hurry. Maintaining a fast pace in answering questions is pointless if it makes you miss questions that you would have gotten right otherwise. Test writers like to include distracting information and wrong answers that seem right. Taking a little extra time to avoid careless mistakes can make all the difference in your test score. Find a pace that allows you to be confident in the answers that you select.

⊘ KEEP MOVING

Panicking will not help you pass the test, so do your best to stay calm and keep moving. Taking deep breaths and going through the answer elimination steps you practiced can help to break through a stress barrier and keep your pace.

Final Notes

The combination of a solid foundation of content knowledge and the confidence that comes from practicing your plan for applying that knowledge is the key to maximizing your performance on test day. As your foundation of content knowledge is built up and strengthened, you'll find that the strategies included in this chapter become more and more effective in helping you quickly sift through the distractions and traps of the test to isolate the correct answer.

Now that you're preparing to move forward into the test content chapters of this book, be sure to keep your goal in mind. As you read, think about how you will be able to apply this information on the test. If you've already seen sample questions for the test and you have an idea of the question format and style, try to come up with questions of your own that you can answer based on what you're reading. This will give you valuable practice applying your knowledge in the same ways you can expect to on test day.

Good luck and good studying!

Nursing Models and Theories

Evidence-Based Practice

CLASSES OF EVIDENCE-BASED PRACTICE

Evidence-based practice is treatment based on the best possible evidence, including a study of current research. Literature is searched to find evidence of the most effective treatments for specific diseases or injuries, and those treatments are then utilized to create clinical pathways that outline specific multi-departmental treatment protocols, including medications, treatments, and timelines. Evidence-based guidelines are often produced by specialty organizations that undertake the task of searching and analyzing literature to produce policies, procedures, and guidelines that become the standard of care for the disease. These guidelines are then used when a patient fits the disease criteria for that guideline.

Evidence-based nursing aims to improve the quality of nursing care by examining the reasons for all nursing practices and determining those that have the most positive outcomes. Evidence-based nursing focuses on the individual nurse utilizing evidence-based observations to influence decision-making.

EVIDENCE-BASED PRACTICE GUIDELINES

The creation of evidence-based practice guidelines includes the following components:

- **Focus on the topic/methodology:** This includes outlining possible interventions and treatments for review, choosing patient populations and settings, and determining significant outcomes. Search boundaries (such as types of journals, types of studies, dates of studies) should be determined.
- **Evidence review:** This includes review of literature, critical analysis of studies, and summarizing of results, including pooled meta-analysis.
- **Expert judgment:** Recommendations based on personal experience from a number of experts may be utilized, especially if there is inadequate evidence based on review, but this subjective evidence should be explicitly acknowledged.
- **Policy considerations:** This includes cost-effectiveness, access to care, insurance coverage, availability of qualified staff, and legal implications.
- **Policy:** A written policy must be completed with recommendations. Common practice is to utilize letter guidelines, with "A" being the most highly recommended, usually based on the quality of supporting evidence.
- **Review:** The completed policy should be submitted to peers for review and comments before instituting the policy.

CRITICAL PATHWAYS

Clinical/critical pathway development is done by those involved in direct patient care. The pathway should require no additional staffing and cover the entire scope of an illness. Steps include:

1. Selection of patient group and diagnosis, procedures, or conditions, based on analysis of data and observations of wide variance in approach to treatment and prioritizing organization and patient needs
2. Creation of interdisciplinary team of those involved in the process of care, including physicians to develop pathway
3. Analysis of data including literature review and study of best practices to identify opportunities for quality improvement
4. Identification of all categories of care, such as nutrition, medications, and nursing
5. Discussion and reaching consensus
6. Identifying the levels of care and number of days to be covered by the pathway

15

7. Pilot testing and redesigning steps as indicated
8. Educating staff about standards
9. Monitoring and tracking variances in order to improve pathways

LEVELS OF EVIDENCE IN EVIDENCE-BASED PRACTICE

Levels of evidence are categorized according to the scientific evidence available to support the recommendations, as well as existing state and federal laws. While recommendations are voluntary, they are often used as a basis for state and federal regulations.

- **Category IA** is well supported by evidence from experimental, clinical, or epidemiologic studies and is strongly recommended for implementation.
- **Category IB** has supporting evidence from some studies, has a good theoretical basis, and is strongly recommended for implementation.
- **Category IC** is required by state or federal regulations or is an industry standard.
- **Category II** is supported by suggestive clinical or epidemiologic studies, has a theoretical basis, and is suggested for implementation.
- **Category III** is supported by descriptive studies, such as comparisons, correlations, and case studies, and may be useful.
- **Category IV** is obtained from expert opinion or authorities only.
- **Unresolved** means there is no recommendation because of a lack of consensus or evidence.

OUTCOME EVALUATION

Outcome evaluation is an important component of evidence-based practice, which involves both internal and external research. All treatments are subjected to review to determine if they produce positive outcomes, and policies and protocols for outcome evaluation should be in place. **Outcome evaluation** includes the following:

- **Monitoring** over the course of treatment involves careful observation and record-keeping that notes progress, with supporting laboratory and radiographic evidence as indicated by condition and treatment.
- **Evaluating** results includes reviewing records as well as current research to determine if outcomes are within acceptable parameters.
- **Sustaining** involves discontinuing treatment but continuing to monitor and evaluate.
- **Improving** means to continue the treatment but with additions or modifications in order to improve outcomes.
- **Replacing** the treatment with a different treatment must be done if outcome evaluation indicates that current treatment is ineffective.

EVIDENCE-BASED NURSING INTERVENTIONS

Evidence-based nursing interventions enable nurses to provide high-quality patient care that is based upon research and knowledge, as opposed to giving care that is based upon tradition or information that is out of date. An evidence-based nursing approach is based on the integration of practical clinical experience with medical and clinical research; it utilizes proven clinical guidelines and assessment practices. Evidence-based nursing interventions allow nurses to make patient care decisions based on cutting-edge research that has been scientifically validated. Studies show that evidence-based nursing practice yields improved patient outcomes, enables nurses to practice up-to-date methods, improves nurse confidence and decision-making skills, and enhances Joint Commission standards.

RESOURCES

There are numerous information resources for evidence-based nursing interventions. These resources include evidence-based textbooks; databases such as CINAHL Plus, COCHRANE library, Mosby's Nursing Index, NursingConsult, and Nursing@Ovid; evidence-based nursing metasites such as the Academic Center for EBN, Joanna Briggs Institute, McGill University, ONS-EBN section, and EBN-University of Minnesota; online

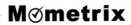

evidence-based nursing journals such as Clinical Nurse Specialist, Clinical Nursing Research, Evidence-Based Nursing, Journal of Nursing Care Quality, Journal of Advanced Nursing, Journal of Nursing Scholarship, Nurse Researcher, Nursing Research, Western Journal of Nursing Research, and Worldviews on Evidence-Based Nursing; and various online tutorials.

OBTAINING RESULTS OF RESEARCH TO USE IN EVIDENCE-BASED PRACTICE

When searching for **current evidence** in print and online literature, the nurse should look for **systematic reviews, analyses, and reports**. PUBMED lists all literature and can be searched for all published articles on a particular subject. These articles can be analyzed to determine treatments that have the best evidence of efficacy. Subject and methodological terms and clinical filters can be used to find necessary information, including a specific medical subject heading (MH), subheading (SH), publication type (PT), and text word (TW). The nurse should also search the National Guideline Clearinghouse, Cochrane Databases, Agency for Healthcare Research and Quality, and US Preventive Services Task Force Recommendations for evidence and guidelines. When trials of a treatment provide evidence of effectiveness, the evidence is weighed for strength and confidence. Those that provide the strongest evidence of efficacy become recommendations and guidelines for use in the field. Research is also done on a smaller scale by specialists who publish in peer-reviewed journals their research results related to the use of a particular intervention.

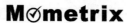

Nursing Theories and Models Significant to Rehabilitation

REHABILITATION NURSING

Rehabilitation nursing was defined in 2000 by the Association of Rehabilitation Nurses as "the diagnosis and treatment of human responses of individuals and groups to actual or potential health problems relative to altered functional ability and lifestyle." Rehabilitation nursing was instituted as a specialty classification in 1964, and the word *rehabilitation* was coined during World War I. However, the field really originated with the practices of **Florence Nightingale** during the Crimean War in the 1850s and **Clara Barton**, founder of the Red Cross, in the Civil War in the United States. The earliest focus was on ways to improve the basic care and conditions of soldiers and gain access to medical supplies for them.

The earliest **textbook** on rehabilitation was published in 1879 and focused on topics such as bedsores and paralysis. By the 1890s and early 1900s, subject matter had expanded to include massage, anatomy, physiology, and eventually occupational and physical therapies.

IMPACT OF EVENTS IN EARLY TO MID-1900S ON DEVELOPMENT OF REHABILITATION NURSING

Immigration, World Wars I and II, and the occurrence of **poliomyelitis epidemics** were the greatest factors in the development of the field of rehabilitation nursing in the early to mid-1900s. Injured men returning from World War I drew attention to the need for rehabilitative care. During the 1920s and 1930s, **physical and occupational therapies** evolved into their own practices, and the nursing field shifted more toward **acute care and diagnosis, education**, and **treatment of children with potential handicaps**. The debilitating injuries suffered by members of the armed forces during World War II increased the awareness of the need for rehabilitative care and functional training. The rehabilitation of patients with poliomyelitis was also important, especially during the peak periods of the disease, which occurred around 1909 and in the early 1950s. **Polio centers and ventilators** were prevalent until the Salk vaccine was introduced in 1954, followed by the Sabin oral vaccine in 1955. These vaccines virtually eliminated polio.

EVOLUTION DURING LAST HALF OF TWENTIETH CENTURY

At the beginning of the last half of the 20th century, rehabilitation nursing was recognized by the publication of a formal **textbook** (Alice Morrissey, 1951), the establishment of various **training programs**, and the founding of the **Association of Rehabilitation Nurses** (ARN, 1974). The bulk of the responsibilities of a rehabilitation nurse shifted more toward addressing the patient's activities of daily life, management of chronic conditions, and the treatment of injuries incurred through sports, work, or automobile accidents. Various **government initiatives** were established to deal with social issues, including reimbursement related to disabilities. The federal department of Social and Rehabilitative Service (SRS) was set up in the 1960s. Medicare began covering rehabilitative services for people with disabilities in 1972. The Education for All Handicapped Children Act was enacted in 1975. In the 1980s, other textbooks, journals, core curriculums, and research projects in the field were started. The key issues during the 1990s were disability rights, addressed primarily with the 1990 Americans with Disabilities Act.

NURSING THEORY RELATED TO REHABILITATION

IMOGENE KING'S THEORY OF GOAL ATTAINMENT

King organizes her **theory of goal attainment** within three systems as follows:

- **Personal systems**: Each individual is a personal system.
- **Interpersonal systems**: Interpersonal systems are the interactions among people.
- **Social systems**: A social system is an organized system of roles, behaviors, and practices.

King's theory states that people come together to help and to be helped. Key concepts of the theory are as follows:

- **Interaction**: Goal-directed communication
- **Perception**: Organizing, processing, storing, and exporting information
- **Communication**: Information-sharing among individuals
- **Transaction**: Observable behaviors of people interacting with their environment
- **Role**: A set of behaviors expected of a person occupying a certain position
- **Stress**: A response to a stressor
- **Growth and development**: Continuous changes which occur in life
- **Time**: The passage of events which move toward the future
- **Space**: A physical area or territory

MARTHA ROGERS' THEORY OF UNITARY HUMAN BEINGS

Nursing theory, according to **Rogers' theory of unitary human beings**, is defined as the phenomenon central to nursing the life process of human beings. Rogers' assumptions are as follows:

- The human being is a unified whole, processing integrity and manifesting characteristics that are more than and different from the sum of his or her parts.
- The person and environment are continually exchanging matter and energy with each other.
- The life process revolves irreversibly and unidirectionally along the time-space continuum.
- Patterns and organization identify individuals and reflect their wholeness.
- Human beings are characterized by their capacity for abstraction and imagery, language, thought, sensation, and emotion.

The **foundational concepts** of Rogers' theory are as follows:

- **Energy field**: An electrical field that is in a continuous state of flux.
- **Openness**: Energy fields are open to exchange with other energy fields.
- **Pattern**: Energy fields have patterns that change as required.
- **Four-dimensionality**: Energy fields are embedded in a four-dimensional space-time matrix.

Rogers' **principles of homeodynamics** are as follows:

- **Integrality**: The continuous, mutual, simultaneous interaction between humans and environmental fields
- **Resonancy**: The identification of human and environmental fields by changing wave patterns
- **Helicy**: The evolving innovative repatterning growing out of the mutual interaction of man and environment

DORTHEA OREM'S THEORY OF SELF-CARE DEFICIT

According to Dorthea Orem, self-care refers to activities that maintain life, health, and wellbeing. The three **categories of self-care fundamentals** are:

- **Universal**: Activities of daily living (ADLs)
- **Developmental**: Specialized activities related to a specific task or event
- **Health deviation**: Activities required by illness, injury, or disease

Self-care deficit refers to the inability to provide complete self-care. Someone with a self-care deficit requires nursing care. Nursing care involves the following:

- Entering into and maintaining the nurse-patient relationship
- Assessing how the patient can be helped
- Responding to patients' needs and requests
- Prescribing, providing, and regulating direct help
- Coordinating and integrating nursing care with other services

Nursing system refers to the amount of nursing care a patient requires, categorized as follows:

- **Wholly compensatory**: Nurse provides all care
- **Partly compensatory**: Nurse and patient collaborate in care
- **Supportive-educative**: Patient provides needed care, while nurse educates and promotes the patient as a self-care agent

ROPER'S MODELS FOR LIVING AND NURSING, GORDON'S FUNCTIONAL HEALTH PATTERNS, AND NEUMAN'S SYSTEM THEORY

Roper and his colleagues developed models for both living and nursing that are essentially based on the ability to perform **activities of daily living (ADLs)**. They also sorted out types of factors that can affect ADLs, such as biological and environmental factors. The model states that all ADLs are interconnected and influence the individual's ability to function.

Gordon describes **functional health patterns (FHPs)** that are also interconnected and related to the whole person, and these FHPs can be employed to treat the patient and those the patient interacts with. Each ADL in the Roper system has one or more FHPs described by Gordon. For example, the ADL sleeping is related to the sleep-rest FHP, and the ADLs breathing, personal cleansing and dressing, and mobilizing are all related to the activity-exercise FHP.

Neuman's systems theory is a multifaceted model developed by Betty Neuman centered on developing the whole person in relation to their environment. She emphasized that the individual is a composite of their environment, experiences, and support systems, and impact on any one of those factors can influence the whole of the individual. For that reason, she believed that treating an individual required the consideration of their system as a whole and was a dynamic process.

SOCIAL COGNITIVE THEORY

Social cognitive theory has been described primarily by A. Bandura. The theory states that **behavioral change** occurs relative to both the **outcome** of the behavior and particularly to the individual's **perception** of their capacity to perform the activity (degree of self-efficacy). For rehabilitation nurses, the use of this theory translates generally into using small, consecutive stages of behavioral modification to increase the individual's confidence. There are a number of other behavior theories as well. **Cultural care theory**, proposed by Leininger and colleagues, emphasizes provision of care within the context of the values and belief systems of the culture of the individual concerned.

ADDITIONAL THEORIES OR MODELS USED IN REHABILITATION NURSING

Since disabilities can be considered chronic illnesses, theories centering on that viewpoint—such as the **chronic illness trajectory model** of Corbin and Strauss or the **reconstruction of self in chronic illness paradigm** of Charmaz—are sometimes utilized. There are a number of theories focused on family systems. One of these is **Anderson's family health system theory (FHS)**, which emphasizes the importance of integrating family and patient health. There are also environmental and ecology models, models based on health and wellness, and models based on alternative approaches to disability and rehabilitation. Many of the latter focus on the stigma associated with disabilities.

DEVELOPMENT OF REHABILITATION SERVICES INTERNATIONALLY

Two major international programs were founded in response to World War I: the **Red Cross Institute for the Crippled and Disabled** (1917) and the **International Society of Crippled Children** (1922). The next major international initiative was not until 1953, when the United Nations established the **Council of World Organizations Interested in the Handicapped**. Later in the 20th century, internationally conducted research, exchange, and training programs emerged. Other countries such as the United Kingdom and Australia have defined policies, research programs, and educational venues for rehabilitation nurses. The World Health Organization (WHO) has played a prime role in defining standard units of measurement and classifications of disabilities. The **International Classification of Functioning, Disability and Health (ICF)** (sponsored by the WHO) became the gold standard in 2001.

WHO's MODEL DISABILITY SURVEY

The WHO's Model Disability Survey seeks to summarize the lifestyles of various populations of individuals with disabilities, comparing various levels of disability to one another in addition to comparing the life of the individual with disabilities to the life of the individual without disabilities. According to the WHO, this survey is necessary because there is a lack of standardized tracking of disability that examines the entirety of a population as it relates to functioning, and there needs to be a tool that helps provide evidence for desired policy changes to better support those with disabilities. The guiding principles of this model are as follows:

- Individuals with disabilities are entitled to participate in their community equally to those without disabilities.
- Disability is more than a functional condition but is also influenced by the individual's interaction with their environment.
- Within the context of disability, there exists a continuum of experiences, from mild to severe; therefore, each individual's case must be considered unique.
- Measuring disability must include contextual barriers (both social and environmental) that may improve or worsen the disability and the individual's overall health.
- Collecting data pertaining to the individual's life experience will help inform policy on methods for improving the individual's overall wellbeing.
- Standardization of this survey across country lines is critical in allowing for the creation of policy that can uniformly be recommended and applied across societies.

INDIVIDUAL AND SOCIAL CONCEPTUAL MODELS OF DISABILITY

There are two primary **individual models of disability**: the Nagi Disability Model (1965) and the WHO International Classification of Functioning, Disability and Health (ICF), which replaced the WHO's original model, the International Classification of Impairments, Disabilities, and Handicaps, in 2001.

- The **Nagi Disability Model** characterizes the subsequent manifestations (impairments) as functional limitations eventually leading to disability, which is restricted capability to perform expected roles and tasks. This model represents the earlier views of disability through a linear biomedical model that limits the definition of disability to a disease of function. It has since been replaced by the more favored WHO ICF.
- The **WHO ICF** moved away from the linear model, viewing disability as a far more complex and dynamic interaction between an individual and their environment. Rather than examining impairment, disability, and handicap, the newer WHO ICF model is more concerned with an individual's disability being a product of their ability to participate in society and the various environmental and personal factors that contribute to their level of disability.

Social models such as the **Independent Living (IL) model** in the United States approach disability as a product of societal mindsets and not the actual functional impairment.

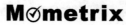

INTEGRATED ICF MODEL OF DISABILITY

The ICF model of disability is a paradigm that amalgamates aspects of both individual and social models. In this paradigm, **disability** is defined as any impairment of either bodily function or structure or ability to engage in **daily activities** (Part I, Functioning and Disability) and/or **personal or environmental dynamics** (Part II, Contextual Factors). Codes for conditions within each part have been developed to describe each factor. Even though social aspects are included, the underlying principle is the actual disease or health condition of the person and its effect on the body. This classification extends the term "disability" in some cases to nontraditional conditions such as stress, genetic conditions, and pregnancy.

OMAHA SYSTEM

The Omaha System is a standardized agenda sanctioned by the American Nurses Association (ANA) for classifying problems, defining intervention schemes and their targets, and rating the outcomes for health issues. Problems are categorized as primarily **environmental, psychosocial, or physiological** in nature, or they are considered **health-related behaviors** (such as substance abuse). The system places interventional approaches into four groups:

- Teaching, guidance, and counseling
- The use of various techniques or procedures
- Case management
- Surveillance

There are over 60 codes for the **targets** of these interventions, ranging from several types of medication use to finances. The **outcomes** of these interventions are also rated in terms of both the level of knowledge attained by the patient and the consistency and appropriateness of the patient's behavior.

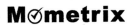

Nursing Process

PURPOSE OF NURSING ASSESSMENT

Nursing assessment evaluates patient data to help in diagnosis and treatment. The nurse assesses baseline health and medical history to be sure the patient will be safe. The nurse also determines what limitations the patient may have in terms of understanding or cooperation. Nursing assessment is an ongoing process, which includes baseline information, information on the patient's response and recovery to the intervention, and continued efforts to maintain the patient's health. The nurse can collaborate with other team members to help in this assessment.

PURPOSE OF NURSING DIAGNOSIS AND PLANNING

Nursing diagnosis is directed at patient comfort and outcome. With a diagnosis, nurses establish nursing interventions that are needed for the patient to be safe and comfortable. The nurse uses the diagnosis to direct therapies and to anticipate potentially needed interventions.

Planning allows the nurse to outline the methods needed to achieve patient goals. This accounts for alternative therapies that may be needed, setting priorities, satisfactory outcomes to be achieved, and expectations for discharge. The nurse needs to document the plan. The plan outlines nursing responsibilities, possible interventions, and expected outcomes.

IMPLEMENTATION OF NURSING PLAN

Implementing the nursing plan requires a measure of fluidity. The original plan is based on initial data. As new data is accumulated, however, the original plan may be modified. There is a need to incorporate individual needs of the patient as the plan proceeds. Different interventions may be called for depending on individual responses or limitations. The nurse needs to continually monitor the patient's response and status to be able to offer appropriate nursing interventions. Documentation is essential at every step of the way. The information can be useful in further treatment of the individual. It can also be used to assess the process so that improvements or adjustments can be made. The documentation may also be used for research purposes to further the knowledge of nursing practice. The record may become necessary for legal purposes as well.

EVALUATION PROCESS

In order to provide the best care for the patient, the nurse must **evaluate** the process in effect. This entails reviewing procedures and interventions in relation to standards of care, quality of care, and patient outcomes. Critical evaluation of the nursing process can lead to changes that may improve the quality of care for patients and/or identify personnel issues that need to be addressed. Modifying care plans is important to maintaining effective patient care. Deficiencies may be noted and can, therefore, be addressed. This underscores the importance of adequate documentation. In order to evaluate the process, the nurse must have access to the documentation to assess the present process. This evaluation may lead to changes that improve the quality of care in the nursing unit.

Related Theories and Models

DEVELOPMENTAL TASKS ACCORDING TO ERIKSON

The developmental tasks according to Erik Erikson:

- **Trust vs. Mistrust (Birth to 1 year):** Trust, faith, and optimism develop if the needs of warmth, food, and love are met. If not, this can result in mistrust.
- **Autonomy vs. Shame/Doubt (Ages 1-3):** The child desires independence in basic self-care tasks and wants choice. If independence is not encouraged, this can lead to doubt and shame. Independence develops self-control and willpower.
- **Initiative vs. Guilt (Ages 3-6):** The child engages in self-directed play and starts activities without outside influence. Imaginative play and competition are introduced. This can lead to guilt or direction and purpose based on how this initiative is supportive.
- **Industry vs. Inferiority (Ages 6-12):** The child values feeling capable and competent and develops a sense of pride and self-worth. They desire to do what is right and good. Social interactions between peers become more important, and comparing achievements can result in feelings of pride or feelings of inferiority if not properly guided.
- **Identity vs. Role Confusion (Ages 12-18):** Parents, teachers, peers, family members, church, culture, and ethnicity all role model and pressure youth to adopt certain behaviors. The task of adolescents is to discover their own identity.
- **Intimacy vs. Isolation (Ages 18-40):** Young people learn to commit to another person in a love or family relationship. They learn the behavior required to maintain this relationship.
- **Generativity vs. Stagnation (Ages 40-65):** Adults have many tasks when they try to find their own interests and niche in the work world. Family, community, and work roles are defined.
- **Integrity vs. Despair (Ages 65+):** Older people ponder their life experiences to put them into perspective. They learn to accept the aging process and begin to think about their own death.

SIGMUND FREUD'S STAGES OF PSYCHOSEXUAL DEVELOPMENT

Sigmund Freud's stages of psychosexual development are listed and described below:

- **Oral stage (Birth to 1 year):** obsessed with oral activities and must have these needs met for proper psychosocial development, very attached to mother.
- **Anal stage (Ages 1-3):** masters toilet training.
- **Phallic stage (Ages 3-6):** child focuses on childbirth and differences between the sexes, develops sexual obsession with parent of opposite sex (Oedipal complex-boy drawn to mother, Electra complex-girl drawn to father).
- **Latency stage (Ages 6-11):** Oedipal or Electra complex wanes, focus is now socialization, begins to gravitate toward the same-sex parent to learn appropriate gender roles.
- **Genital stage (Ages 12 and older):** puberty, attracted to opposite sex, learns to relate to opposite gender and control sexual drive.

PIAGET'S THEORY OF COGNITIVE DEVELOPMENT

Piaget believed that development was progressive and followed a set pattern. He believed the child's environment, his interactions with others in that environment, and how the environment responds help to shape his cognitive development. There are **four stages to Piaget's theory:**

- The **sensorimotor stage (birth to age 2)** is when the child learns to work toward a goal, the relationship between cause and effect, that objects still exist even though they cannot see them, and a sense of self.
- In the **preoperational stage (ages 2-7)**, language skills develop, the child only sees his point of view, he does not think abstractly, and has a difficult time telling fact from fantasy.

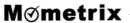

- The **concrete operations stage (ages 7-11)** is when children begin to understand relationships between objects and events, learn to classify and use patterns, understand that some occurrences are reversible, and see others' points of view.
- The **formal operations stage (ages 12 years and older)** is the stage of abstract thinking, better reasoning skills, and forward-thinking.

MASLOW'S HIERARCHY OF NEEDS

Maslow defined human motivation in terms of needs and wants. His **hierarchy of needs** is classically portrayed as a pyramid sitting on its base divided into horizontal layers. He theorized that, as humans fulfill the needs of one layer, their motivation turns to the layer above. The layers consist of (from bottom to top):

- **Physiological**: The need for air, fluid, food, shelter, warmth, and sleep.
- **Safety**: A safe place to live, a steady job, a society with rules and laws, protection from harm, and insurance or savings for the future.
- **Love/Belonging**: A network consisting of a significant other, family, friends, co-workers, religion, and community.
- **Esteem or self-respect**: The knowledge that you are a person who is successful and worthy of esteem, attention, status, and admiration.
- **Self-actualization**: The acceptance of your life, choices, and situation in life and the empathetic acceptance of others, as well as the feeling of independence and the joy of being able to express yourself freely and competently.

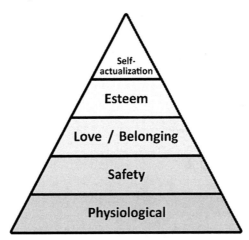

Review Video: **Maslow's Hierarchy of Needs**
Visit mometrix.com/academy and enter code: 461825

BEHAVIORAL THEORIES

Pavlov demonstrated classical conditioning when he found that a dog that would salivate when presented with food would also salivate when the person who normally fed him was present. He paired a bell ringing with the feeding and found that after a time, the dog would also salivate to the ringing of the bell. Consequently, his theory was that learning takes place when a behavior can be produced in response to something totally unrelated to that behavior.

Skinner demonstrated operant conditioning when he found that behavior can be changed depending on the response given to the behavior. If the response to the behavior was positive (praise, a hug), then the behavior would continue or increase in frequency. If the response was negative (a frown, words of criticism), then the behavior would decrease in frequency or cease altogether.

Biopsychosocial Theory of Patient Care

The biopsychosocial theory of patient care recognizes that **biology, psychology, and social circumstances** all interact in the development of an illness, the patient's perception of the illness, and the patient's ability to make a good recovery. In the biopsychosocial care model, a multidisciplinary healthcare team, including nurses, mental health professionals, social workers, and physicians, work together to address all aspects of a patient's health issue—the medical problem, psychological state, and social, cultural, and economic situation—in order to find an integrated solution. For example, adding stress-reduction, exercise, and nutritional programs to the standard medical treatment protocol for cardiovascular disease patients has been shown to be more effective. Many patients with chronic diseases or conditions may benefit from support groups that provide social and psychological benefits that may enhance the effects of drug therapy and surgery.

Biological Theories of Aging

There are a number of biological theories of aging:

- **Wearing down**: The body is compared to a machine that begins to wear down over time because of the damage caused by years of use.
- **Autoimmune reaction**: The body develops an autoimmune reaction against itself with aging, causing damage and destruction to tissues.
- **Free radical accumulation**: Chemicals that bring about aging accumulate in the body.
- **Cellular programming**: The cells of every organism have a predetermined programmed life expectancy beyond which one cannot survive.
- **Mutation**: Mutations within the organism occur over time, and these eventually make changes that are incompatible with life.
- **Homeostasis**: Over time, the body is unable to maintain stable levels of necessary chemicals in the body.

Selye's Theory of Adaptation

Selye developed a theory of adaptation concerning a person's physiologic response to stress called the general adaptation syndrome. This syndrome starts with the classic "fight or flight" response of the body to physiologic stress. Catecholamines are released and the adrenal cortical response begins. This is called the **alarm response** and is short-lived. This immediate response allows the person to respond quickly to stress. Since the alarm response cannot be sustained without resulting in death, the body next shifts into the **resistance stage**. Some cortisol is still being released as the body begins to adapt to the stressor. If the stressor persists, the body becomes exhausted. Changes then occur to the cardiovascular, gastrointestinal, and immune systems, and death can occur. The **exhaustion stage** does not always occur in response to most life stressors. As the body ages, it loses some of its resistance and ability to adapt to stress. This results in exhaustion and death in the elderly more easily than it does in younger people.

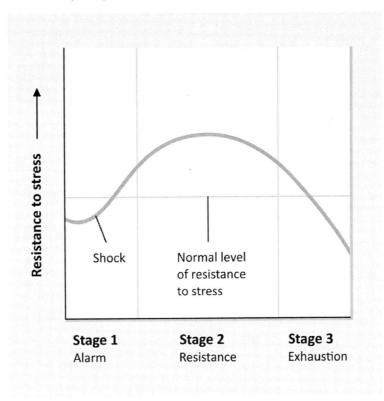

BANDURA'S THEORY OF SOCIAL LEARNING

In the 1970s, Bandura proposed the **theory of social learning,** in which he posited that learning develops from observing, organizing, and rehearsing behavior that has been modeled. Bandura believed that people are more likely to adopt the behavior if they value the outcomes, if the outcomes have functional value, and if the person modeling the behavior is similar to the learner and is admired because of status. Behavior is the result of observation of behavioral, environmental, and cognitive interactions. There are **four conditions required for modeling:**

- **Attention**: The degree of attention paid to modeling can depend on many variables (physical, social, and environmental).
- **Retention**: People's ability to retain models depends on symbolic coding, creating mental images, organizing thoughts, and rehearsing (mentally or physically).
- **Reproduction**: The ability to reproduce a model depends on physical and mental capabilities.
- **Motivation**: Motivation may derive from past performances, rewards, or vicarious modeling.

TRANSTHEORETICAL MODEL OF CHANGE

The Transtheoretical Model of Change puts forth concepts applicable to the process of educating patients and their family members. The **stages of the Transtheoretical Model of Change** include the following:

1. The first stage is **precontemplation**. At this point, the patient is not aware of any need for a change in the health behavior.
2. In the next stage, **contemplation**, the patient begins to realize why the change may be necessary after recognizing that the health behavior in question is unhealthy and weighing the consequences of continuing this behavior.

3. During the stage of **preparation**, the patient imagines making the change at a future time and starts to formulate a plan to do so.
4. The **action** stage occurs when the patient makes specific modifications in health behavior and begins to note the resulting positive changes.
5. During the **maintenance** stage, the patient is able to implement the change over time by utilizing strategies to prevent a return to previously unhealthy behaviors.
6. **Termination** is the stage at which a patient has incorporated the changed behavior into daily functioning, and the patient will not resume the previous unhealthy behavior.

KURT LEWIN

FORCE FIELD ANALYSIS

Force field analysis was designed by Kurt Lewin, a social psychologist, to analyze both the driving forces and the restraining forces for change:

- **Driving forces** instigate and promote change, such as leaders, incentives, and competition.
- **Restraining forces** resist change, such as poor attitudes, hostility, inadequate equipment, or insufficient funds.

The educator can use this force field analysis diagram to discuss variables related to a proposed change in process:

- Write the proposed change in the center column.
- Brainstorm and list driving forces and opposed restraining forces. Score the forces. (When driving and restraining forces are in balance, this is a state of equilibrium or the status quo.)
- Discuss the value of the proposed change.
- Develop a plan to diminish or eliminate restraining forces.

LEWIN'S MODEL OF CHANGE THEORY

Lewin's model of change theory may be used to help some patients make decisions for change. The nurse can educate the patient about the need for change and assist with making alterations in behavior or thoughts in order to better facilitate change; however, only the patient can truly implement the change permanently. Lewin's concept of change theory involves a three-part process:

- **Unfreezing** is the part of the model in which the patient becomes open to change, sees a need for it, and removes the boundaries inhibiting change.
- The patient then makes the **actual change** according to expected outcomes and goals.
- Finally, **refreezing** is the process of maintaining the change so that it becomes a habit, and one that the patient is likely to uphold for a long period of time.

Lewin's theory also involves either driving forces or restraining forces. Driving forces are those outside measures that support the change, while restraining forces inhibit success in implementing the change.

PRINCIPLES OF ADULT LEARNING

Adults have a wealth of life and/or employment experiences. Their attitudes toward education may vary considerably. There are, however, some **principles of adult learning** and typical characteristics of adult learners that an instructor should consider when planning strategies for teaching parents, families, or staff.

- Practical and goal-oriented:
  - o Provide overviews or summaries and examples.
  - o Use collaborative discussions with problem-solving exercises.
  - o Remain organized with the goal in mind.

- Self-directed:
  - o Provide active involvement, asking for input.
  - o Allow different options toward achieving the goal.
  - o Give them responsibilities.
- Knowledgeable:
  - o Show respect for their life experiences/education.
  - o Validate their knowledge and ask for feedback.
  - o Relate new material to information with which they are familiar.
- Relevancy-oriented:
  - o Explain how information will be applied.
  - o Clearly identify objectives.
- Motivated:
  - o Provide certificates of professional advancement and/or continuing education credit for staff when possible.

> **Review Video: Adult Learning Processes and Theories**
> Visit mometrix.com/academy and enter code: 638453

LEARNING STYLES

Not all people are aware of their preferred **learning style.** A range of teaching materials and methods that relate to all three major learning preferences (visual, auditory, and kinesthetic) and that are appropriate for different ages should be available. Part of assessment for teaching involves choosing the right approach based on observation and feedback. Often, presenting learners with different options gives a clue to their preferred learning style. Some people have a combined learning style.

Visual learners learn best by seeing and reading:

- Provide written directions or picture guides, or demonstrate procedures. Use charts and diagrams.
- Provide photos or videos.

Auditory learners learn best by listening and talking:

- Explain procedures while demonstrating and have the learner repeat.
- Plan extra time to discuss and answer questions.
- Provide audio recordings.

Kinesthetic learners learn best by handling, doing, and practicing:

- Provide hands-on experience throughout teaching.
- Encourage handling of supplies and equipment.
- Allow the learner to demonstrate.
- Minimize instructions and allow the person to explore equipment and procedures.

Rehabilitation Standards and Scope of Practice

STANDARDS AND SCOPE OF PRACTICE

The **Association of Rehabilitation Nurses** (ARN) has set standards of care for rehabilitation nursing practice and standards for professional performance. The ARN lists **six standards of care**:

- Assessment: the collection of patient health data
- Diagnosis: use of the health data to identify the problem
- Outcome identification: individualized identification of the expected result
- Planning: development of a care plan
- Implementation: execution of the care plan
- Evaluation: charting of the patient's progress toward the desired result

> **Review Video: Plan of Care**
> Visit mometrix.com/academy and enter code: 300570

The ARN also lists **eight standards of nursing professional performance**:

- Quality of care: evaluation of the quality of the professional's practice
- Performance appraisal: internal evaluation relative to relevant standards and regulations
- Education: keeping up-to-date
- Collegiality: encouragement of peers
- Ethics: conducting business with patients in an ethical manner
- Collaboration: interaction with patient, family, and colleagues for care provision
- Research: use of data from studies
- Utilization: use of principles of safety, efficacy, and cost-effectiveness

REHABILITATION SETTINGS

There are various kinds of rehabilitation settings, depending on the needs of the patient. Once the need for rehabilitation has been determined and the patient has been evaluated regarding specific rehabilitation needs, they can be placed in an appropriate rehabilitation setting. A **long-term acute care hospital** is a rehabilitation facility that is best for patients who are physically and psychologically stable but are receiving medical treatment such as dialysis or ventilation and thus require medical support. A **subacute care unit** is appropriate for patients who require more limited treatment, such as cancer patients. A **comprehensive inpatient rehabilitation facility** is just what the name suggests; it addresses the needs of a broad range of different patients, from burn victims to amputees. The comprehensive rehabilitation center has a team of medical specialists that includes a rehabilitation medicine physician, nurses trained in rehabilitation, occupational therapists, physical therapists, social workers, and speech-language pathologists. **Outpatient rehab** is designed for the high-functioning patient who can return home after rehab sessions.

SPECIALTY PRACTICES

Many rehabilitation programs are offered as **specialty practices** that either concentrate on **specific age groups and developmental levels** or specialize in **specific types of disabilities**. An example of a practice specialized according to age and developmental level would be one geared toward pediatric or geriatric populations. Illustrations of disability type specialty practices include centers that primarily treat patients with strokes or spinal cord injuries. Centers specializing in certain disabilities are generally located in major cities or medical centers, and standards for their operation have been outlined by organizations such as the **Commission on Accreditation of Rehabilitation Facilities (CARF)**.

MODELS OF REHABILITATION CARE

There are various models of rehabilitation care specific to the setting in which they are practiced. **Team-based models** of care approach rehabilitation by utilizing various types of team members to maximize the care of the patient. These members include professionals, such as various therapists, dietitians, doctors, psychologists, social workers, and nurses. Teams may be multidisciplinary, interdisciplinary, or transdisciplinary.

- **Multidisciplinary teams** are composed of specialists from a variety of fields who all communicate with each other regarding their suggestions for patient care and goals. In this way, specialists from different fields are involved in the care of a single patient.
- **Interdisciplinary teams** differ from multidisciplinary teams in that the whole team works together to identify ways to manage the patient; the suggestions are then executed by appropriate team members.
- **Transdisciplinary teams** choose one team member to be the primary caregiver while the other professionals serve as consultants; while this approach can be cost-effective, it also assigns duties to the primary therapist that may be performed better by others, and it obscures roles.

Team approaches have been shown to enhance outcomes, but they are also more expensive than provider-based models.

In **provider-based models** of rehabilitation care, the types of health care providers included are determined by the type of setting and the available payment schemes. There are three types of provider-based models: primary nursing, case management, and advanced practice.

- In the **primary nursing model**, a primary nurse is responsible for a patient, usually under the umbrella of a nursing team; this approach is useful for chronic conditions.
- **Case management** is a system in which there is a team of health care providers, but the patient is referred to a rehabilitation nurse who follows the patient throughout the course of their disability, regardless of setting.
- **Advanced practice nurses**, such as nurse practitioners and clinical nurse specialists, can act as consultants to other nurses for provision of specialized care.

CORE PRINCIPLES OF THE REHABILITATION NURSING RESEARCH AGENDA

In 2019, the Association of Rehabilitation Nurses revised the **Rehabilitation Nursing Research Agenda (RNRA)**, developed in conjunction with the Rehabilitation Nursing Foundation. This manifest speaks to seven areas of desired research:

- Nursing assessments, evaluations, and interventions to promote the function of those with disabilities and/or chronic illnesses
- The experience of disability/chronic illness for both individuals and their families across the lifespan
- The environment of rehabilitation care
- The rehabilitation nurse specialty
- Outcome evaluation
- Evidence-based practice
- Quality and process improvement

MAIN CONCERNS OF RESEARCH PROGRAMS

Rehabilitation nursing research has changed over the years, from an educational and manpower focus in the early 1900s to primarily **outcomes research** in recent years. Currently, there are two main groups involved with research programs for rehabilitation nurses: the ARN Research Committee and the Rehabilitation Nursing Foundation (RNF). The ARN Research Committee was formed in 2017 to help promote the research efforts of the RNF. The RNF provides grants to researchers whose work has the potential to enrich the **quality of care** to patients with disabilities or chronic illnesses; it also disseminates research findings.

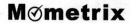

PRIORITIES OF REHABILITATION NURSING RESEARCH OF OTHER NATIONAL ORGANIZATIONS

The American Association of Spinal Cord Injury Nurses has identified a list of research priorities that contain many of the same types of issues outlined in the ARN statement with regard to spinal cord injury; it specifies a few additional issues such as management of pressure sores and caregiver strain. The National Institute on Disability, Independent Living, and Rehabilitation Research (NIDILRR) recognized multiple areas of outcomes research focused primarily on ways to reintegrate the individual with disabilities into the community and workplace, including attitude adjustment, skill improvement, and methods of providing support. The National Institute of Neurological Disorders and Stroke is interested in promoting the discipline of restorative neurology. The National Center for Medical Rehabilitation Research (NCMRR) primarily sponsors research addressing functional improvement and precise measurement techniques. Other sources of research funding include the Centers for Disease Control and Prevention (CDC) and the Department of Veterans Affairs (VA).

COMPETENCY ASSESSMENT TOOLS

Nursing competency assessment tools (**CATs**) are useful for assessing the mastery of knowledge of specific skills or performance areas. Many certifying organizations, like the Joint Commission, require **proof of competency**, so assessment tools meet this requirement. While paper tools can be used, most facilities now use **online platforms** such as HealthStream, making evaluation quick and streamlined and the reporting of compliance to accrediting bodies easier. As changes happen in healthcare and new evidence-based practice guidelines are released, competencies can ensure that all members of an organization are receiving and being tested over new knowledge so that it can be put into practice in a quicker time frame, making health care more up to date, efficient, and supported by the most current evidence-based practice. The ARN offers a multitude of **competency assessment tools** related to rehabilitation, including autonomic dysreflexia, neuropathophysiology and functional assessment, functional transfer techniques, and disability.

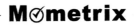

Technology

SMART DEVICES, PERSONAL RESPONSE DEVICES, AND INTERNET SOURCES

Numerous **smart devices** are now available to assist in monitoring a patient's progress and aiding rehabilitation. These devices are available in various forms (watches, bracelets, pendants, patches, leg bands) and can monitor such things as activity levels, falls, and heart rate. They can issue reminders ("Time to stand up and walk around") and automatically contact emergency services if a problem is detected, and some can take and transmit an ECG.

Personal response devices allow the person to signal the need for medical help. Often these are small devices, such as pendants and wristbands, with a button that the individual can push to call for help or that can recognize falls, such as some of the smart devices like the Apple Watch.

Internet sources abound with information about health and wellbeing, but not all sources are accurate or helpful, so individuals should be cautioned to use government sites, such as the CDC and National Cancer Institute, or sites of well-known national health organizations, such as the American Heart Association, rather than blogs, social media sites, or personal web pages.

Nursing Models and Theories

Functional Health Patterns

Restoration and Preservation of Health and Wellbeing

PRINCIPLES OF PHARMACOKINETICS

Pharmacokinetics relates to the route of administration, the absorption, the dosage, the frequency of administration, the distribution, and the serum levels achieved over time.

- The **drug's rate of clearance (elimination)** and **doses needed** to ensure therapeutic benefit are considered. Most drugs are cleared through the kidneys, with water-soluble compounds excreted more readily than protein-soluble compounds.
- **Volume of distribution** (IV drug dose divided by plasma concentration) determines the rate at which the drug passes into tissue. Drug distribution depends on the degree of protein binding and ion trapping that takes place.
- **Elimination half-life** is the time needed for the concentration of a particular drug to decrease to half of its starting dose in the body. Approximately five half-lives are needed to achieve steady-state plasma concentrations if giving doses intermittently.
- **Context-sensitive half-life** is the time needed to reach 50% concentration after withdrawal of a continuously-administered drug.
- **Recovery time** is the length of time it takes for plasma levels to decrease to the point that the effect is eliminated. This is affected by plasma concentration.
- **Effect-site equilibrium** is the time between administration of a drug and clinical effect (the point at which the drug reaches the appropriate receptors) and must be considered when determining dose, time, and frequency of medications.
- The **bioavailability** of drugs may vary, depending upon the degree of metabolism that takes place before the drug reaches its site of action.

PRINCIPLES OF PHARMACODYNAMICS

Pharmacodynamics relates to biological effects (therapeutic or adverse) of drug administration over time. Drug transport, absorption, means of elimination, and half-life must all be considered when determining effects. Responses may include continuous responses, such as blood pressure variations, or dichotomous responses in which an event either occurs or does not (such as death). Information from pharmacodynamics provides feedback to modify medication dosage (pharmacokinetics). Drugs provide biological effects primarily by interacting with receptor sites (specific protein molecules) in the cell membrane. Receptors include voltage-sensitive ion channels (sodium, chloride, potassium, and calcium channels), ligand-gated ion channels, and transmembrane receptors. Agonist drugs exert effects after binding with a receptor, while antagonist drugs bind with a receptor but have no effects, so they can block agonists from binding. The total number of receptors may vary, upregulating or downregulating in response to stimuli (such as drug administration). Dose-response curves show the relationship between the amount of drug given and the resultant plasma concentration and biological effects.

FIRST PASS METABOLISM AND DRUG CLEARANCE

First pass metabolism is the phenomenon that occurs to ingested drugs that are absorbed through the gastrointestinal tract and enter the hepatic portal system. Drugs metabolized on the first pass travel to the liver, where they are broken down, some to the extent that only a small fraction of the active drug circulates to the rest of the body. This first pass through the liver greatly reduces the bioavailability of some drugs. Routes of administration that avoid first pass metabolism include intravenous, intramuscular, and sublingual.

Drug clearance refers to the ability to remove a drug from the body. The two main organs responsible for clearance are the liver and the kidneys. The liver eliminates drugs by metabolizing, or biotransforming, the

34

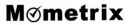

substance or excreting the drug in the bile. The kidneys eliminate drugs by filtration or active excretion in the urine. Drugs use either renal or hepatic methods of clearance. Kidney and liver dysfunction inhibit the clearance of drugs that rely on that organ for removal. Toxicity results from poor clearance.

ENTEROHEPATIC RECIRCULATION OF DRUGS AND RENALLY EXCRETED DRUGS

Enterohepatic recirculation refers to the process whereby a drug is effectively removed from circulation and then reabsorbed. The drug is secreted in bile, which is collected in the gall bladder and emptied into the small intestine, from which part of it is reabsorbed and part excreted in the feces. This reabsorption reduces the clearance of these drugs and increases their duration of action. Generally, drugs susceptible to enterohepatic recirculation are those with a molecular weight greater than 300 g/mol and those that are amphipathic (have both a lipophilic portion and a polar portion).

Renally excreted drugs are metabolized (biotransformed) by the liver to a form that can be excreted by the kidneys. Others are excreted by the kidneys unchanged. Infants with decreased renal function demonstrate decreased urine output or elevated levels of BUN and creatinine. The nurse should avoid using drugs that depend on the kidneys for clearance if the infant has renal impairment, as overdose may result.

ABSORPTION IN RELATION TO ROUTES OF MEDICATION ADMINISTRATION

The absorption rate of a drug depends on its transfer from its site of administration to the circulatory system. Different **routes of administration** have different absorption characteristics:

- **Oral**: Ingested medications pass from the gastrointestinal tract into the bloodstream. Most absorption occurs in the small intestine and is affected by gastric motility and emptying rate, drug solubility in gastrointestinal fluids, and food presence. Orally administered drugs are susceptible to first pass metabolism by the liver.
- **Intravenous**: Medications directly administered to the bloodstream have 100% absorption. Peak serum levels are rapidly achieved. Some drugs are not tolerated intravenously, due to vein irritation or toxicity, and others must be given as an infusion.
- **Intramuscular**: Medications injected into a muscle are absorbed fairly rapidly because muscle tissue is highly vascularized. Drugs in lipid vehicles absorb more slowly than those in aqueous vehicles.
- **Subcutaneous**: Medications injected beneath the skin absorb more slowly because the dermis is less vascularized than muscle. Hypoperfusion and edema decrease absorption further.

EFFECTS OF PHARMACOKINETIC CHARACTERISTICS ON DIFFERENT AGE GROUPS

PEDIATRIC AGE GROUP

Infants, in particular, have unique **absorption profiles** that can dramatically impact the use of drugs in this age group. Babies have very variable rates of absorption, which precludes the use of certain routes of administration. At birth, full-gestational infants generally have a gastric pH near neutral, but after about one day, it drops to the highly acidic range (about pH 1-3). On the other hand, premature babies cannot effectively secrete acid, have a high stomach pH, and empty their stomachs more slowly. Infants also have **immature epithelial barriers** on the skin, making the skin more permeable. Infants have a larger percentage of water weight than adults, making **water-soluble drugs** more effective. However, in turn, their low protein concentrations can depress binding and distribution. Processes involved with elimination are also not fully developed in the infant until he or she is about a year old.

GERIATRIC AGE GROUP

Pharmacokinetics involves four steps: absorption, distribution, metabolism, and elimination. All of these steps are affected by the age of the patient, as the organs involved degenerate from wear and tear:

1. **Absorption** of most drugs occurs in the small intestine. Drug absorption in older adults may be delayed or decreased due to decreased blood flow to the small intestine. This could change the blood levels of drugs achieved in the geriatric patient.

Functional Health Patterns

2. **Distribution** of the drug is altered due to a change in body composition. Elderly patients have decreased total body water and lean muscle mass. This relative increase in total body fat may increase the duration of action of lipid-soluble drugs.
3. Most drugs are **metabolized** by either the liver or the kidneys. Decreased function of these organs leads to delayed metabolism and elimination of certain medications.
4. **Renal function** and **elimination effectiveness** diminish with age, often decreasing the kidney's ability to remove toxins and medications from the body. For this reason, drugs may remain in the body longer, therefore requiring smaller doses among the elderly.

BLOOD DRUG LEVELS

Plasma drug levels are used for **therapeutic drug monitoring** because, although plasma is often not the site of action, plasma levels correlate well with therapeutic (effective) and toxic (dose-related adverse effects) responses to most drugs. The therapeutic range of a drug is that between the minimum effective concentration (level at which there is no therapeutic benefit) and the toxic concentration (level at which toxic effects occur). To achieve drug plateau (steady state), the drug half-life (time needed to decrease drug concentration by 50%) must be considered. Most drugs reach plateau with administration equal to four half-lives and completely eliminate a drug in 5 half-lives. Because drug levels fluctuate, peak (highest drug concentration) and trough (lowest drug concentration) levels may be monitored. Samples for trough levels are taken immediately prior to administration of another dose, while peak samples are taken at various times, depending on the average peak time of the specific drug, which may vary from 30 minutes to 2 hours or so after administration.

SIDE EFFECTS OF MEDICATIONS

All drugs can have side effects, and some are toxic at certain levels or in combination with other drugs. Some side effects will be minor and may go away after a week or two. Others can be severe or life-threatening, such as anaphylaxis. Common side effects include nausea, vomiting, diarrhea, and rashes. Side effects may vary with individuals according to age, gender, and condition and may be related to non-compliance with treatment, incorrect dosage, polypharmacy, or drug interactions. Drug compendiums will list all possible side effects according to system or incidence. Pharmacologically similar medications usually have some common side effects among the drugs in that class. Nursing actions include:

- Always question the patient about allergies or previous drug reactions before administering medication.
- Educate the patient about possible side effects of all medications.
- Watch out for drug-drug and food-drug combinations that are dangerous.

DRUG INTERACTIONS

Drug interactions occur when one drug interferes with the activity of another in either the pharmacodynamics or pharmacokinetics:

- With **pharmacodynamic interaction,** both drugs may interact at receptor sites causing a change that results in an adverse effect or that interferes with a positive effect.
- With **pharmacokinetic interaction**, the ability of the drug to be absorbed and cleared is altered, so there may be delayed effects, changes in effects, or toxicity. Interactions may include problems in a number of areas:
  - **Absorption** may be increased or (more commonly) decreased, usually related to the effects within the gastrointestinal system.
  - **Distribution** of drugs may be affected, often because of changes in protein binding.
  - **Metabolism** may be altered, often causing changes in drug concentration.
  - **Biotransformation** of the drug must take place, usually in the liver and gastrointestinal system, but drug interactions can impair this process.
  - **Clearance interactions** may interfere with the body's ability to eliminate a drug, usually resulting in increased concentration of the drug.

36

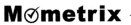

SPECIFIC INTERACTIONS

Some drugs will either increase or inhibit the actions of other drugs. They may interfere with receptor-site binding or the way in which the drug is metabolized or excreted. Certain drugs may cause drowsiness when taken together or with alcohol. Some foods will inhibit drug action, such as the inhibition of warfarin by vitamin-K-containing foods. Other foods may cause toxic levels of a drug to accumulate. Grapefruit juice, for example, is metabolized by the same enzyme that metabolizes about 50 drugs, including digoxin and statins, and this can prevent the liver from breaking down drugs and lead to severe reactions. The nurse should always obtain a complete medication list from the patient, including prescription and over-the-counter medications, herbals, vitamins, minerals, and dietary supplements that are taken regularly and occasionally. All medications taken should be checked for **potential interactions with drugs or foods.**

EXPECTED DEVELOPMENTAL PROFILES AND INTERVENTIONS FOR DISABILITY

INFANCY

Infancy is defined as the period from birth to 1 year of age, although the term **neonate** is often used up to age 1 month. Developmentally, an infant should learn trust, go through stages from sitting to crawling to walking, and explore their various senses and environment. Infants experience separation anxiety and express their emotions through crying and motor activities such as kicking or sucking on their thumb or a pacifier. Infants with disabilities have only a limited ability to explore their environment and do not have proper sensory stimulation. They need to be given appropriate **sensory stimulation**, as much freedom as possible, soothing, and nurturing. There are toys and activities available designed for various disabilities. The parents of a neonate with a disability often feel guilty; they should be encouraged to bond with the child and should be given sufficient information about the disability.

TODDLERHOOD

Toddlerhood is defined as the period from 1 to 4 years of age. This is the time when a child learns various skills such as walking, climbing, drinking from a cup, communicating through language, and using the toilet. It is also the stage when the child develops **independence**, starts to separate from their parents, and develops the ability to think. Toddlers are very egocentric. They tend to cope by insisting on attention, throwing temper tantrums, crying, or other behavioral patterns. If a toddler has a **disability**, the toddler may have restricted mobility and/or elimination difficulties and other problems that force them to be more **dependent**, impeding the toddler's ability to separate from the parents. Suggested interventions include activities that promote independence and mobility, reduce anxiety, set boundaries, and teach the toddler by methods specific to their needs (such as sign language).

EARLY CHILDHOOD

Early childhood or preschool age is the period from 4 to 6 years of age. It is generally the time where the child learns **socialization skills** and the concepts of **right and wrong**. A healthy preschool child can freely discover the wonders of their environment, has developed independent skills related to the activities of daily life, and has mastered thought processes, such as questioning, fantasizing, and fear. The preschooler may interact through routine activities, play, and aggressive actions or words. If the child has a disability, their limitations of mobility, communication, choice, and energy can lead to **disrupted body image** and **overprotection** on the part of the family. A preschooler with disabilities should be given realistic choices and opportunities to act independently. Establishing routines, setting limits, and incorporating play into treatment schedules are useful strategies.

MIDDLE CHILDHOOD

Middle childhood refers to a school-age child between 6 and 12 years of age. This is the time when a large part of the child's environment shifts from the familiarity of home to the school and **increased social interaction and independence**. The child usually learns a number of academic skills, develops a logical pattern of thought, learns new motor skills such as bike riding, and forms friendships. The child also begins to consider the point of view of others. A school-age child who has a disability often misses school, cannot engage in social and

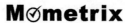

recreation opportunities with peers, and may feel **inferior and dependent**. Such a child may become depressed or act out by withdrawing, using humor, being aggressive toward others, or trying to conceal their illness. Chief among the many intervention strategies are encouragement of regular school attendance and participation in any possible sports or clubs. At home, it is important to include the child in self-care and household responsibilities and offer opportunities for the child to make friends (such as having sleepovers).

ADOLESCENCE

Adolescence, ages 12–18, is generally characterized by rapid and marked changes in physiology (mainly related to puberty), reasoning abilities and abstract thinking, a new viewpoint of personal identity, and increased interest in the opposite sex. It is also the period where the adolescent considers career and personal goals, gets into conflict with parents, and eventually transitions into adulthood. An adolescent with a disability or chronic illness often has a **negative body image** and may have **delayed puberty**. An adolescent with a disability may feel **isolated** from peers, as well as socially—and possibly vocationally—**limited**. Depending on the extent of medical interventions, an adolescent with disabilities may find it hard to be as independent as their peers. They tend to cope by showing resentment or withdrawal. The individual may try to conform or take risks. It is important to allow the adolescent with disabilities to fail, to be as independent as possible, to give them privacy, and to provide social opportunities. An adolescent with disabilities should also be given sexual information just like their peers.

EVALUATION TOOLS FOR PEDIATRIC DISABILITY

The FIM (Functional Independence Measure) has variations called the **WeeFIM** (designed to evaluate functional parameters in children from age 6 months to 16 years) and **WeeFIM II** (for use with children up to age 3). Both are provided by the **Uniform Data System for Medical Rehabilitation (UDSMR)**. These tools take into account developmental age and are mainly used as outcomes measurements for institutions. The **Pediatric Evaluation of Disability Inventory (PEDI)** looks at functional skills related to self-care, mobility, and social functioning in children between 6 months and 7 years of age. It can also be used for older children with functional abilities below their chronological age. In this case, the rehabilitation nurse or other professional interviews the patient about these various functional domains, and the answers are entered and scored through provided software. A **modifications scale** is also provided to assess the child's environment.

GERIATRIC REHABILITATION

NURSING DIAGNOSES AND DESIRED OUTCOMES FOR GERIATRIC REHABILITATION

A common diagnosis for the gerontological patient is **adult failure to thrive**, and desired nursing outcomes are related to improvement of nutritional (including hydration and weight management) or health status, cognitive improvement, and social involvement. Another prevalent nursing diagnosis is **risk for injury**, with the most important risk prevention related to reducing falls. **Disturbed sleep pattern** and **chronic pain** are two other possible nursing diagnoses. Addressing physical and emotional needs (such as elimination patterns and anxiety, respectively) can improve a disturbed sleep pattern. The patient needs to be made comfortable and their symptoms controlled to alleviate pain and stress or depression. **Ineffective coping** is also a possible diagnosis that can be improved by helping the patient learn to cope and get a sense of control. The patient may present with acute or chronic confusion. **Acute confusion** can be caused by temporary or controllable factors, but **chronic confusion** is generally a sign of more permanent problems.

CARE PLANNING FOR OLDER ADULTS

Nurses engaged in gerontological rehabilitation nursing generally deal with patients that are at least 65 years of age. These nurses are often CRRNs. They nurse should perform a complete **physical assessment** similar to that given to any patient, but they should also be attuned to signs that can influence other health issues. A **medication history** is important for this elderly age group because these individuals may be taking many medications and other non-prescription preparations that can interact, are out of date, or are not taken in the proper dosage. **Functional abilities** should be assessed by questioning the patient about the extent to which they participate in ADLs and IADLs (instrumental activities of daily living). The **suitability** of the patient's home and community environment should also be evaluated.

Functional Health Patterns

ASSESSMENT OF GERIATRIC REHABILITATION PATIENTS

The clinician should take the height and weight and look at the general appearance of the patient. The person's head should be examined, including reflexes, acuity, and visual aspects of the eyes, ears, nose, and throat. The patient's cardiac system should be evaluated by taking their blood pressure and pulse in various positions, feeling the carotid and jugular veins, and checking for peripheral edema. The clinician should check the patient's respiratory system by listening for lung sounds, dyspnea, and breathing rhythm and expansion. The abdomen should be checked for firmness, pain, circulation, liver tenderness, and bowel sounds. Rectal and pelvic examinations should be performed; here, the pelvic floor muscle strength is particularly important for incontinence evaluation. A variety of tests for mobility and neurological responses should be done, including screening for balance and gait function and ataxia. Cognitive functions such as comprehension, short- and long-term memory, and ability to express emotion should be evaluated using tools such as the **Mini-Mental State Examination** and the **Geriatric Depression Scale**. The skin should be examined as well.

NORMAL AGING VERSUS PRESENCE OF DISEASE OR CHRONIC ILLNESS

As people age, changes begin to occur in bodily systems regardless of whether the person has a disease or chronic illness. Generally, many **cardiopulmonary functions**, such as the heart's pumping force, work capacity, and chest wall compliance, decrease in older individuals. Older people are at increased risk for arteriovenous (AV) heart blocks, arrhythmias, and other cardiopulmonary diseases and pulmonary infections. However, abnormalities such as hypotension while standing or abnormally low heart rate are usually associated with illness. Many aging individuals have **musculoskeletal issues**, such as decreased height, poor posture, decreased mobility, and rearrangement of body mass, fat, or minerals; however, other problems such as stiff joints or muscle atrophy are disease-related. It is a normal aging response to have diminished short-term memory, response times, or sensory reception, but **neurological problems** such as decreased cerebral blood flow, balance, or coordination indicate an underlying disease process.

There are normal aging changes in bowel, genitourinary, liver, and renal functions. In each case, there can also be **abnormalities** indicating the presence of underlying disease processes. With aging, saliva, gastric juices, absorption, and peristalsis all slow down, affecting bowel function, but the presence of **gastroparesis** or **difficulty swallowing** indicates additional problems. Vaginal atrophy in women and prostatic enlargement in men is to be expected, but the presence of things such as **diverticula** or **elevated post-void residual volume** suggests underlying disease. Liver functions decrease with aging, but **elevated liver enzyme levels** can be associated with chronic illness. Many renal functions and clearance rates are depressed with aging; however, if the person has a **high serum blood urea nitrogen (BUN)** or **creatinine level**, it may indicate some underlying disease. Other systems are similar, such as the endocrine system (assess for hypoglycemia) and integumentary system (note delayed healing time). In addition, sleep patterns incorporating frequent naps may indicate problems.

> **Review Video: AV Heart Blocks**
> Visit mometrix.com/academy and enter code: 487004

FUNCTIONAL STATUS AND REHABILITATION

ADLS

Activities of daily living (ADLs) are a group of activities that are used to evaluate a patient's return to normal function; these are activities that the patient had performed on a daily basis before hospitalization and will be expected to perform once he or she has completed rehabilitation. The **rate** at which the patient accomplishes these activities, in addition to the **level of independence** maintained by the patient when performing the activities, can help caregivers determine the amount of rehabilitation required and can also be used to monitor the progress of the patient during the rehabilitation process. ADLs are grouped into three different areas: **personal or physical**, **instrumental**, and **occupational**.

GROUPING ADLS

The first group of ADLs, the **physical or personal group**, contains those daily activities that relate to the patient's ability to take care of him or herself. Included in this group are activities related to health management, nutritional needs, elimination of bladder and bowel contents, exercise, self-esteem, coping/stress management, cognitive abilities, communication, sexual health and ability, and relationship roles. The second group of ADLs, the **instrumental group**, contains activities such as shopping, answering the phone, and other activities that involve leaving home. The third group, **occupational activities**, includes activities that are required of being a parent, husband, or wife, as well as those required on the job.

ASSESSING POTENTIAL FOR REHABILITATION

There are various factors that are considered when assessing a patient to determine whether he or she will benefit from **rehabilitation**. A patient with the inability to perform any of the ADLs will automatically be considered for rehabilitation. At this point, however, other factors must be considered. First and foremost is whether or not the patient has a **desire to improve his or her functions** through rehabilitation; if the patient is not interested in improvement, the rehabilitation potential is poor. If the patient wants to improve function and increase independence, the potential for rehabilitation is greater. Another factor is whether or not the patient has **support at home**; even if the patient improves greatly during his or her rehabilitation stay, he or she will still most likely need some support at home. If the patient has no support at home, rehabilitation may eventually fail.

DISEASES AND ILLNESSES THAT COMMONLY REQUIRE REHABILITATION

There are some diseases, illnesses, and injuries that almost always require rehabilitation at some point during their course; in these cases, rehabilitation may be initiated before the patient even leaves the hospital to be transferred to a rehabilitation facility. It is important to know which diseases usually require rehabilitation because the sooner evaluation and rehabilitation are initiated, the better the patient's chance of recovery. The following are diseases, illnesses, and injuries that **commonly require rehabilitation**: AIDS, amyotrophic lateral sclerosis (ALS), limb amputation, traumatic or ischemic brain injury, spinal cord injury, burns, Guillain-Barré syndrome, hip or knee replacement, multiple sclerosis (MS), and most types of cancer.

INTERVENTIONS TO CONSIDER WHEN BEGINNING REHABILITATION PROCESS

When a patient is to be considered for rehabilitation, he or she must undergo a rather extensive **evaluation** in order to increase the likelihood that he or she will succeed during rehabilitation. This process of evaluation, which includes various interventions, should take place in the early stages of illness, when the patient is still in the hospital. The goal is to forestall any **secondary complications** that may inhibit the rehabilitation process. These **interventions** include health management, in which the patient and family are educated about his or her disease(s); nutritional status assessment and support; initiation of bowel and bladder management in order to prevent infection; exercises; assessment of cognitive function; and education involving self-esteem, relationship roles, sexual activity, and coping mechanisms.

OCCUPATIONAL THERAPY

Occupational therapy is defined as the use of creative activities in the treatment of individuals with disabilities, whether physical or mental. The purpose of occupational therapy is to provide these individuals with the skills that are necessary to live life as fully and independently as possible; after completion of occupational therapy, the individual should be able to perform at his or her **maximum potential**. The occupational therapist will typically provide the patient with **interventions** tailored to his or her disability. The OT will also visit the patient's home and/or place of employment in order to assess potential problems and provide **adaptive solutions**. As part of occupational therapy, the patient will receive regular **assessments** of his or her skills, as well as specific training. The occupational therapist is also responsible for educating the patient's family, caretakers, friends, and coworkers.

The philosophy of occupational therapy is based on the idea that **occupation** (meaning, loosely, either an activity or activities in which an individual engages) is a **basic human need**, one that is important to an

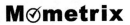

individual's health and overall wellbeing in that it is in and of itself therapeutic in nature. The basic assumptions of occupational therapy are based on the idea of occupational therapy as stated by its creator, **William Rush Dunton**. Dunton states that occupational therapy is a human need because an individual's occupation has an effect on his or her health and general wellbeing. It creates **structure** in the individual's life and allows for him or her to manage and organize time. Another assumption is that individuals have different sets of values and, therefore, will value different occupations; for each person, however, the occupation that he or she chooses is meaningful to him or her.

Areas in Which Occupational Therapy May Be Instituted and Practiced

Although occupational therapy is an important part of the overall rehabilitation process for hospitalized individuals, it is also beneficial in other areas because occupational therapy deals not only with physical disabilities but with **emotional and cognitive disabilities** as well. Occupational therapy as related to **physical disabilities** may be practiced in outpatient clinics, pediatric hospitals or units, acute care rehabilitation facilities, and long-term, or comprehensive, inpatient rehabilitation centers. Occupational therapy as related to **mental disabilities** may be practiced in mental health clinics, acute and long-term psychiatric hospitals, prisons, and gateway or halfway houses. Occupational therapists may also work at schools, childcare facilities, workplaces, or shelters, or they may even work with individuals in their own homes.

Telerehabilitation

With telerehabilitation (telerehab), rehabilitation services are delivered via the internet or other telecommunication devices, using tools such as webcams, videoconferences, and applications on devices such as tablets. Most telecommunication is predominantly **visual communication**. Telerehab is especially beneficial for patients in rural areas and for those with disabilities that make travel difficult. Some fields of rehabilitation are more difficult to use telecommunication in, such as PT and OT, as these usually require more direct supervision and manipulation, as well as physical assistance. Difficulties of telerehab include **reimbursement** for services. While Medicare will cover some telemedicine, it does not cover telerehab, and Medicaid coverage of telerehab is state-based. Private insurance companies vary on what types of telerehab they will cover, and they also vary on restrictions regarding reimbursement, including some policies stating that the patient cannot receive telerehab services at home. Patients should be very aware of what services are covered and what restrictions need to be met so claims will not be rejected. Telerehab services will likely be expanded over the coming years, providing rehab services to vulnerable populations.

Changes of Sexuality Throughout Life

The capacity for sexuality is present throughout life. However, there are changes in children that increase their sexuality or interest in sexual activity as well as their ability to reproduce. For girls, the transformation to **puberty** or physiological maturity typically starts around ages 8–11, prompted by production of **estrogen** and other hormones. For boys, puberty usually begins between ages 9 and 15 and is marked by **testicle, prostate gland, and other organ maturation** and increased production of the hormone **testosterone**. Sexual changes transpire as we age as well. In **postmenopausal women**, hormone levels decrease, interest in or response to sex diminishes, and vaginal atrophy or other losses can occur. As **men** age, testosterone and sperm counts decrease; various sexual organs may atrophy, and ejaculation force may be diminished.

41

STAGES OF SEXUAL RESPONSE

Sexual response depends on an intricate interplay of physiology, neurotransmitters, and psychological factors. There are five phases of complete sexual response:

1. **Desire**: A strong craving for a sexual experience, primarily psychological in nature
2. **Arousal**: Stimulation of sexual desire as evidenced by physiological changes including increased pulse and blood pressure, filling of the blood vessels in genital areas, nipple stiffness, erect penis in men, and vaginal lubrication in women
3. **Plateau:** Further elevation of pulse, blood pressure, and respiratory rate in anticipation of the next stage, orgasm
4. **Orgasm**: Peak of respiratory and heart rate, muscle spasms in bursts in women, ejaculation of sperm in men
5. **Resolution:** Relaxation and reversion to normal physiological levels that existed prior to excitement

NEUROLOGICAL PATHWAYS THAT CONTRIBUTE TO ERECTIONS IN NORMAL MALES

A normal, neurologically intact man can achieve an erection through two pathways.

- The first is a **reflexogenic erection** in which continual touching in the genital area is communicated through the pudendal nerve to the sacral spinal cord at S2 to S4. Parasympathetic efferent nerve impulses are then transmitted via the pelvic and cavernosal nerves to relax the smooth muscle in the penis and cause an erection.
- The other type is a **psychogenic erection**. Here, no tactile stimulation is necessary, only mental impressions or evocation through other senses such as taste or smell. The route is the thoracolumbar sympathetic nerves, T10 through L2, directly to the sexual organ. The sympathetic nervous system is also involved with ejaculation, later reduction in swelling, and tone through control from the hypogastric nerves.

NEUROLOGICAL FOUNDATION OF FEMALE SEXUAL RESPONSE

The female's clitoris and vagina are also innervated by **pudendal nerves**, which when stimulated signal the sacral plexus at S2 to S4. Women also have pelvic nerves present in the vagina, clitoris, and more internal fallopian tubes that receive **parasympathetic signals** from the hypogastric and uterine areas, causing enlargement of the clitoris and vaginal secretions. Responses can also be **psychogenic,** as with one type of male erection. The contraction of muscles in the pelvic floor and vaginal wall is due to activation of somatic pudendal nerves, while sympathetic responses in the ovarian and uterine regions are more controlled by the thoracic and lumbar regions of the spinal cord. In both sexes, maintenance of arousal is also influenced by the brain stem, particularly the hypothalamic-pituitary axis, where production of sexual hormones is controlled.

ASSESSMENT OF SEXUAL FUNCTION

Assessment of sexual function includes a sexual history, a sexual physical examination, and certain diagnostic tests. The purpose of the sexual history is the detection of **sexual problems or erroneous beliefs**. It should include elements such as a medical history of any relevant neurological issues, sexually transmitted diseases, and other germane disorders, such as hypertension, endocrine problems, or diabetes. It should also address current medication usage, sexual function prior to the current problem, physical problems that could influence sexual function (such as paralysis and incontinence), and gender-specific parameters related to sexual response. The **physical examination** ought to include inspection of external genitalia, including neurological assessment of rectal sphincter tone, pelvic and breast examinations in women, and squeezing of the male testicles to look for pain (indicative of psychogenic erections). **STDs** should be diagnosed by means of urine cultures or pap smear. **Neurological capabilities** in the genital area can be appraised using urodynamic testing and, in men, nocturnal penile tumescence testing or intracavernosal injection of drugs to see if erection can be induced.

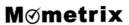

EFFECTS OF NEUROLOGICAL AND OTHER DISORDERS ON MALE AND FEMALE FERTILITY

Men with spinal cord injuries, reduced levels of testosterone due to endocrine problems, or (in some cases) alcoholism, can experience decreased fertility. There are several possible factors that may act in consort. Their semen volume may be low, resulting in a low sperm count or mobility. The endocrine and/or neurological changes may contribute to suppressed libido, changes in secondary sex characteristics, erectile dysfunction, or retrograde ejaculation of semen into the bladder.

Female fertility can be affected by damage to the endocrine system, brain injuries, or disorders that control hormones related to ovarian function, and other reproductive problems such as polycystic ovaries or hypogonadism. It can also be temporarily affected by spinal cord injuries. Birth defects to female genitalia can be caused by alcohol or certain medication use during pregnancy.

CHANGES ASSOCIATED WITH NEUROLOGICAL AND OTHER DISORDERS CONTRIBUTING TO SEXUAL DYSFUNCTION

People with spinal cord and brain injuries, strokes, or other neurological conditions have nerve damage that can cause **sexual dysfunction**. **Musculoskeletal conditions** such as fractures, amputations, or rheumatic disease, in conjunction with **neurological issues** that result in impaired mobility, can also make it difficult to prepare for and perform intercourse. People with neurological conditions usually have altered sensation patterns, which may include decreased or absent sensation in erogenous zones. **Libido** can be suppressed due to pain or fatigue associated with neurological, musculoskeletal, oncological, cardiovascular, respiratory, or digestive disorders; neurological damage can also lead to disinhibition and sexual addiction. Bladder or bowel incontinence associated with neurological deficits (or sometimes cancer-related surgeries) can contribute to sexual dysfunction through increased probability of infection, reflexive actions, and unsightly odors or wetness. Diabetes, alcoholism, hormonal deficits, and neurological problems can lead to impotence and problems with ejaculation or orgasm in men. Inadequate vaginal lubrication due to lack of estrogen and atrophy can occur in women in addition to the possible absence of orgasm.

DRUG TYPES THAT CAN AFFECT SEXUAL FUNCTIONING

Patients with neurological and other disorders generally take a variety of drugs that can also affect their ability to **function sexually**. Many drug classes suppress desire and sexual function in both sexes, including selective serotonin reuptake inhibitors, tranquilizers, tricyclic antidepressants, diuretics, antihistamines, analgesics (particularly narcotics), street drugs, hormones, and H_2 antagonists. In men, **erectile dysfunction** can result from use of many of these; ejaculation difficulties often occur with use of tranquilizers such as diazepam, anticonvulsants such as phenytoin, and hypertensive drugs such as methyldopa. Antihypertensive drugs such as hydralazine can precipitate priapism (prolonged erection) and/or persistent painful erection. **Gynecomastia**, enlargement of the male breast, is generally caused by hormonal imbalances, and also by blood pressure drugs such as methyldopa and diuretics such as spironolactone (also for hypertension). Spironolactone use in women can bring on menstrual changes. Another source of sexual problems in women is **antihistamine** use, which can cause drowsiness and suppress vaginal lubrication. Many drug types can impair arousal or ability to achieve orgasm.

NURSING DIAGNOSES AND INTERVENTIONS AND OUTCOMES APPLICABLE TO SEXUAL FUNCTION

The five possible nursing diagnoses related to sexual function are sexual dysfunction, activity intolerance, disturbed body image or self-esteem, altered sexual role performance, and deficient knowledge related to sexual health. **Sexual dysfunction** issues dictate interventions such as sexual counseling encompassing a variety of areas, including anticipation, self-esteem, body image, and coping, with the desired endpoint being sexual functioning. This diagnosis typically also signals the need for educational counseling on topics such as safe sex, fertility, risk factors, communication, and sexual functioning. If a person cannot **tolerate the activity level**, then interventions are directed toward increasing general exercise and strength training and management of pain and energy use. **Low self-esteem or body image** can be addressed through counseling, socialization and support systems, and teaching ways to avoid incontinence during sex. **Altered sexual role**

Functional Health Patterns

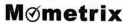

performance implies social isolation, which can be tackled primarily though complex relationship building and socialization techniques.

SEXUAL DYSFUNCTION

TECHNIQUES TO ACHIEVE SEXUAL FUNCTIONING

Patients with sexual dysfunction can often achieve satisfaction using **alternative techniques** such as masturbation, manual or orogenital stimulation, or lubricants. **Erectile dysfunction** can be overcome by techniques such as positioning the soft penis into the vagina with the man on top, by use of external vacuum pumps to engorge the penis, or penile vibrators. At present, the initial recommended therapy for erectile dysfunction is use of oral phosphodiesterase-5 drugs, including avanafil, sildenafil citrate, vardenafil, and tadalafil, which have various effective time ranges. If these drugs do not work or are contraindicated, other options are alprostadil intraurethral suppositories or intracavernosal injection. Papaverine and phentolamine can also be given intracavernosally. All of these relax smooth muscle and allow engorgement. Penile prostheses can also be surgically implanted.

MANAGING OTHER ASSOCIATED ISSUES

Pain control is crucial for sexual functioning in those with several diseases, notably people who have rheumatic diseases or have had recent joint replacement surgery and postmenopausal women. Individuals with **rheumatic diseases** generally need to control joint pain and stiffness before they can enjoy sex; this can be achieved in many ways, including relaxation techniques, range-of-motion exercises, moist heat application, pain medications (including corticosteroid injections), and massage. **Postmenopausal women,** as well as others with nerve or blood vessel issues, may suffer vaginal dryness and discomfort, which can be addressed with lubricants or estrogen creams. **Incontinence** during sex due to autonomic reflexes is common in patients with neurological issues; preparation for this possibility is paramount and includes actions such as prior emptying, scheduling activity relative to bowel programs, and use of protective bed coverings. **Medication** dosage changes or alterations can augment sexual function.

ALLEVIATING SEXUAL DYSFUNCTION IN PATIENTS WITH MOTOR OR SENSORY FUNCTION PROBLEMS

Hypertonicity is the major motor problem in patients with central nervous system impairments as related to sexual function. If the person is **hemiplegic**, the person can lie on the affected side. If the person is **paraplegic** or has apraxia or ataxia, the partner generally must initiate and/or direct movement to achieve sexual response. It is important to recognize **autonomic dysreflexia** in spinal cord injury patients and stop activity if it occurs. A wide variety of sensory changes that may apply to sexual activity can occur in patients with spinal cord injuries, ranging from loss of genital sensation to heightened responses resembling orgasm in other areas (pseudo-orgasm). Effective techniques addressing sensory deficits include visual stimulation (especially for men), touching other areas, and other methods of increasing desire or release, such as mood music or verbal encouragement.

REPRODUCTION ISSUES RELATED TO TRAUMATIC INJURIES OR CHRONIC ILLNESSES

Female fertility is generally affected only transiently by traumatic injuries or chronic illnesses. Women with **spinal cord injuries** can conceive and deliver babies, but they may have problems during labor and delivery due to autonomic dysreflexia. These are usually addressed through use of epidural anesthetics and blood pressure medications. Men can experience **infertility** due to erectile or ejaculation malfunctions, poor thermoregulation to the testicle area, or infections or hormonal imbalances. The latter can affect female fertility as well. A major issue for people with disabilities is **birth control information dissemination and usage**. Individuals with disabilities, especially those of childbearing age, should be informed of options.

PHYSICAL ADJUSTMENTS THAT PATIENTS WITH DISABILITIES MAY NEED TO MAKE TO HAVE SEXUAL INTERCOURSE

Most patients with disabilities can modify the major **sexual positions** of face-to-face (with one or the other on top), side-lying, or rear entry to be comfortable. Patients who have been relatively immobile do need to be

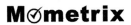

careful to avoid fractures; it is recommended that they use their brace during sex. Positions that put minimal stress on **joints** should be used by individuals with rheumatic diseases. Supportive pillows and side-lying positions are generally recommended for patients with arthritic hip joint issues. It is recommended that patients with spasticity due to spinal cord injuries or other neurological problems assume the **bottom position** due to lack of control. This position is also suggested for people at risk for myocardial infarction, and for these individuals, heart rate should be monitored for about fifteen minutes after intercourse.

INTERVENTIONS RELATED TO PSYCHOSOCIAL ISSUES AND SEXUALITY IN PATIENTS WITH DISABILITIES

The most prominent psychological issues related to sexuality in patients with disabilities are **disturbed body image** and **chronic low self-esteem**. The nurse's roles are to educate the patient about expected changes, retrain them in aspects that might affect body image or self-esteem (such as control of incontinence), and provide a supportive environment. Patients with disabilities often feel **social isolation** as well, which can hamper their ability to foster interpersonal and romantic or sexual relationships. Interventions as simple as clothing or cosmetics that mask the parts affecting body image can alleviate the feeling of social isolation. Patients need to be educated that in most cases lovemaking is still possible. **Sexual rehabilitation** involves development of positive communication patterns with the partner, taking into account that women are more attuned to underlying emotions than men, who are more literal. Healthcare personnel should provide enough privacy for the patient and the patient's partner to at least express affection such as touching, hugging, and kissing.

NURSE'S ROLE AS SEXUAL COUNSELOR FOR PATIENT AND PARTNER

One role of the rehabilitation nurse is **education** of the patient with deficient knowledge. The nurse should be informed, supportive, and respectful of the patient. Some of the patient's needs might require referral to other team members or group classes. The sexual partner also needs to be informed about expected **alterations** in body image and sexual functioning. Several decades ago, a model called **PLISSIT** was proposed by Annon. PLISSIT addresses a logical progression in sexual counseling of the patient, which starts with obtaining permission (P) for discussion, then offering limited information (LI), followed by specific suggestions (SS), and later, intensive therapy (IT) if needed.

PLISSIT MODEL TO ADDRESS SEXUAL ISSUES

The PLISSIT model for communicating about sexuality is as follows:

Level	Intervention	Description
I	Permission	The first step gives the person permission to have feelings or attitudes and to do or not do something. Reassure the person that their feelings are not abnormal. Pointing out consequences of choices is important to put the patient's choices in perspective. Attempt to establish open communication by helping the person to feel comfortable.
II	Limited Information	Information should help to dispel misconceptions and fears and should be specifically related to the needs and concerns of the patient. Information should be factual about the effects of surgery on sexuality.
III	Specific Suggestions	At this point, the person needs to take action or seek treatment with medical guidance. Some specific suggestions might include the use of lubricants, emptying of an ostomy pouch before sexual activity, or using pouch covers.
IV	Intensive Therapy	This involves referral to an appropriate specialist, as the person may, for example, need reconstructive surgery or psychotherapy beyond what the nurse is able to provide.

Functional Health Patterns

45

[Image 0 -> data/images_b/9781609715335_page_054_img_000_29a1cb.png]

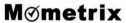

REHABILITATION NURSE'S ROLE IN SEXUAL COUNSELING OF CHILDREN AND ADOLESCENTS

The rehabilitation nurse has a responsibility to provide some sexual education for **children and adolescents with disabilities** if parents cannot do so. This is particularly true when these children are confined to group settings that place them in vulnerable positions. Components of this education should include social skills related to sexuality, specific information related to their age, and information about prevention of sexually transmitted diseases. The age to introduce information about female menses, male nocturnal emissions, puberty changes, sexually transmitted diseases, abstinence, and reproduction is between **8 and 11 years of age**. Between **12 and 18 years of age**, other concepts, such as sexuality within the context of love and communication, birth control, the responsibilities of sexual activity, and condom use should be addressed. The nurse or other educator should be very direct about the consequences of unsafe sex.

DISCUSSING SAFER SEX GUIDELINES WITH PATIENTS WITH DISABILITIES

Safer sex guidelines for patients (with or without disability) should include the following:

- It should be taught that **abstinence** is the only absolutely safe means of birth control and prevention of sexually transmitted diseases (STDs).
- The patient should also be advised that **STDs** are less likely with restriction of the number of sexual partners, mutually exclusive sexual partnering, and prior knowledge about a partner's sexual history.
- High-risk activities should be avoided until **STD status** is known. These activities include unprotected vaginal or anal intercourse and any other activities that can expose the individual to blood, semen, feces, or secretions.
- **Condoms** can greatly reduce the spread of STDs and should be used with oral, anal, or vaginal sexual practices. Condoms should be combined with spermicides, such as octoxynol or nonoxynol-9, for the latter two.
- Lubrication, hygienic practices, and voiding after sex further decrease the likelihood of **infection**.
- People at risk for STDs, especially HIV, should be **tested** and examined periodically.
- If **sexual stimulators** such as vibrators are utilized, they should be cleansed completely before use and used in conjunction with lubricants.

BIRTH CONTROL FOR PEOPLE WITH DISABILITIES

Birth control options with the lowest failure rates (3% or less) are **hormonal-based**, although they may be contraindicated in patients who have additional cardiovascular or other problems. Hormonal-based birth control methods that suppress ovulation come in the form of oral contraceptives, implants, injections, rings, and patches. Depo-Provera, a medroxyprogesterone acetate injection, controls the menstrual cycle. **Barrier methods** include intrauterine devices to prevent implantation, diaphragms to provide a physical sperm barrier, sponges over the cervix, and male condoms. All of these may be used in conjunction with **spermicidal foams or creams,** and the lowest failure rates have been associated with **condoms and diaphragms**. Coitus interruptus (withdrawal prior to ejaculation) and use of natural methods such as rhythm or basal body temperature generally have much higher failure rates. The most effective means of preventing pregnancies is permanent sterilization through **male vasectomy** or **female fallopian tube ligation**.

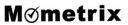

Optimal Psychosocial Patterns and Holistic Wellbeing

ELEMENTS OF THE PSYCHOSOCIAL ASSESSMENT

A psychosocial assessment should provide additional information to the physical assessment to guide the patient's plan of care and should include:

- Previous hospitalizations and experience with healthcare
- Psychiatric history: Suicidal ideation, psychiatric disorders, family psychiatric history, history of violence and/or self-mutilation
- Chief complaint: Patient's perception
- Complementary therapies: Acupuncture, visualization, and meditation
- Occupational and educational background: Employment, retirement, and special skills
- Social patterns: Family and friends, living situation, typical activities, support system
- Sexual patterns: Orientation, problems, and sex practices
- Interests/abilities: Hobbies and sports
- Current or past substance abuse: Type, frequency, drinking pattern, use of recreational drugs, and overuse of prescription drugs
- Ability to cope: Stress reduction techniques
- Physical, sexual, emotional, and financial abuse: Older adults are especially vulnerable to abuse and may be reluctant to disclose out of shame or fear
- Spiritual/Cultural assessment: Religious/Spiritual importance, practices, restrictions (such as blood products or foods), and impact on health/health decisions

HAMILTON ANXIETY SCALE

The Hamilton Anxiety Scale (HAS or HAMA) is utilized to evaluate the anxiety related symptomatology that may be present in adults as well as children. It provides an evaluation of overall **anxiety** and its degree of severity. This includes **somatic anxiety** (physical complaints) and **psychic anxiety** (mental agitation and distress). This scale consists of 14 items based on anxiety produced symptoms. Each item is ranked 0-4 with 0 indicating no symptoms present and 4 indicating severe symptoms present. This scale is frequently utilized in psychotropic drug evaluations. If performed before a particular medication has been started and then again at later visits, the HAS can be helpful in adjusting medication dosages based in part on the individual's score. It is often utilized as an outcome measure in clinical trials.

BECK DEPRESSION INVENTORY

The Beck Depression Inventory (BDI) is a widely utilized, self-reported, multiple-choice questionnaire consisting of 21 items, which measures the **degree of depression**. This tool is designed for use in adults ages 17-80. It evaluates physical symptoms such as weight loss, loss of sleep, loss of interest in sex, fatigue, and attitudinal symptoms such as irritability, guilt, and hopelessness. The items rank in four possible answer choices based on an increasing severity of symptoms. The test is scored with the answers ranging in value from 0-3. The total score is utilized to determine the degree of depression. The usual ranges include: 0-9 no signs of depression, 10-18 mild depression, 19-29 moderate depression, and 30-63 severe depression.

EVALUATION FOR SUICIDAL OR HOMICIDAL THOUGHTS

During a risk assessment two of the most important areas to evaluate are the patient's **risk for self-harm or harm to others**. The staff member performing the assessment should very closely evaluate for any descriptions or thoughts the patient may have concerning these risks. Direct questioning on these subjects should be performed and documented. Close evaluation of any delusional thoughts the patient may be having should be carefully evaluated. Does the patient believe he or she is being instructed by others to perform either of these acts? Safety of the patient and others needs to be a top priority and carefully documented. If the patient indicates that they are having these thoughts or ideas, they must be placed in either suicidal or assault precautions with close monitoring per facility protocol.

47

SUICIDE RISK ASSESSMENT

A suicide risk assessment should be completed and documented upon admission, with each shift change, at discharge, or any time suicidal ideations are suggested by the patient. This risk assessment should evaluate some of the following criteria:

- Would the patient sign a contract for safety?
- Is there a suicide plan? How lethal is the plan?
- What is the elopement risk?
- How often are the suicidal thoughts, and have they attempted suicide before?

Any associated symptoms of hopelessness, guilt, anger, helplessness, impulsive behaviors, nightmares, obsessions with death, or altered judgment should also be assessed and documented. The higher the score the higher the risk for suicide.

ALCOHOL USE ASSESSMENT

The **Clinical Instrument for Withdrawal for Alcohol (CIWA)** is a tool used to assess the severity of alcohol withdraw. Each category is scored 0-7 points based on the severity of symptoms, except #10, which is scored 0-4. A score <5 indicates mild withdrawal without need for medications; for scores ranging 5-15, benzodiazepines are indicated to manage symptoms. A score >15 indicates severe withdrawal and the need for admission to the unit.

1. Nausea/Vomiting
2. Tremor
3. Paroxysmal Sweats
4. Anxiety
5. Agitation
6. Tactile Disturbances
7. Auditory Disturbances
8. Visual Disturbances
9. Headache
10. Disorientation or Clouding of Sensorium

The **CAGE** tool is used as a quick assessment to identify problem drinkers. Moderate drinking, (1-2 drinks daily or one drink a day for older adults) is usually not harmful to people in the absence of other medical conditions. However, drinking more can lead to serious psychosocial and physical problems. One drink is defined as 12 ounces of beer/wine cooler, 5 ounces of wine, or 1.5 ounces of liquor.

- **C** – *Cutting Down*: "Do you think about trying to cut down on drinking?"
- **A** – *Annoyed at Criticism*: "Are people starting to criticize your drinking?"
- **G** – *Guilty feeling*: "Do you feel guilty or try to hide your drinking?"
- **E** – *Eye opener*: "Do you increasingly need a drink earlier in the day?"

"Yes" on one question suggests the possibility of a drinking problem. "Yes" on ≥2 indicates a drinking problem

SCREENING FOR RISK-TAKING BEHAVIOR

The ability to assess outcomes and respond appropriately to risks are part of the decision-making process. Decision making can be impaired in patients with mental health disorders such as depression, anxiety, bipolar disorder, and personality disorders, as well as in patients who have experienced a brain injury or have a dependence on drugs or alcohol. Health care providers should screen patients for the presence of high-risk behaviors. This may be accomplished through a self-administered questionnaire or through a patient interview with a trained clinician. Examples of **high-risk behaviors** include substance use/abuse, high risk sexual behaviors, high risk driving behaviors such as drinking and driving, speeding or riding with a drunk driver, and

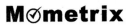

violence related behaviors. Patients with an increased response to risk taking may exhibit signs of impulsivity and sensation seeking. Conversely, other patients may exhibit abnormally cautious behavior.

ASSESSMENT OF UNIQUE NEEDS OF VETERANS

Assessment of **veterans** must include not only the standard assessments appropriate for the patient's age and gender but also assessment of combat-associated injuries and illnesses:

- Shrapnel and/or gunshot injuries: Associated physical limitations, pain
- Amputations: Mobility and prosthesis issues; body image issues
- PTSD: Extent, frequency of attacks, limiting factors, triggers
- Depression, suicidal ideation
- Substance abuse: Type and extent

Because a large number of veterans are among the homeless population, the veteran's living arrangements should be explored and appropriate referrals made if the patient is in need of housing. Veterans may be unaware of programs offered through the US Department of Veterans Affairs and should be provided information about these programs as appropriate for the patient's needs.

BIPOLAR DISORDER

Bipolar disorder causes severe mood swings between hyperactive states and depression, accompanied by impaired judgment because of distorted thoughts. The hypomanic stage may allow for creativity and good functioning in some people, but it can develop into more severe mania, which may be associated with psychosis and hallucinations with rapid speech and bizarre behavior, and then into periods of profound depression. While most cases are diagnosed in late adolescence, there is increasing evidence that some children present with symptoms earlier; especially at risk are children with a bipolar parent. Bipolar disorder is associated with high rates of suicide, so early diagnosis and treatment is critical.

Symptoms may be relatively mild or involve severe rapid cycling between mania and depression.

Treatment includes both medications (usually given continually) to prevent cycling and control depression and psychosocial therapy, such as cognitive therapy, to help control disordered thought patterns and behavior. Psychiatric referral should be made.

DEPRESSION

Depression is a mood disorder characterized by profound feelings of sadness and withdrawal. It may be acute (such as after a death) or chronic with recurring episodes over a lifetime. The cause appears to be a combination of genetic, biological, and environmental factors. A major depressive episode is a depressed mood, profound and constant sense of hopelessness and despair, or loss of interest in all or almost all activities for a period of at least two weeks. Some drugs may precipitate depression: diuretics, Parkinson's drugs, estrogen, corticosteroids, cimetidine, hydralazine, propranolol, digitalis, and indomethacin. Depression is associated with neurotransmitter dysregulation, especially serotonin and norepinephrine. Major depression can be mild, moderate, or severe.

> **Review Video: Major Depression**
> Visit mometrix.com/academy and enter code: 632694
>
> **Review Video: Types of Clinical Depression**
> Visit mometrix.com/academy and enter code: 154589

Symptoms include changes in mood, sadness, loss of interest in usual activities, increased fatigue, changes in appetite and fluctuations in weight, anxiety, and sleep disturbance.

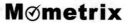

Treatment includes tricyclic antidepressants (TCAS) and SSRIs, but SSRIs have fewer side effects and are less likely to cause death with an overdose. Counseling, undergoing cognitive behavioral therapy, treating underlying cause, and instituting an exercise program may help reduce depression.

ANXIETY AND DEPRESSION DUE TO INTENSIVE CARE STAYS

Anxiety and depression affect over half of patients who are treated in intensive care not only during the stay but also after discharge, especially if care is long-term or if their needs for moderate or high care continue. Additionally, studies have shown that those who suffer depression during and after ICU stays have increased risk of mortality over the next two years. Patients with anxiety may appear restless (thrashing about the bed), have difficulty concentrating, exhibit tachycardia and tachypnea, experience insomnia and feelings of dread, and complain of various ailments, such as stomach ache and headache. Symptoms of depression may overlap (and patients may have both anxiety and depression) and may also include fatigue, insomnia, withdrawal, appetite change, irritability, pessimistic outlooks, feelings of worthlessness, sadness, and suicidal ideation. Brief screening tools for anxiety and depression should be used with all ICU patients and interventions per psychological referral made as needed.

ANXIETY DISORDERS

Anxiety is a human emotion and experience that everyone has at some point during their life. Feelings of uncertainty, helplessness, isolation, alienation, and insecurity can all be experienced during an **anxiety response**. Many times, anxiety occurs without a specific known object or source. It can occur because of the unknown. Anxiety occurs throughout the life cycle, and therefore anxiety disorders can affect people of all ages. Populations that are most commonly affected include women, smokers, people under the age of 45, individuals that are separated or divorced, victims of abuse, and people in the lower socioeconomic groups. An individual can have one single anxiety disorder, experience more than one anxiety disorder, or have other mental health disorders all occurring at the same time.

> **Review Video: Anxiety Disorders**
> Visit mometrix.com/academy and enter code: 366760

GENERALIZED ANXIETY DISORDER

Generalized anxiety disorder can be very insidious and occurs when an individual consistently experiences **excessive anxiety and worry**. This anxiety and worry will be present almost every day and lasts for a period of at least six months. The worry and anxiety will be uncontrollable, intrusive, and not related to any medical disease process. It will pertain to real-life events, situations, or circumstances and may occur along with mild depression symptoms. The individual will also experience three or more of the following symptoms: fatigue, inability to concentrate, irritability, insomnia, restlessness, loosing thought processes or going blank, and muscle tension. The continued anxiety and worry will eventually affect daily functioning and cause social and occupational disturbances.

COMORBIDITIES

Individuals with generalized anxiety disorder (GAD) will often have **other mental health disorders**. When a person has more than one psychological disorder occurring at the same time, these disorders are considered to be **comorbid**. Most patients suffering from GAD will have at least one more psychiatric diagnosis. The most common comorbid disorders can include major depressive disorder, social or specific phobias, panic disorder, and dysthymic disorder. It is also common for these individuals to have substance abuse problems, and they may look to alcohol or barbiturates to help control their symptoms of anxiety.

Functional Health Patterns

LEVELS OF ANXIETY

There are four main levels of anxiety that were named by Peplau. They are as follows:

1. **Mild anxiety** is associated with normal tensions of everyday life. It can increase awareness and motivate learning and creativity.
2. **Moderate anxiety** occurs when the individual narrows their field of perception and focuses on the immediate problem. This level decreases the perceptual field; however, the person can tend to other tasks if directed.
3. **Severe anxiety** leads to a markedly reduced field of perception and the person focuses only on the details of the problem. All energy is directed at relieving the anxiety and the person can only perform other tasks under significant persuasion.
4. **Panic** is the most extreme level of anxiety and associated with feelings of dread and terror. The individual is unable to perform any other tasks no matter how strongly they are persuaded to do so. This level can be life-threatening with complete disorganization of thought occurring.

PHYSICAL SYMPTOMS

Anxiety produces a very physical response and effects the largest body systems, such as cardiovascular, respiratory, GI, neuromuscular, urinary tract, and skin. Symptoms vary and can increase upon a continuum depending upon the level of anxiety the person is experiencing.

- **Cardiovascular symptoms** can include palpitation, tachycardia, hypertension, feeling faint or actually fainting, hypotension, or bradycardia.
- **Respiratory symptoms** can include tachypnea, shortness of breath, chest pressure, shallow respirations, or choking sensation.
- **GI symptoms** can include revulsion toward food, nausea, diarrhea, and abdominal pain or discomfort.

Even though anxiety occurs psychologically, it can produce extreme **physical responses** from the neuromuscular system, urinary tract, and skin. These symptoms can range from mild to severe depending upon the degree of anxiety the person is experiencing.

- **Neuromuscular symptoms** can include hyperreflexia, being easily startled, eyelid twitching, inability to sleep, shaking, fidgeting, pacing, wobbly legs, or clumsy movements.
- **Urinary tract symptoms** can include increased frequency and sensation of need to urinate.
- **Skin symptoms** can include flushed face, sweaty palms, itching, sensations of being hot and/or cold, pale facial coloring, or diaphoresis.

BEHAVIORAL AND AFFECTIVE RESPONSES

Behavioral and affective symptoms along with a multitude of physical symptoms are observable in anxious patients. The effects of these responses can affect the person experiencing the anxiety along with their relationships with others.

- Some **behavioral responses** can include restlessness and physical tension, hypervigilance, rapid speech, social or relationship withdrawal, decreased coordination, avoidance, or flight.
- **Affective responses** are the patient's emotional reactions and can be described subjectively by the individual. Patients may describe symptoms such as edginess, impatience, tension, nervousness, fear, frustration, jitteriness, or helplessness.

COGNITIVE RESPONSES

Anxiety not only produces physical and emotional symptoms, but it can also greatly affect the individual's intellectual abilities. **Cognitive responses** to anxiety occur in three main categories. These include sensory-perceptual, thought difficulties, and conceptualization. Responses that affect the patient's **sensory-perceptual fields** can include feeling that their mind is unclear or clouded, seeing objects indistinctly, perceiving a surreal environment, increased self-consciousness, or hypervigilance. **Thinking difficulties** can include the inability to remember important information, confusion, inability to focus thoughts or attention, easily distracted, blocking thoughts, difficulty with reasoning, tunnel vision, or loss of objectivity. **Conceptual difficulties** can include the fear of loss of control, inability to cope, potential physical injury, developing a mental disorder, or receiving a negative evaluation. The patient may have cognitive distortion, protruding scary visual images, or uncontrollable repetition of fearful thoughts.

> **Review Video: Different Types of Anxiety Disorders**
> Visit mometrix.com/academy and enter code: 366760

PTSD

Patients that experience a traumatic event may re-experience the trauma through distressing thoughts and recollections of the event. In addition, psychological effects of the trauma may include difficulty sleeping, emotional lability and problems with memory and concentration. Patients may also wish to avoid places or activities that remind them of their trauma. These are all characteristics of **post-traumatic stress disorder (PTSD)** and may cause patients extreme distress and significantly impact their quality of life.

Signs and symptoms: Nightmares, flashbacks, insomnia, symptoms of hyperarousal including irritability and anxiety, avoidance, and negative thoughts and feelings about oneself and others.

Diagnosis: PTSD is diagnosed through psychological assessment and criteria defined in the Diagnostic and Statistical Manual of Mental Disorders, Fifth Edition (DSM-5).

Treatment: Pharmacologic therapy may be utilized to help control the symptoms of PTSD. Non-pharmacologic therapy options include group and individual/family therapy, cognitive behavioral therapy, and anxiety management/relaxation techniques. Hypnosis may also be utilized.

PSYCHOSIS

Psychosis is a severe reaction to stressors (psychological, physical) that results in alterations in affect and impaired psychomotor and behavioral functions, including the onset of hallucinations and/or delusions. Psychosis is not a diagnosis but is a symptom that may be caused by a mental disorder (such as schizophrenia or bipolar disease) or a physical disorder (such as a brain tumor or Alzheimer's disease). Psychosis may also be induced by some prescription drugs (muscle relaxants, antihistamines, anticonvulsants, corticosteroids, antiparkinson drugs), illicit drugs (cocaine, PCP, amphetamines, cannabis, LSD), and alcohol. Treatment depends on identifying the underlying cause of the psychosis and initiating treatment. For example, if caused by schizophrenia, then antipsychotic drugs and hospitalization in a mental health facility may be indicated. In most cases of drug-induced psychosis, stopping the drug alleviates the symptoms although some may benefit from the addition of a benzodiazepine or antipsychotic drug until symptoms subside.

> **Review Video: Antipsychotic drugs: Clozapine, Haloperidol, Etc**
> Visit mometrix.com/academy and enter code: 369601

SUBSTANCE ABUSE

Substance abuse is the abuse of drugs, medicines, or alcohol that causes mental and physical problems for the abuser and family. Abusers use substances out of boredom, to hide negative self-esteem, to dampen emotional pain, and to cope with daily stress. As the abuse continues, abusers become unable to take care of daily needs and duties. They lack effective coping mechanisms and the ability to make healthy choices. They can't identify and prioritize stress or choose positive behavior to resolve the stress in a healthy way. Some family members may act as codependents because of their desire to feel needed by the abuser, to control the person, and to stay with him or her. The nurse can help the family to confront an individual with their concerns about the person and their proposals for treatment. Family members can enforce consequences if treatment is not sought.

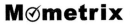

Family members may also need counseling to learn new behaviors to stop enabling the abuser to continue substance abuse.

PATHOPHYSIOLOGY OF ADDICTION

Genetic, social, and personality factors may all play a role in the development of **addictive tendencies**. However, the main factor of the development of substance addiction is the pharmacological activation of the **reward system** located in the central nervous system (CNS). This reward systems pathway involves **dopaminergic neurons**. Dopamine is found in the CNS and is one of many neurotransmitters that play a role in an individual's mood. The mesolimbic pathway seems to play a primary role in the reward and motivational process involved with addiction. This pathway begins in the ventral tegmental area of the brain (VTA) and then moves forward into the nucleus accumbens located in the middle forebrain bundle (MFB). Some drugs enhance mesolimbic dopamine activity, therefore producing very potent effects on mood and behavior.

> **Review Video: Addictions**
> Visit mometrix.com/academy and enter code: 460412

INDICATORS OF SUBSTANCE ABUSE

Many people with substance abuse (alcohol or drugs) are reluctant to disclose this information, but there are a number of **indicators** that are suggestive of substance abuse:

Physical signs include:

- Burns on fingers or lips
- Pupils abnormally dilated or constricted, eyes watery
- Slurring of speech, slow speech
- Lack of coordination, instability of gait, tremors
- Sniffing repeatedly, nasal irritation, persistent cough
- Weight loss
- Dysrhythmias
- Pallor, puffiness of face
- Needle tracks on arms or legs
- Odor of alcohol/marijuana on clothing or breath

Behavioral signs include:

- Labile emotions, including mood swings, agitation, and anger
- Inappropriate, impulsive, or risky behavior
- Lying
- Missing appointments
- Difficulty concentrating, short term memory loss, blackouts
- Insomnia or excessive sleeping; disoriented, confused
- Lack of personal hygiene

ALCOHOL WITHDRAWAL

Chronic abuse of ethanol (alcoholism) can lead to physical dependency. Sudden cessation of drinking, which often happens in the inpatient setting, is associated with **alcohol withdrawal syndrome.** It may be precipitated by trauma or infection and has a high mortality rate, 5-15% with treatment and 35% without treatment.

Signs/Symptoms: Anxiety, tachycardia, headache, diaphoresis, progressing to severe agitation, hallucinations, auditory/tactile disturbances, and psychotic behavior (delirium tremens).

Diagnosis: Physical assessment, blood alcohol levels (on admission).

Treatment includes:

- Medication: IV benzodiazepines to manage symptoms; electrolyte and nutritional replacement, especially magnesium and thiamine.
- Use the CIWA scale to measure symptoms of withdrawal; treat as indicated.
- Provide an environment with minimal sensory stimulus (lower lights, close blinds) & implement fall and seizure precautions.
- Prevention: Screen all patients for alcohol/substance abuse, using CAGE or other assessment tool. Remember to express support and comfort to patient; wait until withdrawal symptoms are subsiding to educate about alcohol use and moderation.

CULTURAL COMPETENCE AND SPIRITUALITY
UNDERSTANDING OF DIVERSE CULTURES

An understanding of diverse cultures is very important when approaching the treatment and management of those with disabilities:

- The way in which the **family structure** is viewed in a particular culture is important to the identification of its support system.
- Communication styles differ between cultural groups, including verbal versus nonverbal clues as well as the language used.
- Various cultures adhere to and are more receptive to certain **health practices**. Their belief systems regarding health and illness color their viewpoints.
- There are many different cultural and religious beliefs and outlooks regarding the **dying process**, as well as diverse **dietary practices** that can affect the acceptance of change.
- Various cultural groups approach **childbearing** or **child care** differently.

All these factors should be taken into account by the nurse when formulating treatment plans. Practices can vary greatly geographically, depending on the proportion of immigrants who settled in the area.

HOLISM AND SPIRITUALITY

Holism is a theory of health treatment that incorporates physical, psychological, and social aspects to achieve health and wellbeing. **Spirituality** is an inner awareness and a relationship with a higher force. This force can be defined by religion, but this is not a prerequisite for spirituality, which is unique to each individual. Spirituality can be part of a holistic approach. Other concepts related to spirituality include soul and spirit. **Soul** refers to the nonphysical aspects of a person that shape their relationships and emotions, and it includes elements such as memory, understanding, and will. Some religions, such as Christianity, contend that the soul continues after death. The **spirit** is the intangible life force of an individual. When patients lose a bond to the higher force they normally embrace, they can experience a spiritual crisis and associated changes detrimental to wellbeing.

HEALING AND FORGIVENESS

Healing is the internal and conscious process of releasing negative attitudes and patterns and the reestablishment of a feeling of wholeness. It is independent of the process of curing or physiological treatment of a disease. The nurse can play an important role in the healing process. One crucial component toward healing is usually **forgiveness**, the act of pardoning oneself and others, and also asking for forgiveness from God or others. Generally, people cannot move on unless they have embraced forgiveness. Another element, often facilitated through forgiveness, is development of a feeling of **serenity or inner peace**.

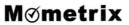

SPIRITUAL ASSESSMENT

Spiritual assessment of a patient is generally done after trust and rapport have been established. Spiritual histories should go beyond questions about religious practices and beliefs. They should also incorporate queries about the person's support system, notions about God or a deity, and how the patient's illness has impacted their spiritual beliefs. There are several **Likert scales** (measuring agreement or disagreement with statements) for spiritual assessment as well. These include the **Spiritual Well-Being Scale (SWBS)**, the **Spiritual Assessment Scale (SAS)**, and others. One of the best scales that minimizes cultural bias is the **Spiritual Involvement and Beliefs Scale (SIBS)**, which has the patient evaluate 26 items on a scale from strongly disagree (1) to strongly agree (7); it also looks at the frequency of five types of behaviors that reflect spirituality.

SPIRITUAL ROLES FOR REHABILITATION NURSES

The rehabilitation nurse can intervene in ways that incorporate a patient's spiritual beliefs without revealing or abdicating their own value system. **Reliance on religion or spirituality** tends to increase greatly during times of illness. The nurse needs to understand that suffering is **personal** and shaped to an extent by the patient's religious or spiritual beliefs. Some people will downplay the severity of their suffering while others will regard it as punishment for their sins. The nursing interventions are mainly **consolation** and **counseling** of the patient in order to create trust, bolster hope, and foster independence. **Being present**, either for support or through touch, is actually the primary spiritual role of the nurse. Spiritual care team members such as the chaplain can also be enlisted. There are also parish nurses who work in the community primarily though some established religious organization. Studies have shown that embracing spirituality during a chronic illness helps a patient to cope.

VALUE OF OTHER NURSING INTERVENTIONS RELATED TO SPIRITUALITY

Instillation of hope or optimism actively enhances coping mechanisms, while a feeling of hopelessness or lack of control impedes them. Hope is entrenched in perception. It also can have two components, a **horizontal** one focused on worldly relationships and a **vertical** one related to eternal goals and connections; the latter can still provide optimism when earthly actions have failed. **Humor** and **laughter** are effective tools for diffusing tension and grief momentarily. The nurse can facilitate the patient's spiritual growth and support the patient in their beliefs by taking the patient to services or providing educational material. There are also several types of **therapy** that have been found to be useful, such as use of music or other arts, bibliotherapy (reading), or reminiscence therapy, in which various strategies are used to invoke previous pleasant memories.

DIAGNOSES, INTERVENTIONS, AND DESIRED OUTCOMES RELATED TO A PATIENT'S SPIRITUALITY

There are five possible nursing diagnoses related to a patient's spirituality.

- The patient may have difficulty **making decisions**. The goal is to establish the ability to process information and make decisions, which can be facilitated by the nurse through goal setting and use of various techniques, such as meditation or relaxation.
- Another potential diagnosis is **dysfunctional grieving**. Here, acceptance and grief resolution are the desired outcomes, which can be aided by working through the grief and guilt.
- **Hopelessness** is a common spirituality-related classification. In order to restore hope and the ability to cope, the nurse should use measures that instill hope and stabilize the patient's mood.
- Some patients can be categorized as **at risk for spiritual distress**, particularly when they are nearing the end of life. In this case, the nurse should employ all means of spiritual support to aid the person in accepting their health-related situation.
- The last designation is a **readiness for enhanced spiritual wellbeing**, which means the nurse should use any available methods to enhance the patient's spiritual or religious beliefs, develop the patient's self-esteem, and help the patient to cope.

Functional Health Patterns

Coping and Stress Management Skills

STRESS
RELATIONSHIP BETWEEN STRESS AND DISEASE

Stress causes a number of physical and psychological changes within the body:

- Cortisol levels increase
- Digestion is hindered and the colon stimulated
- Heart rate increases
- Perspiration increases
- Anxiety and depression occur and can result in insomnia, anorexia or weight gain, and suicide
- Immune response decreases, making the person more vulnerable to infections
- Autoimmune reaction may increase, leading to autoimmune diseases

The body's **compensatory mechanisms** try to restore homeostasis. When these mechanisms are overwhelmed, pathophysiological injury to the cells of the body result. When this injury begins to interfere with the function of the organs or systems in the body, symptoms of dysfunction will occur. If the conditions are not corrected, the body changes the structure or function of the affected organs or systems.

ADAPTATION OF CELLS TO STRESS

The most common stressors to cells include the lack of oxygen, presence of toxins or chemicals, and infection. **Cells react to stress** by making the following changes:

- **Hypertrophy**: Cells swell, leading to an overall increase in the size of the affected organ.
- **Atrophy**: Cells shrivel and the overall organ size decreases in size.
- **Hyperplasia**: The cells divide and overgrowth and thickening of the tissue results.
- **Dysplasia**: The cells are changed in appearance as a result of irritation over an extended period of time, sometimes leading to malignancy.
- **Metaplasia**: Cells change type as a result of stress.

If the stress that caused the cells to change continues, the cells become injured and die. When enough cells die, organ and systemic failure occur.

PSYCHOLOGICAL RESPONSE TO STRESS

When stress is encountered, a person **responds** according to the threat perceived to compensate. The threat is evaluated as to the amount of harm or loss that has occurred or is possible. If the stress is benign (such as with marriage), then a challenge is present that demands change. Once the threat or challenge is defined, the person can gather information, resources, and support to make the changes needed to resolve the stress to the greatest degree possible. Immediate psychological response to stress may include shock, anger, fear, or excitement. Over time, people may develop chronic anxiety, depression, flashbacks, thought disturbances, and sleep disturbances. Changes may occur in emotions and thinking, in behavior, or in the person's environment. People may be more able to adapt to stress if they have many varied experiences, a good self-esteem, and a support network to help as needed. A healthy lifestyle and philosophical beliefs, including religion, may give a person more reserve to cope with stress.

IMPACT OF DIFFERENT KINDS OF STRESS

Everyone encounters **stress** in life and it **impacts** each person differently. There are the small daily "hassles," major traumatic events, and the periodic stressful events of marriage, birth, divorce, and death. Compounded stress experienced on a daily basis can impact health status over time. Stressors that occur suddenly are the hardest to overcome and result in the greatest tension. The length of time that a stressor is present affects the impact with long-term, relentless stress, such as that generated by poverty or disability, resulting in disease more often. If there is **ineffective coping**, a person will suffer greater changes resulting in even more stress.

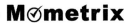

The nurse can help patients to recognize those things that induce stress in their lives, find ways to reduce stress when possible, and teach effective coping skills and problem-management.

GRIEF

KUBLER-ROSS'S FIVE STAGES OF GRIEF

Kubler-Ross taught the medical and nursing community that the dying patient and family welcomes open, honest discussion of the dying process and felt that there were certain **stages** that patients and family go through. The stages may not occur in order, but may vary or some may be skipped. Stages include:

- **Denial**: The person denies the diagnosis and tries to pretend it isn't true. During this time, the person may seek a second opinion or alternative therapies. They may use denial until they are better able to emotionally cope with the reality of the disease or changes that need to be made. Patients may also wish to save family and friends from pain and worry. Both patients and family may use denial as a coping mechanism when they feel overwhelmed by the reality of the disease and threatened losses.
- **Anger**: The person is angry about the situation and may focus that rage on anyone.
- **Bargaining**: The person attempts to make deals with a higher power to secure a better outcome to their situation.
- **Depression**: The person anticipates the loss and the changes it will bring with a sense of sadness and grief.
- **Acceptance**: The person accepts the impending death and is ready to face it as it approaches. The patient may begin to withdraw from interests and family.

> **Review Video: Patient Treatment and Grief**
> Visit mometrix.com/academy and enter code: 648794

GRIEF RELATED TO DISABILITY

Patients with disabilities must cope with almost continuous **grief and loss**, including **primary losses** (spouse, friends, and family) and **secondary losses** (such as companionship and assistance). As losses accumulate, the patient with disabilities may become overwhelmed with grief and unable to cope. Patients may grieve the following losses:

- **Body image**: Physical and psychological as physical condition deteriorates
- **Spouse/partner/friends**: Through death or distance
- **Self-identity and self-esteem**: As roles change
- **Possessions**: If the person moves from a home to an assisted living or other long-term care facility
- **Financial stability**: As income decreases and expenses increase
- **Dignity**: As others care for the person
- **Independence**: As the person is forced to rely on others for assistance
- **Life itself**: Including that of significant others

The ability to **cope** with grief and loss and find hope depends upon one's support system, health status, mental status, and belief system.

LOSS OF INDEPENDENCE ASSOCIATED WITH DISABILITIES

The loss of independence and autonomy associated with disabilities can be profoundly disturbing. Losing the ability to live independently increases overall **dependence** on others, especially if the patient must live with family members or in a long-term care facility. Losing the ability to **drive** can prevent patients from shopping and engaging in social activities. This loss may be devastating to some individuals and may increase symptoms of depression. These individuals may become very angry and resentful. **Role reversal** may occur as adult children may become care providers for their parents and increasingly make decisions for them. This may cause conflicts that are draining to both parties, and some patients with disabilities become increasingly

Functional Health Patterns

57

dependent and demanding. Assistance with **instrumental activities of daily living (IADLs)** and **activities of daily living (ADLs)** is often necessary, but some patients who want to remain autonomous may resist the help.

COPING

Individuals must cognitively appraise a situation before they can decide how to **cope** with it. This appraisal includes a **primary opinion** as to the potential stress evoked, a **secondary appraisal** about possible options, and—if there is additional information—possibly **reappraisal**. People shape their assessments in light of **environmental factors** such as pressures, constraints, and opportunities in the context of their cultural perceptions. They tend to interject **personal variables** as well, such as their goals, beliefs, and personal situation. People have **coping styles** as well. Some use an emotion-based approach, while others are more reflective or more oriented toward problem-solving. The degree of stress invoked by a particular situation or event depends on the person's sense of life as meaningful. Meaning can be either **global**, based on the person's long-term beliefs and goals, or **situational**, shaded by the immediate events. Thus, individual coping mechanisms are extremely personal.

COPING WITH HEALTH ISSUES

Coping is a process of dealing with difficult problems or situations. The manner in which people cope is dependent on their **life experiences** or biography as well as other factors. Central to the ability to cope with health issues is the concept of **wellness** or physical, mental, emotional, and spiritual wellbeing. The physical state of a person alone does not necessarily determine wellness. Other attitudes contribute to wellness as well, such as personal integrity, the feeling of control, and comfort, a comparative measure of contentment. **Personal integrity** is influenced by other perceptions, such as the degree of vulnerability or susceptibility to potentially harmful situations and stressors. **Stress** can be caused by psychological factors, such as past loss, impending threats, or challenges or difficulties that need to be dealt with. Individuals in **dire situations** without choices tend to expend energy just holding themselves together or enduring. If reflection and assessment are added, then the person is experiencing suffering. Constant sadness is referred to as **chronic sorrow**. **Transition** is the evolution from one state through a neutral period into another status.

FACTORS RELATED TO SENSE OF SELF THAT IMPACT THE COPING PROCESS

Many of the factors that impact the coping process are related to the person's **sense of self** and their abilities. These include sense of coherence, self-efficacy, internal locus of control, optimism, hope, hardiness, and resourcefulness. An individual has a sense of **coherence** if the individual responds to stressors with a desire to cope and the perception that they understand and has the available resources to address the challenge. The concept of **self-efficacy**, a belief in oneself that a course of action can be developed and executed, is similar. People with a high **internal locus of control** believe that their own actions can influence outcomes. Optimism and hope are interrelated concepts. **Optimism** is the expectation of a favorable outcome. **Hope** is faith in improvement. Optimistic people generally employ active problem-solving in their coping process, whereas hope is a more emotional concept. **Hardiness** refers to the inherent ability to withstand adversity, and resilience is the capacity for speedy recovery. **Resourcefulness** or ingenuity is a learned process that can aid the ability to cope.

OTHER FACTORS THAT IMPACT THE COPING PROCESS

The **degree of uncertainty**, or lack of predictability of a desired or certain outcome, influences other coping mechanisms. Uncertainty can lead to frustration, hopelessness, aggressive behavior, and a feeling of helplessness in the patient and the patient's family members. **Social support systems** have been found to greatly enhance coping mechanisms in both the patient and family, particularly within the first few months after injury. There have been a number of studies that suggest the ability to cope can be influenced by age, gender, educational level, ethnic background, and the existence of other comorbid conditions.

ASSESSMENT OF INDIVIDUAL'S ABILITY TO COPE WITH HEALTH PROBLEMS

An assessment of an individual's coping effectiveness should include historical, subjective, and objective data, as well as an evaluation of certain physical signs and symptoms. The nurse should ask **historical questions** about the person's previous lifestyle and current circumstances, including things such as health beliefs, developmental stage, and therapies utilized (including perceived effectiveness). Coping effectiveness can be further evaluated by asking a number of questions about issues such as lifestyle and relationship changes, the patient's concerns and difficulties, the amount of control the patient perceives having over the situation, the patient's ability to adhere to a health care plan, and the patient's resources and strengths. The nurse should check for **physical symptoms of stress** such as rapid heart rate, dyspnea, stomach problems, elimination issues, nervous twitching, pain, communication problems, or skin eruptions. **Objective data** should include weight, vital signs, blood pressure, system reviews, inspection for injuries, documentation of all therapeutic items used, ability to describe the precipitating event, and observation of emotional state.

Assessment of Family System and Caregiver Coping

A person with a disability or chronic illness is generally part of a **family system** that must deal with the patient's affliction on a long-term basis. These family members can become overwrought, especially if they assume the role of primary caregiver. This is especially true after the patient leaves the hospital or rehabilitation facility and reenters the community. There are signs of **collapse** that a nurse can look for in family members or other caregivers. These include fatigue, exhaustion, rage, extreme anxiety, sickness or accidents, problems sleeping, depression or thoughts of suicide, substance abuse, presence of an eating disorder, and lack of attention to their own care. The caregiver may express **vexation** about their role and feelings that their choices are limited and/or that their resources are exhausted or unavailable.

Nursing Diagnoses Relevant to Ineffective Coping Mechanisms

NANDA International recognizes a wide variety of nursing diagnoses that reflect **coping or stress tolerance problems**. These diagnoses are primarily relevant to the patient, the family, or the community. Diagnoses pertaining to the **patient** include anxiety, fear, risky behaviors, grieving, lack of hope, low self-esteem, and a number of ineffective coping mechanisms, among others. **Family members** can be diagnosed with other coping- and stress-related issues such as grieving, caregiver role strain, fear, interrupted family procedures or coping, or powerlessness.

Nursing Interventions and Desired Outcomes for Some of the More Prevalent Nursing Diagnoses Related to Coping

Two coping styles, ineffective and defensive coping, indicate **nursing intervention** is needed. For **ineffective coping**, the nurse should provide support that enhances the person's ability to cope, make decisions, and control their anger, and builds self-esteem and enlarges the patient's support system. For **defensive coping**, interventions related to self-awareness and fostering of relationships are important. In each, the desired nursing outcome is the person's **acceptance** of their health status. Another common diagnosis is **hopelessness**, which can be addressed through support groups, therapies, and relationship-building that inspires hope; here the main goal is improvement of mood and enhancement of the patient's will to live. The diagnosis of **impaired social interaction** indicates the need for a number of interventions to improve the patient's environment, resiliency, self-esteem, and awareness. Hopefully, these interventions will lead to an improved social atmosphere and patient involvement. The classification of **chronic sorrow** is generally addressed through facilitation techniques (including support groups) that work through and resolve grief. Nursing interventions for caregiver role strain include **support and respite care** to enhance emotional health and performance.

Promoting Self-Worth and Positive Self-Image in Patients with Disabilities

Strategies to promote self-worth in the patient with disabilities include self-advocacy and self-directed care. **Self-directed care** involves the activities of daily living and modifications that enable the patient to keep chronic issues under control and to decrease the effect that such issues have on physical health status and daily functioning. For example, a patient that suffers from heart failure and who opts for self-directed care may choose to adjust their diet, adhere to a medication regimen, and exercise every day. **Self-advocacy** and self-directed care have been shown to decrease pain, enable shared decision-making about treatment, and enable a sense of control in a patient's life. Another strategy for promoting self-worth is **restorative care,** which

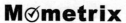

includes activities to improve psychosocial adjustment. The patient is given **short, achievable goals** (e.g., lift a leg, hold a cup) to focus on so that they can see progress and gain confidence. As a goal is achieved, new goals are set. In improving self-image, accepting the disability as part of the body image is associated with high levels of positive self-image. **Spiritual and community groups** are tools that can assist in reaching acceptance of disabilities.

> **Review Video: Patient Advocacy**
> Visit mometrix.com/academy and enter code: 202160

HELPING PATIENTS AND FAMILY MEMBERS COPE WITH ROLE CHANGES

When major disability happens, both the patient and the caregiver may experience unwanted **role changes**. Many caregivers are unprepared for the role of caregiver and lack knowledge about the patient's disease and treatments or strategies to care for the patient. Caregivers should be provided with oral information and, when appropriate, printed information about the basics of the disease process, including what to expect in the future. If the caregiver must carry out medical treatments, they should be instructed with **demonstrations** and should give return demonstrations to show mastery. The cultural needs of the caregivers must be considered. **Role supplementation** can be used preventatively, by discussing and clarifying expectations for new roles for all involved before discharge home from a rehabilitation facility. Encouraging patients to have freedom to grieve the loss of former roles and accept new roles can be beneficial. If patients or caregivers feel themselves insufficient for their new roles, roles may need to be clarified or modified.

COPING ENHANCEMENT

Coping enhancement is a method of helping the patient to adapt to stressors, changes, or threats to their lifestyle. **Active listening** to the person's narrative can help the nurse to develop strategies for coping enhancement. Strategies that have been found to be effective include those aimed at increased patient **self-awareness and/or self-efficacy**. Examples include didactic exercises, feedback or other behavioral techniques, counseling, telephone follow-ups by the nurse, boundary setting, prioritization, detailed planning, development of negotiation skills, recognition of coping sabotage, and use of all available resources. Nursing schemes can target the individual or family as a whole.

COPING WITH STRESS

Patients and family members who are dealing with chronic illness and disability may experience far more **stress** than those without disability and illness. These stressors may include actual and potential stressors, including financial burden, concern for the future, concern over new roles, concern over finding new physicians or other medical services, and concern over time commitments regarding new care needs. Developing **assertiveness** can be a powerful tool for both the patient and the caregiver. Ways to **cope** with stressors include identifying stressors so that they can be responded to, learning money management, making rest and relaxation time for caregivers, asking for help when overwhelmed, being actively involved in making plans for life, getting adequate exercise, eating a healthy diet, and meditation and relaxation techniques. Patients and caregivers should be educated to periodically **evaluate** their stress levels, and find or renew strategies for coping with stress. They should be educated on signs that they are not handling stress well (feeling frustrated, feeling overwhelmed, low self-esteem, physical symptoms) and when to ask for help.

GOAL SETTING

Goal setting should be a mutual process between the patient and the members of the rehabilitation team. If the patient feels that they have a role in establishing goals and making decisions related to their rehabilitation, and that those goals are clear-cut, personally relevant, and achievable, studies have shown that the ability to **cope and work toward these goals** is greatly enhanced. Goals developed should be designed to utilize the strengths of both patient and family and promote the patient's independence. Goals should also be planned with consideration for effective coping, health maintenance, and access to other resources embedded. Strategies should be personal, keeping in mind the cultural preferences and developmental level of the patient.

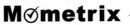

MILIEU THERAPY

Milieu therapy is the utilization of any resources, people, or events in the patient's setting that can enhance **psychosocial functioning**. It is a suggested intervention for people diagnosed with **impaired social interaction**. Milieu therapy involves provision of an environment in the ward conducive to rehabilitation. Milieu therapy includes the following:

- A light-hearted and encouraging atmosphere among the rehabilitation nurses and patients
- Availability of resources and activities such as computers and places for family members to obtain food
- Pleasant use of sounds (piped-in music, nurse's tone of voice, etc.)

HOPE INSTILLATION, COMPLEX RELATIONSHIP BUILDING, AND SUPPORT SYSTEM ENHANCEMENT

Hope instillation is the process of making it easier for a person to develop a positive outlook. It is an individualized process that the rehabilitation nurse can nurture through emphasis on possibilities rather than limitations, the encouragement of every minor success, and the elimination of uncertainties. **Complex relationship building** refers to the development of a mutually beneficial relationship between the patient who has trouble relating and health care workers. This is generally a protracted process of establishing rapport. **Support system enhancement** is the enrichment of the patient's life through interactions with family, friends, and society. The nurse can encourage support system enhancement by having the patient's friends visit them as soon as possible and enrolling the patient in peer support and/or self-help groups.

ROLES ASSUMED BY CAREGIVERS TO PEOPLE WITH INTERRUPTIONS IN HEALTH

Caregivers tend to be one of the following: engaged, conflicted, or distanced.

- Those who are actively **engaged** ascertain the needed care, anticipate the patient's needs, and deliver care skillfully and supportively.
- **Conflicted** caregivers are less engaged and prepared, deliver care primarily only when necessary, and tend to encourage the patient to participate in decisions.
- **Distanced** caregivers make the person being cared for primarily responsible for their own self-care and decisions.

Often the spouse is the caregiver, and again, spouses can assume a variety of roles. Those who are active participants are generally very supportive and positive. Others take on a more regulative role with an authoritative and controlling manner of communication. Spouses might also act in a merely observational manner, in which they are empathetic but relatively acquiescent. Partners can also assume roles that are not particularly helpful to the patient. A partner may, for example, assume a dissociative role in which they are negative and openly reluctant to participate. A partner may also assume an incapacitated position, where despite an interest in helping the patient, the partner has their own issues.

COMPLEMENTARY AND ALTERNATIVE THERAPY

Complementary therapies are often used, either alone or in conjunction with conventional medical treatment. These methods should be included if this is what the patient/family chooses, empowering the family to take control of their plan of care. Complementary therapies vary widely and most can easily be incorporated. The **National Center for Complementary and Alternative Medicine** recognizes the following:

- **Whole medical systems**: Chinese medicine (acupressure, acupuncture), naturopathic and homeopathic medicines, and Ayurveda
- **Mind-body medicine**: Prayer, artistic creation, music and dance therapy, biofeedback, focused relaxation, and visualization
- **Biological medicine**: Aromatherapy, herbs, plants, trees, vitamins and minerals, and dietary supplements

- **Manipulation**: Massage and spinal manipulation
- **Energy medicines**: Magnets, electric current, pulsed fields, Reiki, qi gong, and laying-on of the hands

PRECAUTIONS

The use of alternative and complementary therapies should be thoroughly discussed by patients and their physician. Patients should be encouraged to use therapies that are shown to have a beneficial, complementary effect on conventional medical treatment. These therapies include the use of massage, superficial stimulation, relaxation, distraction, hypnosis, and guided imagery.

- Encourage patients to practice the techniques until they are proficient in their use to give them a chance to prove their value.
- Teach the patient how the therapies work to encourage the patient to believe in them to contribute to the placebo effect.
- Caution the patient against abandoning current medical treatment.
- Inform the patient of the high cost of alternate therapies that can divert needed funds and result in little or no benefit.
- Provide the patient with resources in the form of books, pamphlets, and informative websites that prove the results of scientific research so that they can evaluate alternative therapies for themselves.

WHOLE MEDICAL SYSTEMS

Whole medical systems are different philosophies and methods of explaining and treating health and illness. Some systems include:

- **Homeopathic medicine**: This European system uses small amounts of diluted herbs and supplements to help the body to recover from disease by stimulating an immune response.
- **Naturopathic medicine**: This is a European system that uses various natural means (herbs, massage, acupuncture) to support the natural healing forces of the body.
- **Chinese medicine**: Centers on restoring the proper flow of life forces within the body to cure disease by using herbs, acupressure and acupuncture, and meditation.
- **Ayurveda**: This is an Indian system that tries to bring the spirit into harmony with the mind and body to treat disease via yoga, herbs, and massage.

ESSENTIAL OILS AND CUPPING

Essential oils (concentrated oils from plants) are either inhaled (aromatherapy) or diluted and applied to the skin. Essential oils are believed to reduce stress, aid sleep, improve dermatitis, and aid digestion. Commonly used essential oils include eucalyptus, lavender, lemon, peppermint, rosemary, rose, and tea tree. Oils may cause skin irritation when applied to the skin.

Cupping is an ancient practice still used in Southeast Asia and the Middle East to reduce pain, promote healing, and improve circulation. With dry cupping, cups are heated by placing something flammable (such as paper or herbs) inside the cup and setting it on fire to heat the cup, which is then immediately placed on the back along the meridians (generally on both sides of the spine) to form a vacuum that draws blood to the skin and causes circular bruises believed to heal that part of the body. Wet cupping includes leaving the heated cup in place for three minutes, removing it, making small cuts in the skin, and then applying suction cups again to withdraw blood. Cupping should be avoided in children under 4 and limited to short periods in older children.

ACUPUNCTURE

Alternative systems of medical practice include acupuncture, homeopathy, and naturopathy. **Acupuncture**, an ancient Oriental practice, uses stainless steel or copper needles inserted into superficial skin layers at points where energy or life force called *qi* is believed to occur. The needles are supposed to restore balance and the flow of *qi*. The NIH has recognized the effectiveness of acupuncture for certain side effects of other cancer treatments, such as nausea, vomiting, and pain. However, there is no documented scientific evidence to

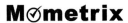

support the principles expounded. Acupuncturists are certified through either formal coursework or apprenticeships, and there is also board certification in this area for physicians. The needles used are classified as class II, which means they have manufacturing and labeling requirements.

USE OF VISUALIZATION

There are a number of methods used for **visualization** to reduce anxiety and promote healing. Some include audiotapes with guided imagery, such as self-hypnosis tapes, but the patient can be taught basic **techniques** that include:

- Sit or lie comfortably in a **quiet place** away from distractions.
- Concentrate on **breathing** while taking long slow breaths.
- **Close the eyes** to shut out distractions and create an image in the mind of the place or situation desired.
- Concentrate on that **image**, engaging as many senses as possible and imaging details.
- If the mind wanders, breathe deeply and **bring consciousness back** to the image or concentrate on breathing for a few moments and then return to the imagery.
- End with positive imagery.

Sometimes, patients are resistive at first or have a hard time maintaining focus, so **guiding** them through visualization for the first few times can be helpful.

RELAXATION EXERCISES

Relaxation exercises can help patients relax and distance themselves from their pain. The **relaxation response** can be generated through other techniques such as self-hypnosis, prayer recitation, deep breathing, muscle relaxation, or specific relaxation exercises. One exercise is the use of **slow, rhythmic breathing**, usually initiated through the abdomen and inspiring and exhaling the same length of time (three counts). **Touch techniques** such as massage with a warm lubricant and/or aromatherapy can promote relaxation. **Visualization and guided imagery techniques**, providing a comfortable environment (incorporating familiar and pleasurable elements such as music or religious programming), and meditation practices can enhance relaxation.

THERAPEUTIC COMMUNICATION
FACILITATING COMMUNICATION

Therapeutic communication begins with respect for the patient/family and the assumption that all communication, verbal and nonverbal, has meaning. Listening must be done empathetically. The following are some techniques that facilitate communication.

Introduction:

- Make a personal introduction and use the patient's name: "Mrs. Brown, I am Susan Williams, your nurse."

Encouragement:

- Use an open-ended opening statement: "Is there anything you'd like to discuss?"
- Acknowledge comments: "Yes," and "I understand."
- Allow silence and observe nonverbal behavior rather than trying to force conversation. Ask for clarification if statements are unclear.
- Reflect statements back (use sparingly): Patient: "I hate this hospital." Nurse: "You hate this hospital?"

Functional Health Patterns

63

Empathy:

- Make observations: "You are shaking," and "You seem worried."
- Recognize feelings:
  o Patient: "I want to go home."
  o Nurse: "It must be hard to be away from your home and family."
- Provide information as honestly and completely as possible about condition, treatment, and procedures and respond to the patient's questions and concerns.

Exploration:

- Verbally express implied messages:
  o Patient: "This treatment is too much trouble."
  o Nurse: "You think the treatment isn't helping you?"
- Explore a topic but allow the patient to terminate the discussion without further probing: "I'd like to hear how you feel about that."

Orientation:

- Indicate reality:
  o Patient: "Someone is screaming."
  o Nurse: "That sound was an ambulance siren."
- Comment on distortions without directly agreeing or disagreeing:
  o Patient: "That nurse promised I didn't have to walk again."
  o Nurse: "Really? That's surprising because the doctor ordered physical therapy twice a day."

Collaboration:

- Work together to achieve better results: "Maybe if we talk about this, we can figure out a way to make the treatment easier for you."

Validation:

- Seek validation: "Do you feel better now?" or "Did the medication help you breathe better?"

AVOIDING NON-THERAPEUTIC COMMUNICATION

While using therapeutic communication is important, it is equally important to avoid interjecting **non-therapeutic communication**, which can block effective communication. *Avoid the following:*

- Meaningless clichés: "Don't worry. Everything will be fine." "Isn't it a nice day?"
- Providing advice: "You should..." or "The best thing to do is...." It's better when patients ask for advice to provide facts and encourage the patient to reach a decision.
- Inappropriate approval that prevents the patient from expressing true feeling or concerns:
  o Patient: "I shouldn't cry about this."
  o Nurse: "That's right! You're an adult!"
- Asking for an explanation of behavior that is not directly related to patient care and requires analysis and explanation of feelings: "Why are you so upset?"
- Agreeing with rather than accepting and responding to patient's statements can make it difficult for the patient to change his or her statement or opinion later: "I agree with you," or "You are right."
- Making negative judgments: "You should stop arguing with the nurses."
- Devaluing the patient's feelings: "Everyone gets upset at times."

- Disagreeing directly: "That can't be true," or "I think you are wrong."
- Defending against criticism: "The doctor is not being rude; he's just very busy today."
- Changing the subject to avoid dealing with uncomfortable topics;
  - Patient: "I'm never going to get well."
  - Nurse: "Your family will be here in just a few minutes."
- Making inappropriate literal responses, even as a joke, especially if the patient is at all confused or having difficulty expressing ideas:
  - Patient: "There are bugs crawling under my skin."
  - Nurse: "I'll get some bug spray,"
- Challenging the patient to establish reality often just increases confusion and frustration:
  - "If you were dying, you wouldn't be able to yell and kick!"

COMMUNICATING WITH PATIENTS WITH DISABILITIES

Guidelines for communicating with individuals with disabilities:

- Do not assume that the person with disabilities also has impaired cognition.
- Always treat the person with respect and dignity.
- Use first names with the patient if asked to do so, but start out formally as with any patient.
- Offer to shake hands even when a prosthesis is present.
- Be patient if communication is impaired.
- Offer assistance, but allow the patient to tell you what is helpful; otherwise, don't assist.
- When a wheelchair is used, sit down so the patient does not have to strain their neck to speak with you.
- If providing directions, consider the obstacles that may be in the way and assist the person to find an appropriate way around them.

COMMUNICATION WITH PATIENTS WITH COGNITIVE DISABILITIES

The person with cognitive disabilities may be easily distracted, so verbal communication should be attempted in a quiet area:

- Address people with dignity and respect.
- Do not try to discuss abstract ideas but stick with concrete topics.
- Keep words and sentences very simple and try rephrasing when necessary. People may have difficulty in distinguishing your spoken words and deriving the meaning from them.
- Be very patient with people's attempts to speak to you since they may have difficulty in processing thoughts and changing them into spoken words.
- Use objects around you and gestures to illustrate your words since the patient may also use pointing and gesturing when unable to find the words to communicate with you. The person may prefer written communication, although some may be unable to read.
- Use touch to convey your regard during communication, as this is recognized by the patient as reassurance of your care and concern for them.
- Give a few instructions at a time as to not overwhelm them.

COMMUNICATING WITH DEAF OR HEARING-IMPAIRED PATIENTS

Communicating with a person with deafness or hearing impairment:

- Try to communicate in a quiet environment if possible.
- Wave or touch the person to let him or her know you are trying to communicate.
- Determine the method the person uses to communicate: sign language, lip reading, hearing devices, or writing.

Functional Health Patterns

65

- Fingerspell or use some signs if able to do so.
- Address the person directly when you speak even though the person may be looking at an interpreter or your lips.
- Look at the person as the interpreter tells you what was said.
- Speak slowly so the interpreter can keep up with you.
- If the person reads lips, face the person and speak clearly and normally, using normal volume.
- If writing a communication, do not speak while writing.
- Do not be afraid to check that the person understands you, and ask questions if you do not understand the person.

COMMUNICATION WITH PEOPLE WITH LOW VISION OR BLINDNESS

Communicating with a person with low vision or blindness:

- Greet the person with low vision or blindness, identifying yourself and others present.
- Always say goodbye when you are leaving.
- Alert the person to written communications, such as warning signs or printed notices.
- Face the person and touch briefly on the arm to let the person know you are speaking to him or her if you are in a group.
- Speak at normal loudness.
- Make any directions given specific in terms of the length of walk and obstacles, such as stairs.
- Use the position of hands on a clock face to give directions (potatoes at 3 o'clock) as well as using *right* or *left*.
- Mention sounds that the person may hear in transit or on arrival at a destination.
- Do not be afraid to use the word *see*, as the person will probably use it as well.

COMMUNICATING WITH A PATIENT ON A VENTILATOR

When a patient on a ventilator is conscious, he or she may still be able to communicate by blinking, nodding, shaking the head, or pointing to a picture or word board:

- If the person is able to write, try to reposition the IV line to leave the dominant hand free to communicate.
- Discuss the need for communication with the physician and ask if a valve or an electric larynx can be used to permit speech.
- Help the patient practice lip reading of single words.
- Remember the patient's glasses or hearing aids when attempting to communicate.
- Enlist the aid of a speech therapist if there is frustration on the part of the patient and family due to communication difficulty.

COMMUNICATING WITH PERSONS WITH SPEECH PROBLEMS DUE TO A STROKE

Methods to communicate with stroke patients with speech problems:

- **Dysarthria**: Patients have problems forming the words to speak them aloud. Give them time to communicate, offer them a picture board or other means of communicating, and give encouragement to family members who are frustrated with the difficulty of trying to communicate.
- **Expressive aphasia**: The patients' efforts at speech come out garbled when they try to say sentences, but single words may be clear. Encourage the patients to try to write and to practice the sounds of the alphabet. Resist the urge to finish sentences for the patients.

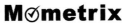

- **Receptive aphasia**: The patients have a problem comprehending the speech they hear. Communicate in simple terms and speak slowly. Test comprehension of the written word as an alternative method of communication.
- **Global aphasia**: The patient has both receptive and expressive aphasia. Use simple, clear, slow speech augmented by pictures and gestures.

COMMUNICATION PROBLEMS OF PATIENTS WITH PARKINSON'S DISEASE

Parkinson's disease causes problems with speaking in the majority (75-90%) of patients. The reason for this is not clear but may relate to increasing rigidity and changes in movement. Speech is often very low-pitched or hoarse, given in a monotone and with a soft voice. Speech production may decrease because of the effort required to speak. **Speech therapy** can develop exercises for the patient that can assist them in remembering to speak slowly and carefully, as patients are not always aware that their **communication** is impaired:

- Allow time for the patient to communicate, asking for repetition if you do not understand the message.
- Help family by teaching ways to facilitate communication with the patient and encouraging them to assist the patient to do the exercises provided by the therapist.
- If speech volume is very low, suggest amplification devices that can be obtained through speech therapy.

COMMUNICATION WITH PATIENTS WITH PSYCHIATRIC PROBLEMS

Persons with psychiatric disorders appreciate being addressed with respect, dignity, and honesty:

- Speak simply and clearly, repeating as necessary.
- Encourage patients to discuss their concerns regarding treatment and medications to improve compliance.
- Use good eye contact and be attentive to your body language messages.
- Be alert, but unless the person is known to be violent, try to relax and listen to them.
- Don't try to avoid words or phrases pertaining to psychiatric problems, but if you do say something inappropriate, apologize honestly to the patient.
- Offer patients outlets for their thoughts and feelings.
- Learn more about their disorder and ways to use therapeutic communication to help them with their problem, such as re-orienting them as needed.

Musculoskeletal Functional Ability

MUSCULOSKELETAL SYSTEM

The musculoskeletal system, comprising over half of an individual's body weight, consists of the bones, cartilage, joints, tendons, fasciae, bursae, and skeletal muscles. The **bone** is the hard part of the skeleton that provides a structural framework to support body weight and shields vital organs. Bones produce red blood cells, and they require calcium and vitamin D for support. The **cartilage** is the strong elastic tissue composed of fibers. **Joints** are the junctions between bones; they contain varying amounts and types of cartilage, ligaments, and synovial fluid, and they determine range of motion. **Ligaments** are relatively tough fibrous tissues that connect the joint area to other structures. **Tendons** are inelastic fibrous bands that connect muscles to bones. Muscles, nerves, and blood vessels are also encased by fibrous tissues called **fasciae**. Pouches containing connective tissue and synovial fluid provide cushioning and are called **bursae**. The **skeletal muscle** is a type of fibrous tissue capable of contraction and extension through its unique organization of threadlike myofibrils and the fluid sarcoplasm.

TISSUES AND STRUCTURES

Bones form the body's basic structure to provide protection and allow us to move. They consist of both highly structured dense tissue called **compact or cortical bone** (the majority) and **spongy or cancellous bone**. Bone formation and degradation is a dynamic process with cells that form bone (**osteoblasts**), reabsorb bone cells (**osteoclasts**), and preserve bone (**osteocytes**). Joints are the connective tissue junctions between bones. The **movable joints**, also called diarthrodial or synovial joints, are responsible for range of motion; they consist of a joint capsule and synovial membrane at each bone terminus and a synovial cavity between them containing plasma or fluid to protect the associated cartilage. There are also **immovable or synarthrodial joints** and somewhat flexible **amphiarthrodial joints** between vertebrae. **Muscle fibers** and associated sensory nerve fibers are also connected to bones and aid in movement through their contractile properties, discussed previously.

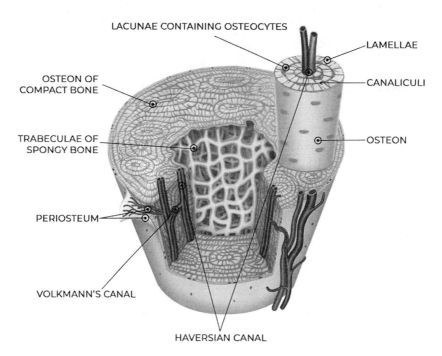

LACUNAE CONTAINING OSTEOCYTES
LAMELLAE
OSTEON OF COMPACT BONE
CANALICULI
TRABECULAE OF SPONGY BONE
OSTEON
PERIOSTEUM
VOLKMANN'S CANAL
HAVERSIAN CANAL

MUSCLE CONTRACTION AND RELAXATION

Initially during contraction, a nerve signal triggers release of the neurotransmitter **acetylcholine**, which transverses the neuromuscular junction and binds to receptors on the muscle fiber. The activated

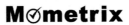

acetylcholine receptors transmit impulses in the muscle and ultimately to the **sarcoplasmic reticulum (SR)**, where calcium ions (Ca^{2+}) are discharged into the **sarcoplasm**. There, the calcium ions bind to **troponin molecules** in the thin myofilaments. The resultant tropomyosin causes the myofilaments to move and uncover active sites on the **actin molecules**. A muscle protein called **myosin** builds cross bridges in the thick myofilaments, binds to actin, and draws the thinner filaments closer to the center of the muscle fiber, using **adenosine triphosphate (ATP)** as the energy source. Eventually, thin and thick filaments slide over each other to cause shortening of the muscle fiber. **Relaxation** occurs when calcium starts being pumped back into the sacs of the SR and is removed from the troponin molecules. **Actin** is blocked and cannot bind to myosin bridges, resulting in a return to normal resting state.

ISOTONIC, ISOMETRIC, AND ISOKINETIC MUSCLE MOVEMENTS

Isotonic movements occur when a muscle is maintained at a constant tension but the muscle length is changed. There are two types of **isotonic movements**, those in which the muscle is lengthened (eccentric) and those where the muscle is shortened (concentric). A related term is muscle tone or firmness while relaxed. **Isometric movements** change the tension of the muscle while maintaining it at a constant length. Such a movement may involve pulling against a force without shortening the muscle. No actual body movement occurs during isometric exercises. There are also other types of movement, most notably **isokinetic**, in which an individual's complete range of motion is utilized through intervention with specialized machinery.

ALTERED MUSCLE MOVEMENT

Altered muscle movements are generally involuntary actions. They are often associated with specific motor defects.

- **Tremors** are slight shaking or trembling movements that are usually rhythmic and unplanned. They are often found in individuals with Parkinson's disease, or they can occur with age, exposure to toxic metals or psychogenic drugs, or injuries to the cerebellum or brain stem.
- **Chorea** refers to arrhythmic, erratic, and forceful unplanned movements.
- **Athetoses** are slow and twisting involuntary movements that occur in distal limbs. Both chorea and athetoses can occur with use of dopamine-related drugs, and chorea can occur in diseases involving increased amounts of or sensitivity to dopamine, such as in Huntington's chorea.
- **Ballism** is the term for very violent and erratic throwing around of the head or arms. It is usually a result of damage to the basal ganglion.

ALTERED MUSCLE TONE

There are a variety of disorders of altered muscle tone:

- A lack of muscle tone is called either **hypotonia** or **flaccidity**. This condition can lead to lack of use and muscle atrophy.
- Increased muscle tone is called **hypertonia** or **spasticity**. Hypertonicity can result in involuntary spasms in muscles often associated with gait defects or inability to move parts of the body. Hypertonic muscles resist stretching and are often found in extremities.
- **Clonus** or **clonic spasm** is the term for rapid repetitive muscle contractions and relaxations usually linked to epileptic seizures. Clonus arises from uninterrupted reflex arcing due to upper motor neuron (UMN) lesions.
- **Rigidity** refers to muscles that are stiff and unbendable as a result of augmented tension between opposing contracting (agonist) and relaxing (antagonist) muscles. Rigidity can result in poor mobility and muscle function.

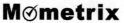

FACTORS THAT SHAPE FUNCTIONAL MOBILITY

INTERNAL

Functional mobility is the ability to perform **activities of daily living (ADLs)** and **instrumental activities of daily living (IADLs)**. It is dependent on both internal and external factors. One internal factor is the **musculoskeletal system,** which forms the basis of muscular strength, range of motion, control of posture and alignment, and joint strength. Both the central and peripheral nervous systems (CNS and PNS respectively) affect functional mobility. The **CNS** controls the auditory, olfactory, tactile, and visual senses, which in turn affect things such as one's ability to feel pain, grasp spatial relationships, and maintain balance. The **PNS** controls descending motor systems that influence reflexes, muscle tone, coordination, and other motor processes. **Cognition perception**, the ability to acquire and assimilate knowledge, is also related to CNS function, and it can be related to impairments of hand-eye coordination, depth perception, inability to perform complex movements, or neglect.

EXTERNAL

In addition to the internal factors, **external factors** can affect functional mobility. The **emotional and psychosocial circumstances** of the patient can influence their attention to self-care and the amount of responsibility the patient takes for their self-care. Self-care can also be discouraged or encouraged by the patient's **environment and access to technology**. If the patient has assistive devices and functions in environments that are accessible and safe, functional mobility is more likely. The **social and cultural beliefs** of the person as well as their **economic situation** can affect the person's ability to trust and seek appropriate services to attain functional mobility. A person's **total health status** and **age or stage of development** can also influence their attainment of functional mobility.

MODELS OF MOVEMENT

SENSORIMOTOR MODELS

Classic movement theories regard motor development as a compilation of developmental milestones reached through maturation directed by the central nervous system. **Life span viewpoints** envision motor behaviors as changeable during life as a result of internal as well as external factors. Sensorimotor models of movement use both of these principles.

- The **Feldenkrais method** is a sensorimotor approach because it touts the reestablishment of lost or changed functional capacity through education and adaptation.
- Another example is the **Bobath approach**, in which the patient actively participates in goal-oriented tasks to improve movement through postural and other changes that enhance their sensations and mobility.
- The **proprioceptive neuromuscular facilitation (PNF) approach** is another example emphasizing special movements of the extremities.

DYNAMIC SYSTEMS MODELS

Dynamic systems models of movement view movement as a **nonlinear process** in which many parts are interconnected in a multifaceted and dynamic manner. Thus, dynamic systems include any of the rehabilitation measures that emphasize tasks to engage use of affected extremities in order to relearn movements. A variant is the **dynamic pattern theory (DPT)**, in which the patient is aided by the nurse in the reestablishment of some measure of function to perform the activities of daily living. This is accomplished through interventions that make it easier for the patient to perform these activities. There are also many **behavioral tactics** that can reduce stress or eliminate pain, such as biofeedback and massage as adjuncts.

PHYSICAL EXAMINATION OF MUSCULOSKELETAL AND NEUROLOGICAL FUNCTIONS

Assessment of musculoskeletal and neurological functions includes a medical history or recording of the patient's ability to perform ADLs. The **physical examination** includes parameters that provide objective assessment of the patient's situation. It should encompass observations related to **musculoskeletal or**

neurological function, such as posture, alignment, skin color and rigidity, gait, and respiratory status. The nurse or other clinician should evaluate **range of motion** and other joint health. The following should also be evaluated: muscle strength, using a manual muscle test to determine ability to flex, relax, and grip; muscle tone, using palpation; motor stretch or deep tendon reflexes, by the striking of specific tendons; cranial function, by assessing vision and eye movements; sensory responses in the trunk and extremities, by dermatome or other mapping; kinesthesia or spatial perception, using a moving finger and/or a tuning fork; balance and coordination while seated or while performing ADLs; gait pattern; and ability of the patient to perform ADLs, by observation.

ASSESSMENT OF MOTOR STRETCH REFLEXES

Motor stretch or **deep tendon reflexes (DTRs)** that should be assessed measure functional responses that are controlled by different portions of the central nervous system. Tendons over specific muscle groups are struck, and then reflexes are evaluated in terms of reflex activity level, symmetry of the reflex, presence of abnormal reactions, and contraction. There are normally 7 motor stretch reflexes that are evaluated. The **biceps, brachioradialis**, and **triceps reflexes** evaluate responses from the upper C5-C6 and C6-C8 (triceps) regions of the spinal cord. The **patellar or knee jerk reflex** measures the lower L2-L4 functions, and the **Achilles or ankle reflex** evaluates the even lower S1-S2 centers. The **abdominal reflex** looks at lower thoracic cord centers and can be used to diagnosis multiple sclerosis. The **plantar or Babinski reflex**, in which the toes should curl up when the sole of the foot is struck, is a measurement of upper motor neuron injury in anyone older than 1 year of age.

SCREENING FOR BALANCE AND GAIT FUNCTION

The **Timed Up and Go Test** is a good, rapid screening tool to assess balance and gait. The patient is seated initially in a chair. They are then requested to get up without using the chair arms for support, briefly stand still, then walk 10 feet, turn, and go back to sitting down in the chair. Nothing should be touched during the sequence, including the chair arms. If the patient is unsteady or must use support, further evaluation is indicated. Another useful screening tool is the **Berg Balance Scale**, which addresses 14 items related to balance. **Ataxia**, lack of muscle control, can be tested by having the patient perform two sequences, finger-to-nose-to-finger and heel-to-shin.

FUNCTIONAL ASSESSMENT TOOLS IN REHABILITATION SETTINGS

The **Barthel Index** and **Functional Independence Measure (FIM)** are validated measurements for ADLs. The **Older American Resources and Services Scale (OARS)** can be administered to assess instrumental ADLs; it is broad-based, with 105 questions. There are several endorsed tools for neurological functions. These include the following:

- The **Glasgow Coma Scale**, which measures level of consciousness (usually after head injuries or strokes).
- The **Mini-Mental State Examination (MMSE)**, which evaluates 7 areas (such as attention and recall) related to mental status.
- The questionnaire developed by the **Center for Epidemiologic Studies Depression Scale (CES-D)**, which evaluates for recent evidence of depression.

The **Medical Outcomes Study (MOS)** is a generic health status and quality-of-life rating tool that addresses physical functioning and a range of sources of limitation. There are additional tools applicable to either nursing home use or community living. These are the **Minimum Data Set (MDS)** and the **Outcome and Assessment Information Set (OASIS)**, respectively.

Functional Health Patterns

FIM INSTRUMENT

The **Functional Independence Measure** (FIM) assesses the ability of the patient to perform ADLs. There are 18 parameters (13 motor and 5 cognitive) that are evaluated at admission, at discharge, and during follow-up:

Motor		Cognitive	
Sphincter control	Bladder	Communication	Comprehension
	Bowel		Expression
Mobility/transfer	Bed to chair or wheelchair	Social cognition	Social interaction
	Toilet		Problem solving
	Shower		Memory
Self-care	Eating		
	Grooming		
	Bathing		
	Ability to dress the upper body		
	Ability to dress the lower body		
	Toileting		
Locomotion	Walk or use a wheelchair		
	Climb stairs		

Ratings are as follows: complete dependence (1–2); modified dependence (3–5, with 5 being supervision with no assistance); modified (device-driven) independence (6); or complete, timely, and safe independence (7). Complete independence for all functions is 126 points. A score of 18 represents absolute dependence for all parameters.

OTHER SCALES FOR FUNCTIONAL ASSESSMENT

The **Barthel Index (BI)** rates patients on 10 functions as independent, requiring assistance (minor or major), or completely dependent. A maximum score of 100 is possible, representing complete independence in terms of ADLs. The parameters evaluated are feeding, grooming, bathing, dressing, bladder and bowel control, capacity to perform wheelchair transfer, ability to walk on level surfaces, and ability to climb stairs. Other scales include the following: the **Katz Index of ADLs**, which only rates 6 tasks for dependency; the **Kenny Self-Care Evaluation**, which evaluates 6 parameters, each on a 5-point scale: the **PULSES Profile**, which covers 6 different functional breakdowns on 4-point scales; and the **Level of Rehabilitation Scale (LORS)**, which evaluates dependence level based on patient interviewing. An additional tool is the **Patient Evaluation Conference System (PECS)**, which plots 7 levels of dependence for 15 different categories, such as rehabilitation medicine, ADLs, medication, pain, and psychology.

PRINCIPLES OF BODY MECHANICS IN THE CONTEXT OF EXERCISE AS SELF-CARE

The principles of body mechanics describe the optimal ways of standing, moving, and lifting to prevent injury. They are especially important when prescribing exercise as a self-care technique. At the core of the principles is **good posture**, which means a straight back with knees slightly bent, weight concentrated over one's center, and a wide base of support. Bending should be done from the hips and knees, not the back. Interactions should be performed by moving closer instead of reaching. The body should not be twisted or pivoted to make a turn. Lifting should be avoided and smooth pulling or pushing actions used instead. **Props** such as mechanical lifts or carts, as well as safety devices such as gait belts or transfer boards, should be used. The environment should be surveyed for safety hazards before movements are initiated. Injuries should be reported and treated promptly.

MUSCULOSKELETAL PROBLEMS

COMMON PROBLEMS

Osteoporosis is the result of bone resorption outpacing bone formation, making the bones brittle and susceptible to breakage. **Osteopenia** also refers to low bone mass but is less severe than osteoporosis.

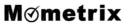

Osteoporosis can cause vertebral compression fractures of bones in the spinal column, resulting in spinal curvature.

Spinal deformities are another common musculoskeletal problem, and are classified as follows:

- **Kyphosis**, an outward curving of the upper spine (resulting in a hunched back)
- **Lordosis**, an inward curving in the lower spine
- **Scoliosis**, a marked sideways curvature of the spine

There are also abnormal curvatures in the knee area; **genu varum** is outward bowing, while **genu valgum** is characterized by inward bowing or so-called "knock-knees."

> **Review Video: Osteoporosis**
> Visit mometrix.com/academy and enter code: 421205

Functional Health Patterns

CONDITIONS THAT CAN PRODUCE SECONDARY MUSCULOSKELETAL PROBLEMS

The most common conditions that produce secondary musculoskeletal problems are strokes and spinal cord injuries. People who have experienced a **stroke** often cannot move one side of their body and develop upper extremity pain for a variety of reasons, including rotator cuff tears, spastic shoulder muscles, and nerve impingement. Some of the more common complications are **hemiplegic shoulder subluxation** (dislocation) and **complex regional pain syndrome** (CRPS), characterized by unremitting sharp and worsening pain, skin changes, and motor problems in the extremities. Musculoskeletal complications from **spinal cord injuries** are numerous, most notably spasticity (which can lead to bone fractures, tissue damage, and contractures), overuse syndrome of the shoulders, problems with bone remodeling due to loss of calcium in the urine, and deposition of new bone in joint areas. Muscle atrophy can also occur secondary to the use of glucocorticoids in patients with autoimmune diseases such as systemic lupus erythematosus or rheumatoid arthritis.

DIAGNOSTIC TESTS

Typical blood tests performed to glean data regarding musculoskeletal problems include **red and white blood cell counts** to look for anemia or inflammation and infection. **Cultures** of appropriate fluids are collected to identify infectious agents. **Immunoglobulin levels**, some of which are elevated with inflammation or infection, are also assessed. Other inflammatory markers include **C-reactive protein** and **erythrocyte sedimentation rate**, which are both generally elevated in conditions such as rheumatoid arthritis. **Electrolyte levels** should be taken, especially calcium concentrations, because levels are a reflection of bone health. Other laboratory tests include alkaline phosphatase, creatinine phosphatase, uric acid levels, or analysis of joint fluids. **Diagnostic scanning modalities** include dual-energy x-ray absorptiometry (DEXA) for bone mineral density, contrast discography, and radioactive scintigraphy of specific bone areas.

NURSING DIAGNOSES AND TREATMENT INTERVENTIONS AND GOALS

The most common nursing diagnoses in patients with musculoskeletal disorders are pain, activity intolerance, self-care deficit, impaired mobility, and/or a poor body image. The nurse's role for a patient with pain is to **manage** and eventually develop a program to **control** that pain. **Activity intolerance** generally indicates both pain and fatigue, which means the nurse's main job is to institute a process of energy management to conserve the person's vigor. If the patient cannot perform **self-care tasks**, then the nurse is responsible for assisting the patient with these until they can perform activities of daily life. There are several **interventional components** if the person has impaired physical mobility, all involving exercise therapy or promotion. **Therapy** includes exercises that promote joint mobility and ability to walk. Strength training should be incorporated. The eventual goals of therapy are active functionality and ability to either walk or use a wheelchair. If the person has a **poor body image**, any technique that might enhance that image should be attempted, be it behavioral interventions (exercise, strength training), or emotional/cognitive interventions. The nurse might find other issues to address as well, such as depression or other psychosocial issues, cognitive defects, compromised skin integrity, or sexual problems.

DYSPRAXIA AND APRAXIA

The terms "dyspraxia" and "apraxia" both refer to the inability to perform complex movements, especially as a result of brain damage. Dyspraxia is a partial loss of function, whereas apraxia is the complete loss of function (usually of gross and/or fine motor skills). This damage is often due to a stroke. There are five main types of apraxia: ideomotor, conduction, disassociation, ideational, and conceptual.

Ideomotor apraxia is the inability to process the sequential and spatial relationships of movement. There is a posterior form, resulting from damage to the left parietal cortex, in which the person has trouble responding to commands and discriminating their performance level; there is also an anterior form, occurring further forward in the same area, that is less severe. **Conceptual apraxia** arises from damage to the bilateral frontal and parietal areas and is characterized by an inability to recall how to use certain tools or mechanical objects. The brain defect area of the remaining three types of apraxia is uncertain. Individuals with **conduction apraxia** can comprehend movements and gestures but have difficulty performing them; those with **disassociation apraxia** can perform well with objects but have poor verbal responses, and people with **ideational dyspraxia** cannot carry out an idea or sequence of actions properly.

GAIT DISORDERS

Functional movement disorders are defined as an involuntary, abnormal movement of part of the body in which pathophysiology is not fully understood. Functional tremors are the most frequent type of functional movement disorder. Dystonia, myoclonus, and Parkinsonism are other types of functional movement disorders. Functional gait disorders are another type of functional movement disorder and are common in the elderly. Gait disorders can manifest as a dragging gait, knee buckling, small slow steps or "walking on ice," swaying gait, fluctuating gait, hesitant gait, and hyperkinetic gait in which there is excessive movement of the arms, trunk, and legs when ambulating. Patients with gait disorders are at an increased risk of falling. Gait disorders are diagnosed by a thorough clinical examination (including a neurologic assessment) and health history. Treatment for functional gait disorders includes strength and balance training. Assistive devices such as walkers and canes may also be utilized.

POST-POLIO SYNDROME

Post-polio syndrome (**PPS**) is the term for a set of symptoms experienced by individuals with previous acute poliomyelitis. These symptoms include tiredness, low energy, lack of concentration, areas of joint or muscle pain, muscle degeneration, and often cognitive defects. These symptoms appear in the same muscle groups several decades after the original poliomyelitis virus infection has resolved, but there is no evidence of viral reactivation. **Neural stress and immunological or inflammatory mechanisms** have been postulated as contributors. Generalized **fatigue** in PPS is addressed with energy conservation techniques, weight loss, or use of braces. These measures can also help with pain and joint instability. Anti-inflammatory drugs may be incorporated. Strengthening exercises, rest sessions between activities, and use avoidance are recommended for the muscle weakness. These patients may use nocturnal and other positive-pressure ventilation and should be educated in swallowing techniques if their bulbar muscles are weak. Upper extremity exercises are used for cardiopulmonary conditioning.

MUSCULAR DYSTROPHY

Muscular dystrophies are genetic disorders with gradual degeneration of muscle fibers and progressive weakness and atrophy of skeletal muscles and loss of mobility. **Pseudohypertrophic (Duchenne) muscular dystrophy** is the most common form and the most severe. It is an X-linked disorder in about 50% of the cases with the rest sporadic mutations, affecting males almost exclusively. Children typically have some delay in motor development with difficulty walking and have evidence of muscle weakness by about age 3. Pseudohypertrophic refers to enlargement of muscles by fatty infiltration associated with muscular atrophy, which causes contractures and deformities of joints. Abnormal bone development results in spinal and other skeletal deformities. The disease progresses rapidly, and most children are wheelchair bound by about 12 years of age. As the disease progresses, it involves the muscles of the diaphragm and other muscles needed for respiration. Mild to frank mental deficiency is common. Facial, oropharyngeal, and respiratory muscles weaken

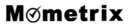

late in the disease. Cardiomegaly commonly occurs. Death most often relates to respiratory infection or cardiac failure by age 25. Treatment is supportive.

REPETITIVE MOTION INJURIES

When muscle groups are used **repetitively**, such as while exercising, engaging in sports, or performing the same task at work, the muscle fibers involved can tear and form relatively inelastic **scar tissues**. When certain bones are repeatedly stressed, they can form **thicker outer layers** or develop **fractures**. Sports injuries are among the most common type of repetitive motion injuries. For example, runners can develop a host of injuries including damage to the calf or Achilles tendon, knee pain, shin splints, stress fractures, and more. The probability of sports-related injuries can be diminished by incorporation of **strength training and range-of-motion exercises** into a routine. One of the most common job-related injuries to the musculoskeletal system is **carpal tunnel syndrome**, in which pressure on a median nerve within the carpal tunnel of the hand causes lack of sensation or tingling and eventual muscle wasting. Repetitive or sudden hand movements can also cause **ganglion cysts**, swollen pockets of tissue that can be painful or limit activities.

LIMB AMPUTATION

Amputation is the surgical removal of all or part of a limb or other body appendage in order to eliminate tissues that are infected or not receiving an adequate blood supply, while conserving healthy vascularized tissues and some functional limb length. Amputations are done after traumatic accidents as well as in severe cases of peripheral vascular disease, conditions such as in advanced diabetic neuropathy and when there is excessive dead and gangrenous tissue. The types are defined in terms of location. Lower extremity amputations include **below-the-knee (BKA), above-the-knee (AKA), foot and ankle (Syme's), foot below the ankle bone (Hey's or Lisfranc's)**, and **hip disarticulation at the hip joint**. There is also a rare critical procedure called **hemicorporectomy** in which half the body is removed, including the pelvic and lumbar areas. Upper extremity amputations include **hand or isolated digits, arm above the elbow (A/E), arm below the elbow (B/E)**, and **shoulder disarticulation at the shoulder joint**.

TREATMENT AFTER SURGERY

After surgical amputation, the residual limb is initially **wrapped** with a soft elastic bandage to shape the stump and decrease swelling. For a lower limb, the **figure-eight method** of wrapping is generally used. Wrapping proceeds from vertical to lateral to oblique coverage of the residual portion, then around the hip, and back to anchor the bandage with safety pins on the front of the stump. **Bandage pressure** is always applied upward and outward on the residual portion. There are also more rigid **plaster cast sockets** that can be used temporarily right after surgery. A temporary (and later permanent) **prosthesis** or artificial limb is not developed until the residual limb has healed and swelling is minimal.

GOALS AND ADLS FOR LACK OF COORDINATION OR LIMB AMPUTATION

The main goals of rehabilitation for patients who lack coordination are **safety and independence** within an environment that lessens their anxiety. The patients' ADLs should be performed slowly and methodically in order to conserve energy. A good tactic is to prop their upper limbs on a solid surface for **stabilization**. These individuals tend to also need **gait training**. They should slide items instead of lifting them. Recommendations for individuals who have had upper limbs amputated are similar to those with hemiplegia. If a lower limb has been amputated, then the patient will need to use specialized **dressing techniques** such as bridging while lying down, dressing while seated, or dressing while rolling on the bed. They may need to use **assistive devices** designed to put on shoes or socks.

POSITIONING PATIENTS WHO HAVE HAD AMPUTATION OF A LOWER EXTREMITY

Patients who have had a lower extremity amputated present unique **positioning issues. Positioning aids** such as pillows under the hip, knee, or back, or between the thighs, should not be used when the patient is lying down, and the bed end should not be raised. The legs should not be allowed to spread outwards while the patient is on their back. The residual limb should not lean into the affected one, nor should it be allowed to rest on the side of the bed or chair. The upper body is generally strengthened using an **overhead trapeze**. When

Functional Health Patterns

75

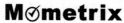

the patient is seated, the affected limb should never be bent and should instead be extended straight and propped up with a **leg rest** or **limb board**. When the patient is standing, they should not be allowed to support their affected limb on the **walker bar** or **crutch grip**. The limb should remain straight, pointing toward the ground, and close to the unaffected leg.

HIP REPLACEMENT OR HIP FRACTURE

Total hip replacement (THR), also called total hip arthroplasty, is routinely done on many people with various types of arthritis (most commonly, osteoarthritis), hip fractures, bone tumors, and other musculoskeletal disorders. Hemiarthroplasty involves the replacement of the femoral head. A THR involves the replacement of the femoral head and the acetabular cup. There are various ways of performing THR, including insertion of various pins or screws or use of hip prosthetic devices. These hip prostheses can be cemented in place, or they can be made of porous materials such as ceramics that permit bone growth into the device. After surgery, the patient is **positioned** on the bed on their unaffected side, with a foam wedge or pillow secured with Velcro between the legs and hips. The affected hip is **flexed** somewhat, and the knees should not touch each other. The nurse should also watch for signs of **infection** at the surgical site, such as drainage, redness, edema, or soreness, that might require wound care or IV antibiotics.

ARTHRITIC DISORDERS

Arthritis is a general term for conditions that impact the joints, resulting in pain, swelling, and stiffness. It can have a variety of causes. Arthritic disorders are classified as inflammatory, degenerative, or metabolic joint diseases.

- There are two main types of arthritis characterized by **inflammation**: rheumatoid arthritis and juvenile rheumatoid arthritis. There are also a number of rheumatoid-like disorders and spondyloarthropathies of the spine.
- The main **degenerative joint disease (DJD)** is **osteoarthritis (OA)**. OA can be either **primary** (also known as idiopathic), in which the cartilage in many joints is destroyed, or **secondary**, occurring in specific joints as a result of trauma or other mechanical stressors.
- There are also a number of metabolic disorders that manifest partially as arthritic problems; **gout** is the major example.

> **Review Video: <u>Immunomodulators and Immunosuppressive Agents</u>**
> Visit mometrix.com/academy and enter code: 666131

RHEUMATOID ARTHRITIS AND JUVENILE RHEUMATOID ARTHRITIS

Both rheumatoid arthritis (RA) and juvenile rheumatoid arthritis (JRA) are systemic, inflammatory processes. **RA** typically begins around age 20 or later, mostly in women, while **JRA** occurs in the teenage or younger population. Genetic or pathogenic factors such as **viruses** probably trigger each type, though their etiology remains unknown. People with RA have prolonged morning stiffness affecting many joints on both sides of the body; this is due to progressive inflammation enhanced by cytokines such as interleukins and tumor necrosis factor, plus thickening, granulation, and adhesions in joint structures. Somewhat nonspecific diagnostic indicators such as rheumatoid factor (RF), erythrocyte sedimentation rate (ESR), platelet counts, and C-reactive protein levels can be used for diagnosis. ESR and C-reactive protein levels may only be elevated during the acute phase of RA. Children with JRA present with unrelenting pain in selected joints as well as fever and skin rashes. RF, or another test called antinuclear antibody (ANA), may be positive in these children; they may also have an elevated ESR and white blood cell counts, and decreased hemoglobin levels.

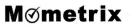

Possible Nursing Diagnoses, Interventions, and Desired Outcomes for RA

Generally, there are 3 possible nursing diagnoses for the patient with RA.

- The first, **chronic pain** related to joint inflammation, requires nursing interventions such as giving prescribed drugs as directed and analgesics when needed, providing heat application to increase blood flow to joints, using alternative therapies for pain relief, and documentation. The goal here is reduction of joint pain.
- Another nursing diagnosis is **impaired physical mobility** related to fatigue, pain, and inflammation. This is addressed through interventions such as reinforcing the importance of joint and muscle exercises prescribed by the physical therapist, getting the patient to walk and do other recreational exercises, underlining the importance of ambulatory aids, and focusing on the patient's strengths, with the objective of getting them to ambulate independently.
- The third possible diagnosis is a **partial self-care deficit** related to fatigue, pain, stiffness, and joint deformity. Many techniques, assistive devices, muscle training exercises, pain interventions, or teaching processes can be used to get patients to independently perform ADLs.

Differences in Hand Appearance for Rheumatoid Arthritis and Osteoarthritis

The hand of a person with RA typically shows **subcutaneous nodules or protuberances** on the top of the hand near the joints where digits connect. An individual with RA also usually has **ulnar drift** or bowing of the fingers toward the outside and the ulnar bone. A person with OA has neither of these hand abnormalities. Instead, an individual with OA may have **Bouchard's nodes** and/or **Heberden's nodes**, which are swollen areas above the joints—in the center or near the nail, respectively—on each digit. In addition, while morning stiffness is usually experienced by both of these types of patients, it tends to last longer and show less improvement with movement in the RA patient.

Rheumatoid-Like Inflammatory Disorders

Rheumatoid-like inflammatory disorders include scleroderma, systemic lupus erythematosus (SLE), Lyme disease, and polymyositis. All of these are **systemic vascular diseases** with inflammatory and connective tissue involvement. **Scleroderma** is characterized by thickening and hardening of the skin, but it also affects the lungs, GI tract, and other tissues. **SLE** presents initially as short-lived treatable arthritis but can progress to joint deformity, inflammation of kidney and heart cells, rashes, and other symptoms. **Lyme arthritis** is a late-stage manifestation of untreated or unresponsive Lyme disease caused by the bacteria of Lyme disease entering the joints, usually affecting the knees. Lyme disease is acquired through tick transmission of the bacterium *Borrelia burgdorferi*.

Gout and Other Metabolic Disorders That Can Lead to Arthritic Problems

Gout is a metabolic disorder in which **uric acid salts** are deposited in some part of the joints. Most patients with gout are males over the age of 30 who are obese, alcoholic, heavy red meat eaters, or hypertensive, or who have renal problems or are taking diuretics. Joints are painful, swollen, and eventually deformed, and gout sufferers can develop blood clots and hypertension. Gout can also develop in elderly men or women. There are also other **metabolic disorders** with arthritic components, including amyloidosis (high accumulation of the protein amyloid), hyperlipidemia (high accumulation of lipids), and CPPD (deposition of calcium pyrophosphate dihydrate crystals).

Spondyloarthropathies

Spondyloarthropathies are chronic inflammatory types of arthritis that involve the **spinal column** and appear to have a genetic component (human leukocyte antigen HLA-B27) that is activated by environmental factors. The most common example is **ankylosing spondylitis**, which is characterized by back pain, limited movement from the neck down the back and ribs, posture problems, spinal fractures, weakness in lower limbs, and elimination problems. Some of these spondyloarthropathies are considered **reactive arthritis**. **Reiter's syndrome** is an example caused by a genitourinary or gastrointestinal infection that activates the HLA-B27 gene (found in about 80% of these patients). The individual develops arthritis as well as conjunctivitis,

Functional Health Patterns

77

urethritis, and other involvement. **Psoriatic arthritis** is another type affecting the skin and nails, in which rheumatoid factor is not observed.

CONDITIONS SOMETIMES CONFUSED WITH ARTHRITIS

A relatively common condition affecting primarily women is **fibromyalgia syndrome (FMS)**, which is chronic muscle (not joint) pain in a variety of sites. The etiology of FMS is unclear and may involve a genetic component. Symptoms vary and can include restless leg syndrome, low back pain, or irritable bowel syndrome. **Spinal stenosis**, the tapering of part of the spinal canal, can also mimic arthritis by generating pressure on nerves and causing pain or numbness in the back or lower extremities. **Fractures** or other traumatic injuries acquired through motor accidents, falls, or punctures may have consequences that can affect musculoskeletal function. These can include cerebral or spinal cord injury and bone damage.

TREATMENT AND MEDICATION OPTIONS FOR MAIN TYPES OF ARTHRITIS

OA is generally managed by promoting **joint mobilization** and **moderate exercise**. The management approach to the major inflammatory types, RA and JRA, is different. Adults with RA may have their joints immobilized or splints applied as needed, while children with JRA are generally advised to rest and perform within their capabilities. Typical medication regimens for all three include use of **NSAIDs**. **Steroids** may be injected into the site in patients with OA or used systemically in RA, but they are generally not utilized in children with JRA. Osteoarthritis is also treated with hyaluronan or Hylan G-F.

PHARMACOLOGICAL MANAGEMENT OF RA

The American College of Rheumatology recommends the used of **disease-modifying antirheumatic drugs (DMARDs)** in the initial and ongoing treatment of RA. This category of drugs includes nonbiologic drugs (specifically immunosuppressants such as methotrexate), biologic drugs (which are produced to target the cytokine response, such as monoclonal antibodies and TNF inhibitors), and targeted synthetic drugs. DMARDs are recommended in conjunction with anti-inflammatory drugs (NSAIDs or, in severe cases, corticosteroids) because DMARDs require time upon initiation for effectiveness. Analgesics, such as acetaminophen, tramadol, and opioids, are generally not recommended unless the patient is in the end stage of the disease.

ANTI-INFLAMMATORY DRUGS TO TREAT AUTOIMMUNE DISEASES, REDUCE PAIN, OR IMPROVE MOBILITY

Anti-inflammatory drugs are either nonsteroidal drugs or steroids. **Nonsteroidal anti-inflammatory drugs (NSAIDs)** are used for relief of a variety of diseases and conditions, including rheumatoid arthritis and ankylosing spondylitis (autoimmune diseases), dysmenorrhea, pain, inflammation, osteoarthritis, fever, and gout. There are many NSAIDs, including ibuprofen (Advil), naproxen (Aleve), indomethacin (Indocin), nabumetone (Relafen), and the subclass of COX-2 inhibitors of which celecoxib (Celebrex) is a member. COX-2 inhibitors are effective against more acute pain than other NSAIDs. **Corticosteroids** are also used to treat inflammatory disorders, and they are also effective against pneumonia and the autoimmune disease systemic lupus erythematosus (SLE). There are many available corticosteroids, including dexamethasone, hydrocortisone, and prednisone.

DRUG CLASSES IN MANAGEMENT OF OSTEOPOROSIS

Osteoporosis can be addressed through use of various drug classes. **Bisphosphonates** such as Fosamax, which inhibit bone resorption, are the drug class of choice for prevention and treatment, specifically in women. The patient must take these drugs in the morning with plenty of water when sitting upright; eating or lying down must be avoided for at least half an hour. Another category utilized is **selective estrogen receptor modulators (SERMs)**, which act by selectively binding to estrogen receptors on cells; SERMs include raloxifene (Evista), the recommended drug, and tamoxifen (Soltamox). **Teriparatide** (Forteo) is a drug sanctioned for actual treatment of osteoporosis through promotion of bone formation; it contains calcitonin-salmon. Hormone replacement therapy is no longer suggested, as it may promote breast cancer and cardiovascular disease.

THERAPEUTIC POSITIONING

An individual with limited mobility needs to **change position** regularly to avoid discomfort and a range of problems, including edema, pressure ulcers, contractures, and loss of sensation. There are four basic optimally therapeutic positions. The nurse can aid the patient in changing to these positions.

- The first is **lying on the back** (or the supine position) with a small pillow under the head, neck, and shoulders and a trochanter roll under the hips, which maintains proper hip alignment.
- Another is the **lateral or side-lying position**, which uses several pillows to support the body at the head and neck, at the upper arm, in front of the lower leg (where the higher leg is supported), and behind the back.
- In the **prone position**, the patient is positioned on their abdomen and their head is turned to one side for breathing. The head, knees, hips, toes, and feet are propped up with pillows.
- In the **thirty-degree lateral position**, the patient is positioned on their back with the body turned approximately 30 degrees to the bed (using wedges or pillows) and the limbs flexed. Pillows may be placed between the knee and leg area, beneath the top arm, and behind the head.

POSITIONING AIDS

Pillows or folded towels are commonly used to relieve pressure and align and stabilize the patient. There are also specially designed positioning aids. These include **trochanter rolls**, designed to prevent outward rotation of the hip while prone; **hand rolls** or **hard cones**, which are placed under the hand to keep it in place and prevent it from contracting; and **abductor wedges** or pillows, which keep the prosthesis in position after total hip replacement surgery. A variety of **splints or orthotic braces** are available that either give support without allowing movement (static) or permit some motion (dynamic). These include short and longer leg braces, walkers, specialized shoes, and orthoses made specifically for particular conditions. **Casts** are more rigid supports made of plaster, plastic, or fiberglass. They are used for fractures, as well as prevention of cardiopulmonary complications in postural conditions such as scoliosis, or contractures due to issues such as burns, rheumatoid arthritis, or limp muscles.

ASSISTANCE WITH PERSONAL CARE ACTIVITIES OF DAILY LIVING

There are various aspects of personal care activities of daily living that individuals with disabilities may require temporary or permanent assistance in executing:

- Patients of various levels and types of disability generally have difficulty **washing their hair**. If patients can sit, they can use a shower seat for this task; if they cannot, a pan can be used for rinse water when lying down.
- **Nail care** is very difficult for a person with balance and range-of-motion issues. Since many patients are elderly or diabetic, nail care is crucial, necessitating intervention. Patients can wear a magnifying glass around their neck for inspection purposes. Individuals with diabetic neuropathy may require a professional to do nail care in order to prevent cuts that could result in dangerous infection.
- **Grooming actions**, such as shaving for men, application of makeup for women, and use of deodorant, may need to be performed using creative measures.
- People with functional disabilities commonly suffer from neglect of **oral hygiene**; the nurse can assist them with creative modifications in dental aid use and scheduling dental services.
- For women with disabilities of **menstrual age**, management of their menstrual period is problematic because they may lack the sensation, strength, or functional mobility to change menstrual pads or tampons. They can make the task easier by manipulations such as sitting on a raised toilet seat or forward in a wheelchair, bracing against the back of the wheelchair, using a mirror, or holding on to a grab bar or locked wheelchair.

GOALS AND ADLS FOR PATIENTS WITH LIMITED RANGE OF MOTION AND STRENGTH

Patients with limited range of motion and strength, such as those with arthritis, should incorporate measures into their daily routine that conserve energy, lessen their pain, and offset their reduced capacity for mobility.

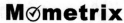

These measures include **modifications for daily living** such as use of the following: shoe fasteners, stocking aids, and easy closers (e.g., large buttons or Velcro); assistive devices for reaching; dietary aids (e.g., utensils with large handles, cup modifications such as attachable straws or bottom suction cups), easily opened jars or openers, and foods that have been pre-prepared and stored in containers; and devices that enhance grooming and toileting (e.g., electric toothbrushes and razors, tub grab bars and handheld showerheads, carrying bags attached to walkers).

DRESSING ISSUES FOR PATIENTS WITH RESTRICTED RANGE OF MOTION

Patients with a restricted range of motion need to develop **routines** that enable them to dress themselves. If they cannot stand, they can use a technique called **bridging**, in which they flex their unaffected knee and push down on the bed to raise their hips. Then they can use their good hand and arm to pull on their pants. If they can stand and balance, the patients can start by sitting and using their unaffected hand to elevate and cross the affected leg over the other one. They can then begin to draw the pants leg up over the affected limb, uncross the legs, insert the good leg into the other side of the pants, and then pull up the pants and zip the pants with their unaffected hand. For women, putting on a bra is difficult. While seated, a woman generally puts the bra on backwards at the waistline and then switches it to the front. Using her unaffected hand, the woman then places the affected arm into the bra strap first and then fits in the other arm and adjusts the bra with her good hand. Alternatives to hook-type bras include ones with Velcro closures or stretch bras that can be pulled either down from overhead or up after stepping into them.

SAFETY GRAB BAR INSTALLATION IN BATHROOM OF PATIENT WITH DISABILITIES

For patients who need to use a grab bar for balance when using the toilet, there are several possible configurations. The bar can be installed **diagonally** at a 45-degree angle on the wall near the patient's strong hand. If necessary, a raised toilet seat may be used to facilitate use. Typically, a 33-inch bar is used (although there are other lengths); the lower and upper ends of the bar are about 35 and 60 inches from the floor respectively, and the bar projects 2–4 inches from the wall. There are a number of primarily **right-angle configurations** for bathtub or shower grab bars commercially available as well. Alternatively, a one-piece right-angle bar can be mounted from a point on the person's stronger side. A typical height for a right-angle bar is 31 inches. Various **transfer boards** and **bathtub seats** are also sold.

ASSISTIVE DEVICES FOR PREAMBULATION

A physical therapist often plans the isometric and therapeutic exercises to prepare a patient for **standing and ambulation**. The nurse often implements these plans. **Preambulation exercises** usually include isometric exercises to strengthen the trunk and extremities, adapted sit-ups and push-ups done in bed, exercises for the arms done in a seated position, and passive standing activities if possible. **Passive standing** can be assisted through use of either a tilt table or standing frame. The patient is strapped to a **tilt** with their feet on a footrest. The table is then adjusted from about a 15–20° angle at small increments until the patient can stand for about 10 minutes to a half hour. It is important to measure parameters such as blood pressure, heart rate, and swelling in the lower limbs prior to beginning and during the use of the tilt table. Another method makes use of a **standing frame or table**, which uses stabilizers in front of and behind key support areas (such as the knee, abdominal, pelvic, and buttock regions) to directly move the patient from a sitting to a standing position.

ASSISTIVE DEVICES FOR AMBULATION

The most commonly used assistive devices for ambulation are the cane, walker, and crutches. In order to be effective, these devices must be properly fit to the individual patient.

- A **cane** should be held in the opposite hand of the side of injury. When the patient is holding the cane in neutral position, the elbow should be bent at about a 15-degree angle. When the patient is holding the cane straight down to the side of the body, the top of the cane should be in line with the crease of the wrist.

- The same is true of a **walker**; the elbow should be bent at 15 degrees when standing up straight and grasping the handles, and the handle grasps should be in line with the crease of the wrists. The patient should be able to move the walker forward without leaning over.
- **Crutches** should be properly fitted to the patient before attempting ambulation. The correct height is one hand-width below the axillae. The handgrips should be adjusted so that the patient's body weight is supported comfortably with elbows slightly flexed rather than locked in place. The patient should not bear weight under the axillae as this can cause nerve damage. Instead, they should hold the crutches tight against the side of their chest wall. The type of gait used depends on the type of injury.

AMBULATING A PATIENT WITH CRUTCHES
FOUR-POINT TECHNIQUE AND THREE-POINT TECHNIQUE

The **four-point technique** (displayed below) for crutch walking is the preferred method of ambulation for a patient with poor lower body strength who is ambulating with crutches. While the patient is standing, instruct them to move the left crutch forward first, followed by the right foot. The right crutch should then be moved forward, followed by the left foot. The advantage of this method of ambulation is that the patient has at least three points of contact with the ground at all times, offering the most stability; the disadvantage is that it requires a slow movement speed.

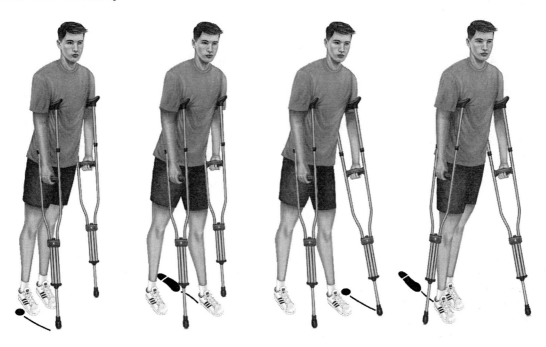

The **three-point technique** (displayed below) is recommended for patients who are unable to bear weight on one foot while ambulating with crutches. While in a standing position, the patient should move both crutches and the affected limb forward. Then, while placing their weight on the crutches, the patient should move their strong leg forward until it is even with the affected extremity.

Functional Health Patterns

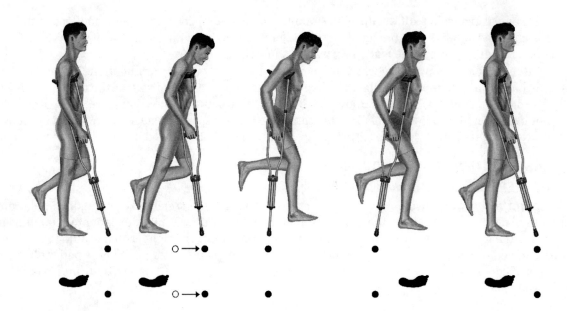

SWING-TO METHOD AND SWING-THROUGH METHOD

The **swing-to and swing-through methods of crutch walking** are intended for patients who have decreased lower body strength. Both methods are advantageous in that they are easy to learn and allow for a quick gait. The disadvantage is that both methods require strong upper body strength. In the swing-to method, both crutches are moved forward and placed at the length of a step in front of them. The patient then places their weight upon the crutches and swings their body forward until the feet are equal to the crutches. In the swing-through method, both crutches are moved forward. Placing their weight upon the crutches, the patient swings their lower body forward and places their feet slightly in front of the crutches.

TRANSFERRING PATIENT FROM CHAIR OR SITTING POSITION TO STANDING POSITION USING CRUTCHES

While the patient is sitting in the chair, instruct them to hold both crutches in one hand by gripping the handgrips. Instruct the patient to scoot their hips to the edge of the chair and stretch the non-weight-bearing foot out straight. Help the patient rise to a standing position, using the arm of the chair to support one of the patient's arms and the crutches to support the other. Once the patient has balanced their weight on one foot, instruct the patient to move one of the crutches to the opposite side and place their hands on the handgrips.

TRANSFERRING PATIENT FROM STANDING TO SITTING POSITION USING CRUTCHES

To move from a **standing to a sitting position**, instruct the patient to approach the chair until they are one step away from the front of the chair. Instruct the patient to carefully turn using their weight-bearing leg and the crutches until their back is to the chair. Assist the patient in finding their balance before transferring one of the crutches to the opposite side. Instruct the patient to grip both crutches by the handgrips. Help the patient to reach back with the free hand to find the arm of the chair. Instruct the patient to stretch the non-weight-bearing foot forward. Assist the patient with slowly lowering their weight into the chair.

AMBULATING PATIENT WITH A WALKER

A patient who is learning to ambulate with a **walker** should wear a gait belt at all times. Instruct the patient to stand in the middle of the walker, holding it by the handgrips. Instruct the patient to move the walker forward until the back legs are even with the toes. While keeping their weight on the strong leg, the patient should then take a step forward with the weaker leg, until it is in the center of the walker. Then, instruct the patient to place their weight upon the handgrips while taking a step forward with the strong leg. Once the patient has regained balance, repeat the process.

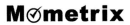

ASSISTING PATIENT FROM SITTING POSITION TO STANDING WITH WALKER

While the patient is sitting in the chair, open the walker and place it in front of the patient. Make sure the patient is wearing a gait belt. Instruct the patient to scoot forward until they are sitting on the edge of the chair. Instruct the patient to place both hands on the arms of the chair. On the count of three, assist the patient into a standing position. While providing support for the patient, instruct them to move their hands, one at a time, from the arms of the chair to the handgrips of the walker. Wait a moment to ensure the patient is not dizzy before beginning to ambulate.

AMBULATING A PATIENT WITH A CANE

While ambulating a patient who is learning how to walk with a **cane**, always provide the patient with a gait belt. Instruct the patient to hold the cane in their strong hand. As the patient takes a step forward with the affected extremity, advance the cane forward, keeping the cane even with the leg and the patient's full weight upon their strong leg. Once the weakened leg and the cane are in place, instruct the patient to place their weight upon the cane while taking a step forward with the unaffected extremity. Allow the patient a moment to regain balance before repeating the process.

POSITIONING CONSIDERATIONS FOR PATIENTS USING A WHEELCHAIR

Patients capable of using a wheelchair should be seated with their feet level on the floor, footstool, or footrests, preferably with their shoes on for additional safety. Their weight should be symmetrically balanced over the hips. It is important to use a wheelchair that conforms well to the patient's body in terms of correct, firm seat cushions and back supports. Pressure exerted on the patient by the chair should be spread out evenly. Any cushions that could cut off circulation or compromise skin integrity should not be used. Adjustments or pillows or armrests for support may be needed. If a patient needs a permanent wheelchair, it should be custom ordered.

HOW PATIENTS CONFINED TO A WHEELCHAIR CAN PUT ON PANTS OR UNDERWEAR

Patients with neurological syndromes who are confined to a wheelchair can put on pants or underwear while seated. The patient should lock the wheelchair and then move to the front of it while bracing against the back of the seat. The patient then pulls each leg of the pants up to their knee in sequence while flexing the leg, and collects as much material as possible. The patient then briefly raises up their buttocks, thighs, and eventually the pants, and afterward sits further back in the seat. While holding the waist of the pants, the patient repeats a pattern of sliding into the pants and lifting as before until the pants are in the correct position. In order to take off the pants, the patient again sits forward, unfastens the waistband, and then pushes up to allow the pants to slide down.

ORTHOTICS, BRACES, PROSTHETIC DEVICES, AND OTHER TECHNIQUES TO AID AMBULATION

An orthotic is any type of brace or other device that can assist mobility. **Orthotics** range from corrective shoes and inserts to various types of braces. **Leg braces** are often used by individuals with the inability to move on one side. A brace may be either a knee-ankle-foot (long) orthosis or a shorter leg brace. The brace may be connected to the shoe to discourage pronation of the ankle. **Prosthetic devices** are customized apparatuses to replace body parts after surgery. A patient is fitted for a permanent prosthesis after shrinkage of the remaining portion of the affected limb has concluded.

ASSISTIVE DEVICES TO HELP PATIENTS CARRY OUT SELF-CARE ACTIVITIES

The array of available assistive devices to aid patients in independent self-care activities is plentiful. The rehabilitation nurse or therapist selects appropriate devices and teaches the patient to use them. Some of these devices also **conserve energy**, such as long-handled shoehorns that can be used from a seated position, long-handled curved brushes that the patient can use for bathing, or reachers that alleviate the need to bend (useful for total hip replacement patients). Another assistive device for total hip replacement patients is a **raised commode seat**. There are also **motor-driven prostheses** such as the Motion Control (MC) Elbow, the MC Taska Hand, or the Boston Digital Arm System, which controls a variety of devices. Some assistive devices are

Functional Health Patterns

much simpler, such as elastic shoelaces or Velcro closures, but they are still quite useful in helping the patient to perform self-care activities.

MAINTAINING MOBILITY USING RANGE-OF-MOTION EXERCISES IN PATIENTS WITH DISABILITIES

The nurse can help the patient maintain mobility by helping them perform range-of-motion (ROM) exercises. The **isotonic ROM movements** can be used to help maintain flexibility, tone, strength, and functional mobility; the nurse should measure the angle of flexion if possible. The nurse can manipulate the patient's joints (passive ROM), help the patient perform the exercises, or teach the person to actively carry out exercises independently (active ROM). **Modifications** can be made in specific instances, such as using unaffected extremities to aid paralyzed limbs. **Isometric exercises** that engage the patient should also be done. Usually, the patient tenses or contracts certain muscles for 10 seconds before releasing them; typical muscle groups of focus are abdominal, gluteal, and quadriceps. **Resistive-type isometric exercises** such as flexing the plantar of the feet against a board would also be recommended. **Kegel exercises** and **oral-facial exercises** are recommended for incontinence and Parkinson's disease respectively. Any type of exercise program that the patient can safely participate in should be used, while unsafe exercises are not recommended. For example, patients with osteoporosis should not do spinal flexion movements.

IMPORTANCE OF PERFORMING RANGE OF MOTION ON PATIENTS

Patients who are bed bound are at an increased risk of muscle deterioration from lack of use. Lack of regular exercise also places patients at risk for developing contractures, a painful condition that results in the permanent shortening of the muscle or tendon. **Range-of-motion exercises** can be performed to maintain muscle tone during periods in which the patient lacks the strength to perform other forms of activity. Patients may also be assisted with performing range-of-motion activities if they are unable to do so themselves, such as in cases in which patients are sedated or comatose.

MOVEMENTS USED DURING RANGE-OF-MOTION EXERCISES

Specific **movements** used during ROM exercises can be described using the following terms:

- **Flexion** refers to bending at a joint, resulting in a decrease in the angle of the joint. For example, when the arm is bent at the elbow, it is flexed.
- **Extension** refers to the straightening of a joint, or increasing the angle of that joint. For example, when the arm is straightened, it is extended.
- **Abduction** refers to the movement away from the trunk. For example, when the arm is moved away from the body, such as during jumping jacks, it is abducted.
- **Adduction** refers to a movement that brings a limb closer to the trunk. For example, when the arm moves back toward the body, it is adducted.
- **Rotation** occurs when a part of the body pivots on a central axis. For example, when the head turns from side to side, it is considered to be rotating.

How to Perform Range of Motion on Patients

Range-of-motion exercises are typically performed during the patient's bath. They can also be performed while the patient is sitting in a chair or lying in bed. Each exercise should be performed 10 times to ensure it is effective. The procedure is as follows:

1. Wash hands and explain to the patient what is going to be done.
2. Raise the level of the bed until it is a comfortable height.
3. Begin by performing range-of-motion exercises on the patient's head; instruct the patient to rotate the head from one side to the other. This exercise should not be performed on patients who have suffered neck or spinal cord injuries.
4. Work on the arms next. Flex and extend both arms at the elbow then abduct and adduct the arm. Flex and extend both wrists and all fingers.
5. Range of motion of the legs includes flexion and extension of the leg at the knee, as well as abduction and adduction of the leg.
6. Finally, flex and extend the ankles and toes.

Active Range of Motion and Passive Range of Motion

Active range of motion (AROM) occurs when patients are able to perform range-of-motion activities by themselves. Though they may receive directions from the nurse, the patient performs the bulk of the exercise.

Passive range of motion (PROM) consists of the same exercises that are performed during AROM. PROM occurs when the nurse is performing range-of-motion activities on a sedated or comatose patient to prevent muscle weakness. PROM may also be performed on patients whose muscle weakness is so pronounced that they require assistance in order to perform the activity.

Functional Health Patterns

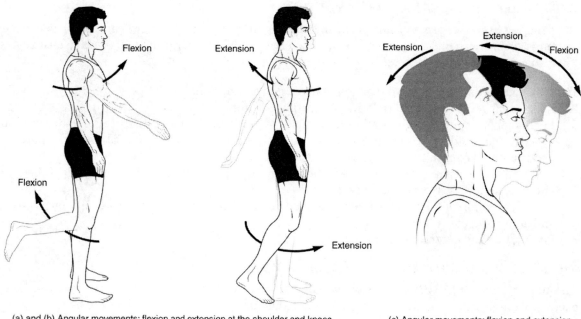

(a) and (b) Angular movements: flexion and extension at the shoulder and knees

(c) Angular movements: flexion and extension of the neck

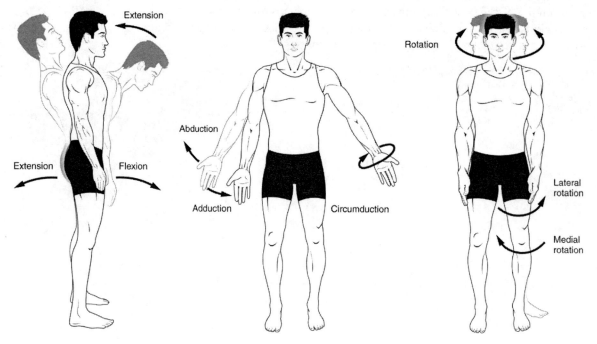

(d) Angular movements: flexion and extension of the vertebral column

(e) Angular movements: abduction, adduction, and circumduction of the upper limb at the shoulder

(f) Rotation of the head, neck, and lower limb

ABNORMAL FINDINGS

Range-of-motion exercises should be performed at least once or twice every day to make sure the patient's joints do not become **contracted**. Stiffness or the inability to move the joint may be an indication of the onset of contractures; if either of these symptoms is noticed, they should be reported to the nurse immediately. While performing range of motion, the nursing aide should monitor for any signs of **swelling or inflammation** in the joints. If the patient experiences **sudden severe pain** or **respiratory distress** while performing range of motion, the nurse should be notified immediately.

PATIENT MOVEMENT WHILE IN BED

While in bed, a patient needs to turn, change positions to alleviate pressure, move to different spots on the bed, or if possible, sit up on the bed. Patients capable of assisting in these **position changes** can use side rails, cords attached to various areas, or trapezes to help them. If a caregiver is needed to move the patient, then the bed needs to be **locked** into place at about hip height. Usually, two people are needed to move a patient, one to support the patient's **upper back** with two arms and another to position their arms to hold up the **lower back**. Each person stands with slightly bent knees and one foot in front of the other, in other words, using good body mechanics. One strong person can help a patient to move if the latter assists or if the caregiver approaches the task in sections. In order to turn a person, the caregiver should stand on the **side to which the patient is to be turned** and swiftly transfer the weight from one leg to the other, using hand pressure behind the shoulder and hips.

LOGROLLING A PATIENT WITH A NECK OR SPINAL CORD INJURY

Logrolling is a procedure that is performed whenever the patient has sustained a neck or spinal cord injury. Ideally, patients with this type of injury should be turned as little as possible until the neck or spine has been stabilized. In certain cases, turning cannot be avoided, such as if the patient has become incontinent. If the patient must be moved, the head, neck, and back must be kept in a stable position to prevent further injury. This requires good communication among the caregivers who are moving the patient to ensure that their movements are coordinated to maintain proper alignment.

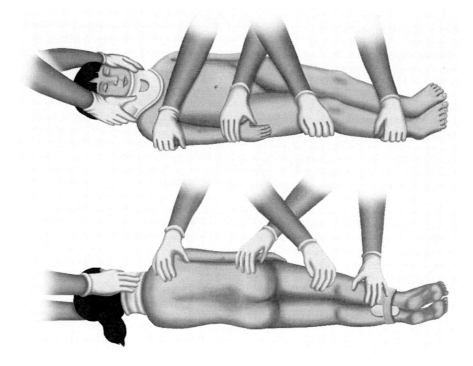

Logrolling a patient requires a minimum of three people in order to be performed successfully. The procedure is as follows:

1. Wash hands, don a pair of gloves, and explain what is going to be done.
2. Have one person positioned at the patient's head and two others on the side in which the patient is to be facing.
3. Grasp the draw sheet and turn the patient. The person at the head of the bed should keep the patient's head midline with the rest of the body, while the people at the side of the bed keep the back and hips in alignment.

Functional Health Patterns

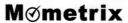

4. Perform the necessary procedures and then return the patient to their back. It is imperative that the patient's head, neck, and back are kept in alignment.
5. Position the patient for comfort and wash hands.

PATIENT TRANSFERS

TRANSFERRING A DEPENDENT PATIENT FROM THE BED TO OTHER LOCATIONS

Dependent patients who need to be transferred to other locations, such as a wheelchair, toilet, or bathtub, can be assisted in several ways.

- The first is by use of a **mechanical device** such as a pneumatic lift, which picks up the patient in a seated position and then delivers and lowers the patient onto the other site.
- Two nurses or other caregivers can lift transfer a patient from the bed to a chair together by **synchronizing the transfer** while one supports the patient under the arms, grasping opposite wrists, and the other holds up the patient's feet and legs.
- A **pivot transfer** involves initially sitting the patient on the side of the bed and then assisting transfer by having the patient hold on and supporting the patient's lower back.

TECHNIQUES FOR PATIENT TRANSFER WITH INDIVIDUALS CAPABLE OF SOME INDEPENDENCE

Patients capable of some independence may be able to change positions by doing a pivot transfer, by doing an independent standing transfer, or by using a transfer board. In this version of the **pivot transfer**, the brace is locked in place, and then the patient pivots and uses their unaffected leg to supply support and balance for things such as toilet use. A hemiplegic patient can usually perform the **independent standing transfer** from a wheelchair close to the head of the bed by locking the chair parts and then rising to a standing position by using their good foot and an armrest to push up. The patient then uses their unaffected arm as support on the bed and takes short side steps until they can sit on the side of the bed. A useful device for relatively independent patients is a **transfer board**, which is used for bed-wheelchair transfers with both at the same height. The patient shifts to place their buttocks on the board and then uses the upper limbs to help them scoot across it. Paraplegics with a lesser degree of loss of use can use their upper extremities for transfer assistance.

ENERGY CONSERVATION TECHNIQUES FOR PATIENTS WITH ACTIVITY INTOLERANCE

There are general energy conservation techniques for individuals with activity intolerance due to musculoskeletal issues. Many require the person to plan ahead or maintain an agenda. The patient should always take their time and incorporate rest breaks into activities. This means that the patient should **rest** every 10 minutes per hour of activity or 30–45 minutes after eating. The patient should feel free to ask the caregiver for help and be attuned to signs of **stress** such as chest pain or shortness of breath during the activity. Energy conservation may mean that the patient needs to **adapt** their activities so that they can be done from a seated position or with the use of a rolling cart. The person should avoid **temperature extremes**, both hot and cold, and **extra movements** for ADLs and other activities. Items that are used often should be close at hand and at arm level. The patient is instructed to use **good posture** (standing or sitting tall without crossing their legs) and **body mechanics** (two-handed flowing movements, pushing instead of pulling, etc.).

PRINCIPLES OF CARE FOR PATIENTS WITH IMPAIRED PHYSICAL MOBILITY

The nurse should institute **joint mobility exercises** that protect the joints by incorporating activities that reduce effort and stress on the joints. Only the bigger and stronger joints should be utilized. These joints should be used in secure positions. Positions should be changed often, pain should not be ignored, and periods of rest should be interspersed with work. **Strength training** should be integrated as well. The nurse is also responsible for specific interventions, such as regular skeletal pin site cleansing with chlorhexidine, periodic assessment of the affected extremities, and training of the patient and potential caregivers in use of assistive devices or newer lightweight automatically controlled prostheses.

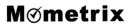

SURGICAL INTERVENTIONS FOR ADDITIONAL MUSCULOSKELETAL PROBLEMS

Total knee replacements, in which some sort of internal prosthetic implant is substituted, are common. Recovery is generally rapid through postsurgical use of **continuous passive motion machines** and exercises to improve **range of motion and mobility**. Surgical procedures that either replace vertebral discs or decrease pressure on spinal nerves include the following:

- **Laminectomy**, in which a portion of the lamina is removed.
- **Discectomy**, in which some or all of a ruptured intervertebral disc is excised.
- **Foraminotomy**, which widens the foramen portion to make room for the spinal nerve.
- **Spinal fusion**, in which several vertebrae are stabilized by insertion of bone grafts and sometimes other devices.
- **Spinal decompression**, where bones or tissues are taken out to eliminate pressure on the spinal nerves.

POSSIBLE POSTSURGICAL COMPLICATIONS

A rehabilitation nurse is responsible for surveillance of postsurgical complications after a patient has had a musculoskeletal surgery. A rehabilitation nurse constantly monitors the patient's circulation, sensation, movement, and firmness at the surgical site and looks for signs of swelling or bleeding. After surgery, anemia and cardiopulmonary problems may occur. There are also several syndromes that can transpire. One is **compartment syndrome**, in which site pressure from an external case or dressing or internal swelling or bleeding cuts off circulation to the area. This can lead to loss of viability of the affected limb and function if undiscovered, with the possibility of eventual infection, deformity, or amputation. One rare complication is **fat embolism syndrome**, in which fat globules from the bone marrow area are discharged into the vascular system, causing blockage. The patient develops hypoxia, cardiac problems, chest pain, alterations in mental status, and other symptoms.

DEEP VENOUS THROMBOSIS

Deep venous (or vein) thrombosis (**DVT**) is thrombus or blood clot formation in the deep venous system of the legs, resulting in either **thrombophlebitis** (inflamed vein) or **phlebothrombosis** (no inflammation). Blood clots form due to stoppage of blood flow, hypercoagulability of the blood due to increased levels of coagulation factors such as fibrinogen, and/or vessel wall injury. A **thrombus** begins at the outer edges of the blood vessel and organizes inward to fill and occlude (block) the vessel. Inflammation often occurs because inflammatory cells, white blood cells, and immune cells, as well as fibroblasts, are recruited to the area. Circulation may be shunted to superficial veins. However, if the iliofemoral or axillary veins are occluded, only **limited collateral circulation** can occur, causing increased venous pressure, distension of blood vessels, edema (fluid accumulation), and fluid and electrolyte abnormalities.

> **Review Video: DVT - Prevention and Treatment**
> Visit mometrix.com/academy and enter code: 234086

PROPHYLAXIS OF VTE IN HOSPITALIZED MEDICAL PATIENTS

Venous thromboembolism (VTE) refers to a vein blocked by a blood clot or thrombus that has detached from its original site. Most hospitals have protocols in place for **prophylaxis of VTE** in the hospitalized medical patient. Criteria for risk include reduced mobility plus at least one VTE risk factor. Common risk factors include age over 40 years, previous history of VTE, and related diseases such as thrombophilia, collagen-vascular disorder, varicose veins, and inflammatory disorders. Other risk factors are obesity, admission to the intensive care unit, central venous line or catheter, non-hemorrhagic stroke, heart failure, cancer, chronic lung disease or respiratory failure, and pneumonia or other serious infection. If the patient has hypersensitivity to heparin or thrombocytopenia induced by it, active bleeding, uncontrolled hypertension, a clotting disorder, recent cranial or eye surgery, or recent spinal tap or epidural anesthesia, they are given **intermittent pneumatic**

89

compression. Otherwise, at-risk individuals are usually given **subcutaneous enoxaparin** (40 mg daily) or **unfractionated heparin** (5000 international units every 8 hours).

RISK FACTOR ASSESSMENT

The risk of developing deep venous thrombosis increases with age (at least 41 years of age), history of prior surgeries, obesity, an acute myocardial infarction, COPD, swollen legs, sepsis, and—for women—recent pregnancy, abortion, premature birth, or hormone use. It is even more likely if the patient is at least 60 years old, has undergone certain surgeries such as arthroscopy or laparoscopy, is currently in a cast, or has central venous access. Risk is compounded for people who are over 75 years old, have prior history of DVT or pulmonary embolism, or who have certain serum markers. These markers include things such as positive prothrombin variants, elevated homocysteine, anticardiolipin antibodies, and positive lupus anticoagulant. If a patient has had a recent hip, pelvic, or leg fracture; a stroke; trauma; or spinal cord injury, they are at great risk for DVT. Risk factors are additive, and prophylaxis generally depends on the **cumulative risk level**.

SIGNS AND POSSIBLE NURSING DIAGNOSIS AND INTERVENTIONS

Signs of DVT are generally acute pain, edema, and deep muscle tenderness related to inflammation. Fever, lethargy, a high white blood cell count, elevated sedimentation rate, and swollen feet and/or ankles are other possible signs. If larger veins are involved, **systemic reactions** may occur, resulting in high fever. DVT must be detected and managed early in order to prevent **pulmonary embolism**. DVT can be diagnosed using the D-dimer test, duplex ultrasound, or contrast venography (either gadolinium with MRI or ascending). The possible nursing diagnoses are ineffective peripheral tissue perfusion, anxiety, or ineffective therapeutic regimen management. Primary interventions are to stop the clotting through use of anticoagulants such as heparin or warfarin, dissolve existing clots, thwart the migration of clots to other sites, support the patient, and in some cases actually remove the blood clot. Other nursing interventions are provision of pain medications, elevation of the extremity, providing antiembolism stockings, and maintaining as much patient range of motion and mobility as possible.

CONTRACTURES

A contracture is the permanent tightening or shortening of a body part such as a muscle. They result from **joint immobilization** and are compounded by conditions such as plasticity, paralysis, or areas of muscle disparity. There are three types of muscle contractures:

- An **arthrogenic contracture** is the multidirectional stiffening caused by injury to cartilage, synovium, or the joint capsule.
- **Soft tissue contractures** involve unidirectional loss of range of motion due to damage to the periarticular, subcutaneous, or cutaneous tissues.
- When muscle fibers are replaced with collagen during inflammatory, neurological, or traumatic events, a **myogenic contracture** can occur. These contractures leave the extremity in a flexed position.

SERIAL CASTING AND DYNAMIC SPLINTING

Serial casting and dynamic splinting are methods of maximizing stretching, range of motion, and movement in patients with contractures.

- In **serial casting**, a well-cushioned cast is applied to the joint area in extremities right after the joint has been stretched. Within 2 or 3 days, the cast is removed, the skin integrity is evaluated, and another similar casting is done; the process is repeated for up to about 5 days.
- **Dynamic splinting** is routinely performed after orthopedic surgery, particularly to upper limbs. It allows a fair amount of movement while using tension to stretch the joint. There is usually a **continuous passive motion (CPM) device** attached that promotes joint mobility and prevents tightening of muscles.

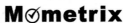

Respiratory Functional Ability

RESPIRATORY TRACT

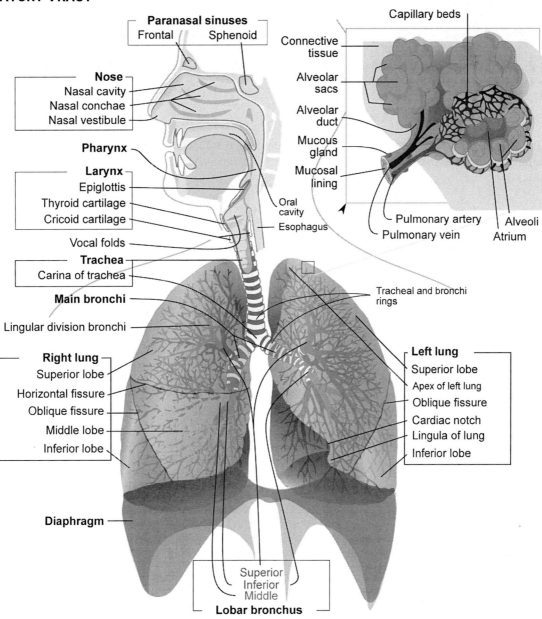

There are two types of respiratory structures in the respiratory tract. The **conducting airways** are channels that carry air from the nose through the pharynx, larynx, trachea, and branches of the bronchus, and ultimately to the terminal bronchioles. In the nasopharyngeal region, there are many blood vessels that warm up and humidify the inspired air, as well as ciliated mucous membranes to entrap particles. As part of normal function, the epiglottis closes off to protect the airway during swallowing. The **terminal bronchioles** are another type of airway known as **respiratory units** because their primary function is the exchange of gases. Respiratory units are composed of respiratory bronchioles, alveolar ducts, and the alveoli, where gas exchange occurs.

> **Review Video: What Is the Pulmonary Circuit?**
> Visit mometrix.com/academy and enter code: 955608

ASSESSMENT OF THE RESPIRATORY SYSTEM

If significant respiratory distress is present, one must stabilize the patient before doing a **respiratory history** or ask family if available:

- Question the patient about risk factors, such as smoking, exposure to smoke or other inhaled toxins, past lung problems, and allergies.
- Ask the patient about symptoms of respiratory problems, such as dyspnea, cough, sputum production, fatigue, ability to do ADLs and IADLs, and chest pain.
- Determine how long symptoms have been present, the length of periods of dyspnea, aggravating and alleviating factors, and the severity of symptoms.

When performing a **physical assessment**, one should assess vital signs, posture, pulse oximetry, check nails for clubbing, do a skin assessment, listen to lung sounds via auscultation and percussion, and look for accessory muscle use, signs of anxiety, and edema. Depending on condition, blood may be drawn for arterial blood gases, electrolytes, and CBC. Sputum cultures may be obtained.

PRIMARY AND SECONDARY MUSCLES USED FOR BREATHING

Muscles used for breathing are separated into primary and secondary muscle groups.

- The **primary muscle groups** are those that are used in normal, quiet breathing. When patients are in respiratory distress and breathing is more difficult, secondary muscle groups become activated. The muscles considered primary for breathing are the diaphragm and the external intercostal muscles. These muscles act by changing the pressure gradient, allowing the lungs to expand and air to flow in and out.
- The **secondary muscle groups** include the sternocleidomastoid, scaleni, internal intercostals, obliques, and abdominal muscles. These secondary muscle groups work when breathing is difficult, both in inspiration and expiration, in cases such as obstructions or bronchoconstriction. Use of these secondary muscle groups can often be seen on exam and may be described as see-saw or abdominal breathing (when the abdominal muscles are being used during exhalation) or retractions as the muscles activate and can be seen between rigid structures such as bone.

VENTILATION/PERFUSION RATIO

In order to maintain homeostasis, the respiratory and cardiac systems need to maintain a careful balance. The **ventilation/perfusion ratio** indicates that ventilation of the lungs and perfusion to the lungs are within a normal balance. A normal ventilation/perfusion ratio is equal to 0.8. A ventilation/perfusion ratio higher than normal is indicative of ventilation that is too high, perfusion that is too low, or some combination of the two. This can occur because of hyperventilation (either physiological or caused by healthcare practitioners due to incorrect ventilator settings), pulmonary embolism, or hypotension. Essentially, a high ventilation/perfusion ratio means that there is more ventilation than perfusion. If the ventilation/perfusion ratio is lower than normal, then ventilation is too low, perfusion is too high, or some combination of the two. This can be caused by atelectasis, pneumonia, or lung disease. Whatever the cause, a low ventilation/perfusion ratio indicates that there is more perfusion than ventilation.

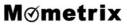

NORMAL AND ABNORMAL BREATH SOUND TERMS

Normal breath sounds can be divided into three types. Vesicular breath sounds are low, soft sounds that can normally be heard over the peripheral lung space. Bronchovesicular breath sounds are moderate pitch breath sounds that are normally heard in the upper lung fields. Tracheal breath sounds are higher in pitch and heard over the trachea. Abnormal breath sounds are also known as adventitious lung sounds. Wheezes are high-pitched, expiratory sounds caused by air flowing through an obstructed airway. Stridor is also high-pitched, but is usually heard on inspiration in the upper airways. Coarse crackles are caused by an excessive amount of secretions in the airway and can be heard on inspiration and expiration. Fine crackles occur late in the expiratory phase and usually occur when the peripheral airways are being "popped" back open.

> **Review Video: Lung Sounds**
> Visit mometrix.com/academy and enter code: 765616

DIAGNOSTIC PROCEDURES AND TOOLS USED DURING ASSESSMENT OF PULMONARY TRAUMA/DISEASE

The diagnostic procedures and tools used during assessment of **pulmonary and thoracic trauma/disease** will vary according to the type and degree of injury/disease, but may include:

- **Thorough physical examination** including cardiac and pulmonary status, assessing for any abnormalities.
- **Electrocardiogram** to assess for cardiac arrhythmias.
- **Chest x-ray** should be done for all those with injuries to check for fractures, pneumothorax, major injuries, and placement of intubation tubes. X-rays can be taken quickly and with portable equipment so they can be completed quickly during the initial assessment.
- **Computerized tomography** may be indicated after initial assessment, especially if there is a possibility of damage to the parenchyma of the lungs.
- **Oximetry and atrial blood gases** as indicated.
- **12-lead electrocardiogram** may be needed if there are arrhythmias for more careful observation.
- **Echocardiogram** should be done if there is apparent cardiac damage.

AIRWAY CLEARANCE

Normal airway clearance is caused by various aspects of the respiratory system. A thin layer of mucus lines the airways as a protective mechanism against debris and helps trap foreign objects before they enter the lower airways. Proper hydration keeps the mucosa adequately moist so it can trap foreign debris. As this debris lands in the mucus, the cilia in the respiratory tract act as an "elevator" to push the debris up to the larynx, where it can either be coughed up or swallowed and digested. An intact cough reflex is necessary for the debris to stimulate the cough, and normal muscle strength and nerve innervation of the diaphragm is required to produce a sufficiently forceful cough.

INEFFECTIVE AIRWAY CLEARANCE

Individuals with ineffective airway clearance cannot discharge secretions or obstructions from their respiratory tract. Patients with neuromuscular diseases generally have **weak respiratory muscles**, predisposing them to ineffective airway clearance. A person needs enough muscle strength to take a deep breath before they cough and to create enough **intrathoracic pressure** to clear the airways. Ineffective clearance can also be due to **excessive secretions**, which are commonly found in people with chronic bronchitis, cystic fibrosis, bronchiectasis, or lower respiratory tract infections (LRTIs). Usually, these patients have complaints about chest congestion, inability to cough up secretions, shortness of breath, tiredness, or anxiety. Physical examination generally shows abnormal breath sounds such as wheezing and crackling, and sputum is thick and not clear.

Functional Health Patterns

93

CHEST PHYSIOTHERAPY TO AID INEFFECTIVE AIRWAY CLEARANCE

Chest physiotherapy refers to any maneuver that can enhance movement of airway secretions from distal airways to more central passages for eventual expectoration or other removal. One type of chest physiotherapy is **chest percussion**, in which a health care worker thumps appropriate areas of the patient's chest with a cupped hand. Percussion is usually used in tandem with coughing techniques or other forms of chest physiotherapy. One of the other forms is **chest vibration**. Here the clinician uses a flat hand against the chest area to be cleared during expiration; the clinician alternates tension and relaxation in the arm to create vibrations in the patient's chest wall. There are devices available that similarly enhance clearance, such as the **flutter valve** or a number of appliances that use **positive expiratory pressure**. Another common modality is **postural drainage**, in which the patient is placed in a position (12 are possible) to drain affected lobes and airway segments.

COUGHING TECHNIQUES

Patients with ineffective airway clearance (excluding those with airway collapse) may benefit from use of the controlled cough, huff cough, or pump cough.

- In a **controlled cough**, the person breathes in slowly and holds the breath for a few seconds before coughing several times.
- The **huff cough** is a variation of the controlled cough that saves the patient energy; the patient leans forward while holding a pillow during inspiration and then says the word *huff* during expiration to keep the glottis open. A variant is the **pump cough**, in which the patient says three rapid huffs followed by three brief coughs during expiration.

Patients with neuromuscular diseases and undermined respiratory muscles are often taught either the quad cough or the glossopharyngeal breathing (GPB) method.

- The **quad cough** is an assisted cough in which a helper pushes against the patient's epigastric region with their hand at the xiphoid process while the patient tries to cough. Sometimes the patient can do a quad cough independently by leaning forward and using a pillow to push.
- In **GPB**, the patient entraps air in the mouth, pushes it to the posterior with the tongue, and keeps the mouth closed until air is in the trachea.

INTERVENTIONS IN PATIENTS WITH TRACHEOSTOMY

A tracheostomy is a hole cut in the trachea to unblock the airway and/or suck out secretions. Patients who have had a tracheostomy usually have a tube inserted that can also prevent aspiration due to an impaired gag reflex or serve as a conduit for mechanical ventilation. The **tracheostomy tube** may be one of the following: a soft, flexible, cuffed tube that is inflated and does not allow air leakage; a fenestrated tube with openings for airflow to the larynx to allow the person to speak; or an uncuffed plastic or metal tube for longer use in patients with an operative epiglottis. Tubes should be removed as soon as the patient can independently sustain ventilation, cough, and expel secretions. **Suctioning** is typically done at about 60–80 mmHg pressure. In order to prevent encrustation of the tube, **humidity** can be introduced via a collar with a heated nebulizer. The tube needs to be cleaned based on facility or manufacturer's protocol. The insertion site should also be cleansed with hydrogen peroxide followed by saline.

OTHER MODALITIES TO AID INEFFECTIVE AIRWAY CLEARANCE

In order to aid ineffective airway clearance, **hydration levels** should be kept in the normal range without pushing fluids or using diuretics. **Humidifiers** with heat and moisture exchangers (HME) that can be briefly connected to a tracheotomy tube until the patient coughs up secretions or needs suctioning are often used. Droplets of water vapor or drugs are often administered as **aerosols** through inhalers or nebulizers as small particles that can theoretically reach airway passages. Airway or nasotracheal **suctioning** is done by lubricating the suctioning catheter with a water-soluble gel and then inserting a cone into the nasal cavity. The patient takes breaths of oxygen while suction pressure is applied through a catheter to suction out secretions.

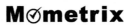

Other techniques include **deep breathing exercises** (ideally while standing) and **incentive spirometry**. The ultimate goal of any of these interventions is airway patency, ventilation, and normal gas exchange.

PHARMACOLOGIC AGENTS

Pharmacologic agents are used to treat ineffective airway clearance and inflammation by decreasing the effort needed to breathe. There are four types of common agents utilized.

- **Bronchodilators** relax the airway passages. There are several drug classes that serve as bronchodilators: (1) β2-agonists, used to control bronchospasm in asthmatics and individuals with COPD or bronchiectasis; (2) anticholinergics, which prevent contraction of respiratory smooth muscle and suppress oversecretion; and (3) methylxanthines, which act by improving diaphragm function and dilation of local blood vessels and are used for stable cases of COPD or asthma.
- **Inhaled corticosteroids** are given for their anti-inflammatory properties.
- When there is some evidence of infection, such as purulent sputum, sinusitis, or pneumonia, **antibiotics** are indicated.
- An associated immunologic approach to reducing infections is **vaccination** for diseases such as influenza and pneumococcus.

INEFFECTIVE BREATHING PATTERN

An ineffective breathing pattern is one in which adequate oxygen needed for cellular requirements cannot be maintained. The most common signs are shortness of breath and fatigue. Proper ventilation cannot be sustained due to obstructive defects, restrictive defects, a combination of both, or other factors such as the hyperventilation and low carbon dioxide pressures that occur in high altitudes or during anxiety attacks. **Obstructive defects** like COPD usually cause alveolar hypoventilation with high levels of CO_2; this mismatch can also occur in children with bronchopulmonary dysplasia. People with **restrictive defects**, in particular those caused by weakened respiratory muscles in neuromuscular diseases, also can develop alveolar hypoventilation. Different neuromuscular diseases show evidence of ineffective breathing at different times. The main example of **combined obstructive/restrictive defects** is cystic fibrosis, in which thick enzyme-containing secretions not only block passages but also destroy tissues, impair transport, and encourage infection.

BREATHING TRAINING TECHNIQUES

The goals for a patient with an ineffective breathing pattern are the optimization of ventilation and improved airway flow. Ventilation can be improved by **retraining** the person to breathe differently and control their breathing. One method is **pursed-lip breathing**, in which the expiratory phase of the breath is controlled by blowing out slowly through pursed or partially sealed lips while seated and bending forward. The inspiratory phase is also relatively slow. This technique increases resistance, lowers respiratory rate and minute ventilation, improves the oxygen to carbon dioxide ratio, and clears the lung of trapped air. Another technique, **diaphragmatic breathing**, is often taught to people with a somewhat paralyzed diaphragm, such as those with spinal cord injuries. Here the health care worker aids the patient's breathing by putting their hand on the diaphragm. Other breathing methods include **GPB** and **segmental breathing**.

VENTILATORY SUPPORT DEVICES

Noninvasive rocking beds and pneumobelts were once used for patients with neuromuscular diseases, but have since been replaced by noninvasive positive-pressure ventilation (NPPV) systems such as CPAP and BiPap. Invasive devices are usually mechanical ventilators that apply either negative or positive pressure. A **negative-pressure ventilator (NPV)** utilizes negative pressure at the thorax to generate a pressure gradient in the thoracic cavity and aid airflow to the lungs. It is appropriate for patients with neuromuscular diseases but is rarely used currently. Most modern ventilators are **positive-pressure ventilators (PPVs)**—either a pressure-cycled ventilator that mechanically inflates the lungs to a certain pressure during inspiration and then allows reflexive expiration, or a volume-cycled ventilator that uses a programmed volume during

Functional Health Patterns

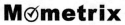

inhalation. An adjunct is **diaphragmatic pacing**, in which radio frequencies are directly delivered as stimulus to the phrenic nerve.

Review Video: <u>Medical Ventilators</u>
Visit mometrix.com/academy and enter code: 679637

EXERCISES USED IN PULMONARY REHABILITATION

Supervised or home-based exercises to strengthen certain muscle groups form the basis of pulmonary rehabilitation. A typical program might be 20–30 minutes of exercise 3–5 days a week at about 60% of the maximum possible workload. Depending on the patient, the exercise training periods could be nonstop or interspersed with rest intervals. One of the main goals of **upper extremity exercises** is to increase the person's endurance upon lifting their arm without support. Usually, light weights are elevated from waist to shoulder level with or without support. Exercises utilizing the **lower extremities** are usually of the aerobic variety and include such exercises as walking or stair climbing, which beneficially decrease parameters such as oxygen consumption and heart and respiratory rates. A newer type of exercise training is **inspiratory muscle training**, in which the patient uses a special resistive device to breathe in and out. The device induces high and normal airway pressures during inspiration and expiration respectively, theoretically strengthening the respiratory muscles. This has proven beneficial in patients with COPD.

OTHER INTERVENTIONS

The patient should be taught **energy conservation methods**. For example, shortness of breath can be reduced by bending over and exhaling through pursed lips while raising the chest and inspiring while lifting arms to the side or above. Breathing can also be facilitated by placing the hands on the hips during inhalation. Various adaptive equipment and behavioral modifications can help conserve energy. If the patient has sleep problems, such as apnea or snoring, techniques such as application of **positive pressure** during sleep through a mask (CPAP) can be used. Individuals with chronic lung diseases tend to experience **anxiety or depression**. These can be alleviated through interventions from rehabilitation team members such as social workers or psychiatrists, peer groups, relaxation techniques, or pharmacologic agents. Other interventions include protocols for **smoking cessation** and use of **drugs** such as bronchodilators before sexual activity if applicable.

RESTRICTIVE AND OBSTRUCTIVE LUNG DISEASES

Restrictive lung diseases are characterized by a diminution of lung expansion exacerbated by certain neuromuscular diseases, spinal cord injury or deformation, bony deformities in the chest wall, or interstitial pulmonary fibrosis. Clinically, patients present with a breathing pattern in which they use their chest wall muscles and diaphragm in tandem to breathe because their muscles are weak. The weak diaphragm is also evidenced by inward displacement of the abdomen when the patients breathe in (called paradoxical breathing), especially while lying down. Obstructive lung diseases are characterized by an increased resistance to airflow due to chronic bronchitis, emphysema, asthma, BPD, or cystic fibrosis. Patients with obstructive lung disease have an increased respiratory rate that is further amplified during an exacerbation or respiratory failure. During exacerbations, the patient's minute ventilation (V_E) declines and their breathing pattern becomes quick and shallow. Pulmonary function tests can be used to distinguish between restrictive and obstructive disease, particularly the FEV_1/FVC ratio, which is high or low respectively.

IMPAIRED GAS EXCHANGE
ASSOCIATED RESPIRATORY DISEASES

Impaired gas exchange is altered oxygen or carbon dioxide exchange in the lungs or intracellularly. Usually, there is low blood oxygen (also known as hypoxemia) due to a disparity between ventilation and perfusion. Impaired gas exchange is common in patients with chronic lung diseases, and it also occurs in individuals with restrictive lung problems secondary to infection or spinal cord issues. **Chronic lung diseases** displaying poor gas exchange are COPD, interstitial lung disease, asthma, and bronchopulmonary dysplasia (BPD) in infants. In COPD, all airways and associated vasculature are inflamed, most commonly due to inhalation of smoke,

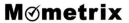

occupational irritants, or genetic predisposition (notably α1-antitrypsin deficiency). This causes abnormalities in ventilation and perfusion and ultimately insufficient oxygen, excessive CO_2, and/or pulmonary hypertension. In **interstitial lung disease**, airway and vascular structures are disrupted through contact with occupational or environmental irritants. Inflammatory and immune cells are recruited, and restrictive and gas exchange impairments occur. **Asthma** results in chest tightness, coughing, and difficulty breathing, caused by allergens or irritants that induce mucous accumulation in the bronchi and bronchioles.

> **Review Video: Respiratory Diseases**
> Visit mometrix.com/academy and enter code: 973392

INTERVENTIONS

The primary intervention for a patient with impaired gas exchange is some type of **oxygen therapy**. Otherwise, many of the modalities discussed for alleviation of ineffective airway clearance may be utilized, and if the person smokes, some sort of program to assist the individual in quitting is indicated. Oxygen therapy lessens cardiopulmonary workload and improves many parameters, such as lung functions, exercise capacity, mental sharpness, and blood characteristics, but it does not address the underlying defect. Quantitative goals of oxygen therapy are an **oxygen pressure (P_aO_2) of 60–65 mmHg** or a **minimum saturation level of 90–92%**. Oxygen therapy may be administered on an inpatient basis or at home, using compressed gas from tanks or cylinders, liquid oxygen units, or oxygen concentrators that use power to pull oxygen from the air and concentrate it. Nasal cannulas and oxygen masks are usually used for introduction of the oxygen and exhalation of other gases. The oxygen can also be introduced directly into the trachea through a tracheostomy.

PEDIATRIC INCLINATION TOWARD RESPIRATORY COMPROMISE

Children have anatomical and physiological differences from adults that can place them at higher risk of respiratory compromise. **Anatomical differences** include relatively small airways, slower development of the distal respiratory passages, immature cartilage and intercostal muscle support until about age 5, a larynx that is further forward than in adults, a proportionately larger tongue, and relatively cartilaginous ribs. **Physiological differences** include immature CNS breathing control (especially in infants), fewer alveoli to facilitate gas exchange, and increased oxygen consumption. Young children also tend to breathe through their noses, which can become obstructed, and the pediatric population in general has a higher rate of **respiratory infection** than adults. All of these factors contribute to high rates of respiratory compromise in children.

BRONCHOPULMONARY DYSPLASIA IN CHILDREN

Bronchopulmonary dysplasia (BPD) is a chronic lung disease characterized by alveolar damage resulting from abnormal development with inflammation and development of scar tissue. Risk factors include:

- Prematurity of >10 weeks prior to due date
- Birthweight <2.5 lb or 1000 g
- Hyaline membrane disease or respiratory distress syndrome (RDS) at birth
- Long-term ventilatory support/oxygen

Most of the infants with BPD have immature lungs with inadequate surfactant to allow the lungs to expand properly, so they cannot breathe without assistance. **Symptoms** include severe respiratory distress and cyanosis. Usually, infants improve within 2-4 weeks with treatment, but some progress from RDS to BPD. Their lungs often have fewer but enlarged alveoli with inadequate blood supply. BPD is usually diagnosed if respiratory symptoms do not improve after 28 days.

Supportive **treatment** provides oxygenation, protects vital organs, and allows the lungs to mature. Treatment includes:

- Surfactant
- Nasal continuous positive airway pressure (NCPAP)

- Mechanical ventilation or high-frequency jet ventilation (HFJV)
- Supplemental oxygen
- Bronchodilators (albuterol) to open airways
- Furosemide (Lasix) to reduce pulmonary edema
- Antibiotics as indicated
- Gastric/enteral feedings or total parenteral nutrition (TPN)

Complications: Most infants are hospitalized for about 4 months but may need treatment for months or years at home. Most will eventually develop nearly normal lung function as new lung tissue grows and takes over the function of the scarred tissue. Some long-term complications may occur:

- Increased risk of bacterial and viral infections, such as RSV and pneumonia
- Chronic or recurrent pulmonary edema
- Pulmonary hypertension
- Side effects related to long-term use of diuretics, such as hearing deficits, renal calculi, and electrolyte imbalances
- Slow growth patterns

MECHANICAL VENTILATION USED AT HOME

There are electrical, battery, and gas-powered **mechanical ventilation systems** that can be used in the home. The home is prepared to provide a safe operational environment; electrical stipulations must be adequate, and schedules with vendors and support staff—such as home health care aids—must be set up. Emergency or adjunct equipment also needs to be available. This includes such things as self-inflating resuscitation bags (in the event the unit fails) and provisions for cuffed tracheostomy tubes. The latter need to be inflated during eating, and for a few hours after, to avoid aspiration. Patients other than those with severe neuromuscular diseases are often weaned from ventilator use. **Pulmonary function parameters** are used to determine the possibility of weaning. If the patient has a respiratory-rate-to-tidal-volume ratio (also known as the rapid shallow breathing index, or **RSBI**) of ≤80 breaths/minute/liter, they can generally be weaned. During the **removal process**, breathing can be supported by pressure support, use of a T-piece that delivers humidity and oxygen, CPAP (which provides positive pressure to keep alveoli open), or synchronized intermittent mandatory ventilation (SIMV). The weaning should occur during rest periods, and the patient must be monitored.

CLASSES OF DRUGS USED TO ENHANCE PULMONARY FUNCTION

Drugs used to enhance pulmonary function are bronchodilators, anticholinergics, anti-inflammatory drugs, mediator-release inhibitors, and smoking cessation drugs, as well as combination drugs.

- **Bronchodilators**, which relax the main airway passages and are used to treat either bronchospasm or chronic obstructive pulmonary disease (COPD), generally fall into the category of β-adrenergic drugs. Some, such as albuterol, are dispensed primarily by means of inhalers. Others, such as epinephrine or terbutaline, are given subcutaneously or intramuscularly.
- **Anticholinergics** used in the respiratory setting include ipratropium and tiotropium.
- **Anti-inflammatory drugs** used to enhance pulmonary function are all corticosteroids and are used primarily for asthma maintenance or to treat allergic rhinitis. These drugs include beclomethasone and triamcinolone.
- The main **mediator-release inhibitor** is cromolyn sodium, which prevents release of histamine from mast cells and is used for asthma maintenance. Montelukast (Singulair) is a leukotriene modifier.
- **Smoking cessation drugs**, mainly nicotine substitutes, also enhance pulmonary function.

Cardiovascular Functional Ability

ASSESSMENT OF THE CARDIOVASCULAR SYSTEM

Cardiovascular assessment includes questioning the patient for any family history of death at a young age or other cardiovascular diseases. Elderly African American males are at the highest risk for cardiovascular problems. One must question the patient about edema, chest pain, dyspnea, fatigue, vertigo, syncope or other changes in consciousness, weight gain, and leg cramps or pain. If chest pain is a symptom, one must ask about the intensity, timing, location, and quality of the pain; whether there is any radiation of the pain; any factors that aggravate or alleviate the pain; and nausea, dyspnea, diaphoresis, or any other accompanying symptoms. Physical assessment includes assessment of vital signs, heart and lung sounds, skin assessment, pulse checks (radial, popliteal, and pedal pulses), circulation and sensation of extremities, and auscultation of the cardiac, renal, iliac, and femoral arteries for bruits. Blood should be taken for a lipid profile and electrolytes. The patient must be helped to modify risk factors such as hypertension, smoking, diabetes, obesity, hyperlipidemia, inactivity, and stress.

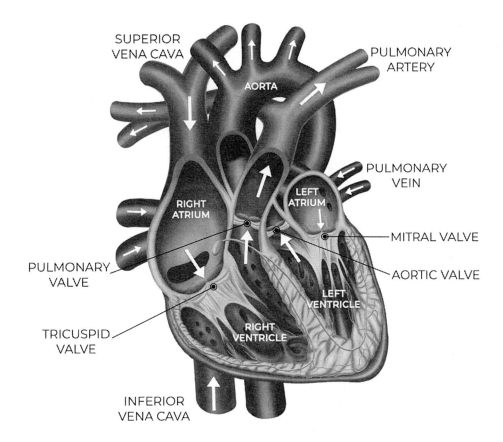

Functional Health Patterns

Review Video: **Cardiovascular Assessment**
Visit mometrix.com/academy and enter code: 323076

Review Video: **Cardiovascular System**
Visit mometrix.com/academy and enter code: 376581

Review Video: **Heart Blood Flow**
Visit mometrix.com/academy and enter code: 783139

CORONARY ARTERY PERFUSION

Blood is supplied to the heart muscle through two **coronary arteries** arising from the right and left sides of the aorta. The **perfusion**, or amount of circulation of this blood, is primarily related to the heart rate, the cardiac cycle, and the diastolic intraventricular pressure. **Diastole** is the rhythmic expansion and filling with blood of heart chambers, whereas systole is the contraction of the heart and pumping out of blood. If perfusion is altered, patients experience **acute coronary syndrome (ACS)** due to an inadequate blood supply, most often signaled by chest pain. ACS includes stable or unstable angina or infarctions with or without Q-wave involvement. The biggest factor is usually an increased heart rate with subsequent shortened filling time and depressed perfusion. **Elevated circulating blood volumes**, as seen with congestive heart disease, can reduce blood flow to more distant subendocardial areas of the heart due to high diastolic interventricular pressure, also resulting in ACS. Abnormalities seen with **myocardial ischemia** include chest pain, dyspnea, cough, stenotic lesions, infarctions, and elevated heart rate.

SINUS BRADYCARDIA

There are 3 primary types of **sinus node dysrhythmias**: sinus bradycardia, sinus tachycardia, and sinus arrhythmia. **Sinus bradycardia (SB)** is caused by a decreased rate of impulse from sinus node. The pulse and ECG usually appear normal except for a slower rate.

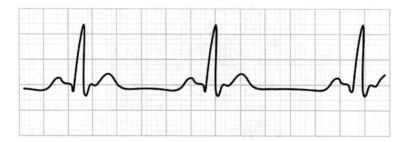

SB is characterized by a regular pulse <50-60 bpm with P waves in front of QRS, which are usually normal in shape and duration. PR interval is 0.12-0.20 seconds, QRS interval is 0.04-0.11 seconds, and P:QRS ratio of 1:1. SB may be caused by several factors:

- May be normal in athletes and older adults; generally not treated unless symptomatic
- Conditions that lower the body's metabolic needs, such as hypothermia or sleep
- Hypotension and decrease in oxygenation
- Medications such as calcium channel blockers and β-blockers
- Vagal stimulation that may result from vomiting, suctioning, defecating, or certain medical procedures (carotid stent placement, etc.)
- Increased intracranial pressure
- Myocardial infarction

Treatment: involves eliminating cause if possible, such as changing medications. Atropine 0.5-1.0 mg may be given IV to block vagal stimulation or increase rate if symptomatic.

SINUS TACHYCARDIA

Sinus tachycardia (ST) occurs when the sinus node impulse increases in frequency. ST is characterized by a regular pulse >100 with P waves before QRS but sometimes part of the preceding T wave. QRS is usually of normal shape and duration (0.04-0.11 seconds) but may have consistent irregularity. PR interval is 0.12-0.20 seconds and P:QRS ratio of 1:1.

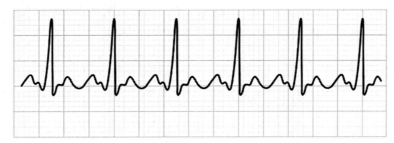

The rapid pulse decreases diastolic filling time and causes reduced cardiac output with resultant hypotension. Acute pulmonary edema may result from the decreased ventricular filling if untreated. ST may be **caused** by a number of factors:

- Acute blood loss, shock, hypovolemia, anemia
- Sinus arrhythmia, hypovolemic heart failure
- Hypermetabolic conditions, fever, infection
- Exertion/exercise, anxiety, stress
- Medications, such as sympathomimetic drugs

Treatment: eliminating precipitating factors, calcium channel blockers and β-blockers to reduce heart rate.

HYPOTENSION

Hypotension is defined as a systolic pressure of 90 mmHg (millimeters of mercury) or lower and a diastolic pressure of 60 mmHg or lower. Hypotension can be caused by reduced blood volume (hypovolemia), decreased cardiac output in the presence of normal blood volume, or excessive vasodilation. There are a number of **hypotensive syndromes**, including orthostatic hypotension, neurocardiogenic syncope, and postprandial hypotension.

- **Orthostatic hypotension** occurs following a change the position of the body, usually from sitting to standing. Treatment includes educating the patient to rise slowly and sit back down immediately if feeling lightheaded, identifying and correcting hypovolemia if present, wearing compression stockings, and using medications such as volume expanders (fludrocortisone) or short-acting vasoconstrictors (atomoxetine).
- **Neurocardiogenic syncope** occurs as a result of an increase in the activity of the vagus nerve. It usually doesn't require intervention, only identification and avoidance of triggers.
- **Postprandial hypotension** occurs 30–75 minutes after a heavy meal. Symptom management includes eating smaller/more frequent meals, staying seated for 30–60 minutes post eating, having caffeine, and exercising between meals.

Orthostatic hypotension and postprandial hypotension occur most commonly in those older than age 65.

CLASSIFYING A PATIENT AS STABLE ENOUGH FOR CARDIAC REHABILITATION OR SUITABLE FOR ACTIVITY PROGRESSION

In order to be deemed stable enough to start cardiac rehabilitation, a patient must meet certain **criteria**. In the previous 8 hours, the patient should not have had any new or recurring chest pain or significant changes in heart rhythm or electrocardiogram (ECG). The patient should not display any fresh signs of **uncompensated failure**, generally defined as chest pain while resting with bibasilar rales. Laboratory testing of **creatine kinase (CK) or troponin** should show no rise in levels. Once the patient has begun an activity and exercise program, there are also guidelines for progression to higher levels related to heart activity parameters. The **heart rate** should be sufficient, there should be no evidence of **novel rhythm or ST changes**, and new symptoms of **cardiac problems** such as palpitations, shortness of breath, or chest pains should not be present. In addition, the patient's **systolic blood pressure** should elevate 10–40 mmHg above resting levels during activity. Precautions against DVT or pulmonary emboli must be in place during exercise.

METs REQUIRED FOR CARDIAC PATIENTS

METs refer to **metabolic equivalents**. One MET is equal to 3.5 mL O_2/kg/min , which is the concentration of oxygen in terms of body weight a person needs while standing at rest. Different activities or exercises typically expend more METs. For example, there are **2-MET activities** where twice the oxygen and energy are expended. A healthy person can perform activities requiring more METs than a person initially undergoing cardiac rehabilitation, who might typically be able to achieve only 5 METs. One of the goals of cardiac rehabilitation is to eventually **increase the number of METs** at which the patient can exercise, suggesting improvement in cardiac parameters. Elderly patients or those with other chronic or restrictive conditions usually work in lower MET ranges.

RISK STRATIFICATION FOR CARDIAC EVENTS DURING EXERCISE PARTICIPATION

A **cardiac risk assessment** includes documentation of age, gender (including female menopausal status), tobacco use, physical activity level, history of hypertension, nutritional status, psychosocial background (including depression), hostility level, and family history. Some specific **tests** are also conducted, including a lipid profile, body mass index and other anthropometric measurements, and factors indicative of diabetes such as fasting blood glucose. According to the American Association of Cardiovascular and Pulmonary Rehabilitation (AACVPR), **risk stratification** should also involve measurement of things such as functional capacity, rest ejection fraction, presence of congestive heart failure (CHF), and evidence of arrhythmias, angina, dyspnea, or dizziness upon exertion. Patients are then classified as low, intermediate, or high risk. **Low risk** means that all of the risk factors such as angina or CHF are absent, functional capacity is ≥7 METs, rest ejection fraction is ≥50%, and the myocardial infarction or revascularization procedure was uncomplicated. **Intermediate-risk patients** exhibit symptoms, some silent ischemia, a functional capacity of less than 5 METs, and a rest ejection fraction of 40–49%. **High-risk patients** have further abnormalities.

INPATIENT CARDIAC REHABILITATION

The AACVPR divides **cardiac rehabilitation** into three stages: (1) **inpatient**, begun during hospitalization, (2) **early outpatient**, a supervised program for up to 2 months after release, and (3) **lifetime maintenance**. Their guidelines for inpatient cardiac rehabilitation include early evaluation and mobilization, identification of cardiac and self-care risk factors, education of patient and family, and an all-inclusive discharge session including plans for transition. Inpatient rehabilitation is only about 3–4 days, beginning shortly after myocardial infarction or cardiovascular surgery. Before starting, a patient must be deemed stable. A cardiac rehabilitation team member must determine baseline heart rate, blood pressure, cardiac rhythm, heart and lung sounds, musculoskeletal strength and range of motion (ROM), and self-care potential. Depending on the severity of the cardiac problem, a supervised, progressive exercise program is begun, usually consisting of low- to moderate-intensity strength training, ROM exercises, walking, and possibly other aerobics.

> **Review Video: Myocardial Infarction**
> Visit mometrix.com/academy and enter code: 148923

IDEAL CANDIDATES FOR CARDIAC REHABILITATION

There are many types of cardiac disease. Not all cardiac patients are **ideal candidates for rehabilitation**, but the candidate pool has enlarged in recent decades due to changing views on treatment. According to the Agency for Healthcare Research and Quality, the best candidates are those who have survived a myocardial infarction (MI), people with stable angina, patients who have had coronary artery bypass graft surgery (CABG) or percutaneous transluminal coronary angioplasty (PTCA), patients who have had heart valve replacement/repair, and patients with chronic/congestive heart failure. Participation is also affected by presence of risk factors and comorbidities.

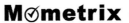

OUTPATIENT CARDIAC REHABILITATION PROGRAM
PATIENT ADMITTANCE

Before a patient is admitted to an outpatient cardiac rehabilitation program, the healthcare team must take a medical history and administer a physical examination, resting ECG, and exercise test. The exercise test usually consists of a treadmill exercise protocol to determine risk stratification and a suitable exercise program. If the patient can walk at 70% of their age-predicted rate, the patient is considered a candidate. Exercise nuclear imaging, echocardiography, pharmacological stress testing, arm crank ergometry, stationary cycling, and the 6-minute walk test are other possible forms of exercise testing. The patient is also stratified for risk of cardiac events and undergoes a psychosocial evaluation to identify depression, lack of self-esteem, or other factors that might affect their participation.

> **Review Video: How Does the Six Minute Walk Test Work?**
> Visit mometrix.com/academy and enter code: 444929

EXERCISE PROGRAM

Outpatient cardiac rehabilitation exercise programs are individualized prescriptions (usually determined by an exercise physiologist) for a specific patient. Walking is the most common prescription, but arm ergometry, aquatic exercises, rowing, jogging, cycling, or low-intensity weight training may be incorporated. A typical **session** consists of a warm-up (5–15 minutes) including stretching and ROM exercises, an individualized conditioning portion (20–30 minutes), and a cool-down period (5–10 minutes). Usually there are 3–5 sessions per week. An individual is closely monitored by ECG during the program, which is terminated if certain parameters fall into undesirable ranges, such as diastolic blood pressure ≥110 mmHg, systolic blood pressure rising more than 10 mmHg, significant dysrhythmias, heart block, or symptoms of chest pain or shortness of breath.

MAINTENANCE PHASE OF CARDIAC REHABILITATION

Cardiac rehabilitation maintenance starts 2–3 months after a cardiac incident and should continue throughout the person's life. It can be done at a hospital or clinic, in a community-based exercise facility, or (in some cases) at home. Generally, a big part of the maintenance phase is evaluation for and facilitation of a return to work. A treadmill test is done to determine the number of METs at which a patient can operate. During this stage, there may be other relevant nursing diagnoses, such as ineffective coping, grieving, unsuccessful role performance, social isolation, or noncompliance. Interventions include continued rehabilitative cardiac care and patient support, such as emotional support, support groups, counseling, anxiety reduction, role promotion, and family integration.

NURSING DIAGNOSES AND THERAPEUTIC OBJECTIVES

According to NANDA-I, nursing diagnoses common to both inpatient and early outpatient cardiac rehabilitation are risk for activity intolerance, anxiety, and deficient knowledge. Further categories applicable to early outpatient settings include risk-prone health behavior, ineffective health maintenance, and sexual dysfunction. The nurse is responsible for helping manage the patient's symptoms, improve their functional abilities, develop the patient's exercise tolerance, and temper the patient's cardiac risk factors through lifestyle modifications. The latter includes implementation of an exercise program, weight management, diet changes to lower cholesterol, cessation of smoking and alcohol use, stress and coping strategies, and control of blood pressure and diabetes if present. Therapeutic objectives include cardiac care, rehabilitation cardiac care, anticipatory guidance, anxiety reduction, and education of both patient and family about the exercise program, the disease process, risks, lifestyle modifications, and other factors.

EVALUATION OF CARDIAC REHABILITATION SERVICES

Cardiac rehabilitation services should be evaluated in terms of both the process and the outcome. Program **standards** and desired **competencies** for professionals are available to compare for process evaluation. There are also **nursing outcomes** expected for assessment of the end product. Some nursing outcomes apply to all

103

Functional Health Patterns

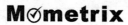

phases of cardiac rehabilitation, such as cardiac disease management and control of risk to cardiovascular health. Many apply primarily to the inpatient phase, such as circulation status, fluid balance, response to medication, and cardiac tissue perfusion, while others are relevant later, including the control of depression and adherence to health-seeking behaviors. Some change focus slightly. For example, a patient should rest during the inpatient phase but concentrate on energy conservation later. Various studies have shown that cardiac rehabilitation can improve functional capacity and decrease mortality rates.

QUALIFICATIONS FOR CARDIAC REHABILITATION CARE PROFESSIONALS

Cardiac rehabilitation programs are generally comprehensive and long-lasting, incorporating various facets, including medical evaluation, exercise regimens, risk factor adjustments, education, and counseling. There is usually a **health care team** comprising a supervisory doctor, a registered nurse, a program coordinator (who may be either a nurse or another type of allied health professional), and various consultants (dietitian, cardiologist, physical therapist, etc.). In their *Guidelines for Cardiac Rehabilitation and Secondary Prevention Programs*, the AACVPR set **minimum qualifications** for each of these team members: a bachelor's degree or licensure in an appropriate field (such as exercise science), training and experience in cardiovascular rehabilitation, knowledge of areas such as exercise physiology and nutrition, and completion of a course in basic life support. The AACVPR also prefers completion of an advanced cardiac life support course and professional certification.

CARDIOVASCULAR PHARMACOLOGY

CLASSES OF DRUGS TO TREAT CARDIOVASCULAR DISEASE

The following classes of drugs are used to treat cardiovascular diseases, in particular congestive heart failure.

- **ACE inhibitors:** Captopril (Capoten), enalapril (Vasotec), and lisinopril (Prinivil). Decrease afterload/preload and reverse ventricular remodeling; they also prevent neuropathy in DM. Contraindicated with renal insufficiency, renal artery stenosis, and pregnancy.
  - Side effects include cough (#1), hyperkalemia, hypotension, angioedema, dizziness, and weakness.
- **Angiotensin receptor blockers (ARBs):** Losartan (Cozaar) and valsartan (Diovan). Decrease afterload/preload and reverse ventricular remodeling, causing vasodilation and reducing blood pressure. They are used for those who cannot tolerate ACE inhibitors.
  - Side effects include cough (less common than with ACE inhibitors), hyperkalemia, hypotension, headache, dizziness, metallic taste, and rash.
- **β-Blockers:** Metoprolol (Lopressor), carvedilol (Coreg) and esmolol (Brevibloc). Slow the heart rate, reduce hypertension, prevent dysrhythmias, and reverse ventricular remodeling. Contraindicated in bradyarrythmias, decompensated HF, uncontrolled hypoglycemia/diabetes mellitus, and airway disease.
  - Side effects: bradycardia, hypotension, bronchospasm, may mask signs of hypoglycemia.

CALCIUM CHANNEL BLOCKERS

Calcium channel blockers are primarily arterial vasodilators that may affect the peripheral and/or coronary arteries.

- Side effects: Lethargy, flushing, edema, ascites, and indigestion.
- Nifedipine (Procardia) and nicardipine (Cardene) are primarily arterial vasodilators, used to treat acute hypertension. Diltiazem (Cardizem) and Verapamil (Calan, Isoptin) dilate primarily coronary arteries and slow the heart rate, thus are used for angina, atrial fibrillation, and SVT. *Note:* Nifedipine (Procardia) should be avoided in older adults due to increased risk of hypotension and myocardial ischemia.

Review Video: Ca Channel Blockers
Visit mometrix.com/academy and enter code: 942825

DIURETICS

Diuretics increase **renal perfusion and filtration**, thereby reducing preload and decreasing peripheral and pulmonary edema, hypertension, CHF, diabetes insipidus, and osteoporosis. There are different types of diuretics: loop, thiazide, and potassium sparing.

LOOP DIURETICS

Loop diuretics inhibit the reabsorption of sodium and chloride (primarily) in the ascending loop of Henle. They also cause increased secretion of other electrolytes, such as calcium, magnesium, and potassium, and this can result in imbalances that cause dysrhythmias. Other side effects include frequent urination, postural hypotension, and increased blood sugar and uric acid levels. They are short-acting so are less effective than other diuretics for control of hypertension.

- **Bumetanide** (Bumex) is given intravenously after surgery to reduce preload or orally to treat heart failure.
- **Ethacrynic acid** (Edecrin) is given intravenously after surgery to reduce preload.
- **Furosemide** (Lasix) is used for the control of congestive heart failure as well as renal insufficiency. It is used after surgery to decrease preload and to reduce the inflammatory response caused by cardiopulmonary bypass (post-perfusion syndrome).

> **Review Video: Diuretics**
> Visit mometrix.com/academy and enter code: 373276

THIAZIDE DIURETICS

Thiazide diuretics inhibit the **reabsorption of sodium and chloride**, primarily in the early distal tubules, forcing more sodium and water to be excreted. Thiazide diuretics increase secretion of potassium and bicarbonate, so they are often given with supplementary potassium or in combination with potassium-sparing diuretics. Thiazide diuretics are the first line of drugs for treatment of **hypertension**. They have a long duration of action (12-72 hours, depending on the drug) so they are able to maintain control of hypertension better than short-acting drugs. They may be given daily or 3–5 days per week. There are numerous thiazide diuretics, including:

- Chlorothiazide (Diuril)
- Bendroflumethiazide (Naturetin)
- Chlorthalidone (Hygroton)
- Trichlormethiazide (Naqua)

Side effects include, dizziness, lightheadedness, postural hypotension, headache, blurred vision, and itching, especially during initial treatment. Thiazide diuretics cause sensitivity to sun exposure, so people should be counseled to use sunscreen.

POTASSIUM-SPARING DIURETICS

Potassium-sparing diuretics inhibit the **reabsorption of sodium** in the late distal tubule and collecting duct. They are weaker than thiazide or loop diuretics, but do not cause a reduction in potassium level; however, if used alone, they may cause an increase in potassium, which can cause weakness, irregular pulse, and cardiac arrest. Because potassium-sparing diuretics are less effective alone, they are often given in a combined form with a thiazide diuretic (usually chlorothiazide), which mitigates the potassium imbalance. Typical side effects include dehydration, blurred vision, nausea, insomnia, and nasal congestion, especially in the first few days of treatment.

- **Spironolactone** (Aldactone) is a synthetic steroidal diuretic that increases the secretion of both water and sodium and is used to treat congestive heart failure. It may be given orally or intravenously.
- **Eplerenone** is an antimineralocorticoid similar to spironolactone but with fewer side effects.

ANTI-HYPERTENSIVE MEDICATIONS

The classes of anti-hypertensive medications are as follows: Diuretics, sympatholytics, vasodilators, calcium channel blockers, and angiotensin-converting enzyme inhibitors (ACE inhibitors).

- Diuretics include hydrochlorothiazide, chlorthalidone, chlorothiazide, indapamide, metolazone, amiloride, spironolactone, triamterene, furosemide, bumetanide, ethacrynic acid, and torsemide.
- Sympatholytics are clonidine, methyldopa, guanabenz, guanadrel, guanethidine, reserpine, labetalol, prazosin, and terazosin.
- Vasodilators include diazoxide, hydralazine, minoxidil, and nitroprusside sodium.
- Calcium channel blockers include amlodipine, nimodipine, isradipine, nicardipine, nifedipine, bepridil, diltiazem, and verapamil.
- ACE inhibitors include benazepril, captopril, enalapril, fosinopril, lisinopril, moexipril, quinapril, ramipril, and losartan.

> **Review Video: What are the Side Effects of ACE Inhibitors and ARBs?**
> Visit mometrix.com/academy and enter code: 525864

DRUGS THAT INDIRECTLY INFLUENCE CARDIOVASCULAR FUNCTION

Drugs can indirectly influence cardiovascular function either by acting to suppress platelets or coagulation or by lowering cholesterol. Medications with **antiplatelet activity** include aspirin and clopidogrel (Plavix). Platelets are involved in the clotting process, which can interfere at times with blood flow. The most prominent **anticoagulant** is warfarin or Coumadin, which is also used to manage atrial fibrillation. **Cholesterol-lowering agents** are either HMG-CoA reductase inhibitors such as atorvastatin (Lipitor) or simvastatin (Zocor), or fibric acid derivatives (which break down fibrin) such as colestipol (Colestid) or niacin. High levels of cholesterol can predispose an individual to atherosclerosis, or plaques on arterial surfaces that can obstruct blood flow.

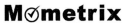

Neurological Function

NERVOUS SYSTEM

The human nervous system is divided into the central nervous system (CNS) and the peripheral nervous system (PNS).

- The **CNS** is composed of the brain and spinal cord and is located in the dorsal cavity. The brain is protected by the skull, while the spinal cord is protected by the vertebrae.
- The **PNS** is made of those structures of the nervous system not contained in the dorsal cavity, such as long nerves (neuron axons). The PNS is divided into the somatic nervous system and the autonomic nervous system. The autonomic nervous system is further divided into the sympathetic nervous system and the parasympathetic nervous system.

> **Review Video: Nervous System**
> Visit mometrix.com/academy and enter code: 708428

SOMATIC NERVOUS SYSTEM

The somatic division of the PNS is involved in the coordination of body movements. It is composed of peripheral nerve fibers that receive sensory information and carry this information into the spinal cord. It also contains motor nerve fibers that connect to skeletal muscle. The somatic system employs an afferent nerve network to carry sensory information to the brain and an efferent nerve network with motor nerves that transmit information from the brain to the skeletal muscles. The somatic nervous system regulates activities that are under the individual's conscious control, processes sensory information, and executes voluntary movements. The somatic nervous system does not control reflex arcs.

AUTONOMIC NERVOUS SYSTEM

The **sympathetic division** of the PNS is involved in the "fight-or-flight" response and is activated in times of danger or stress. Signs and symptoms of sympathetic stimulation are an increased heart rate (tachycardia), vasoconstriction and rise in blood pressure, dilation of the pupils (mydriasis), goose bumps on the skin (piloerection or cutis anserina), increased sweat secretion (diaphoresis), and feelings of excitement. These reactions are due to the release of adrenaline (epinephrine).

The **parasympathetic nervous system** is in charge when the individual feels relaxed or is resting. The parasympathetic system is responsible for constriction of the pupil, slowing of the heart rate, dilation of blood vessels, and stimulation of the digestive tract and genitourinary system. The neurotransmitter at work is acetylcholine.

DORSAL CAVITY

The dorsal cavity contains the brain and spinal cord, which are the organs of the central nervous system (CNS). Like the ventral cavity, the dorsal cavity is divided into two smaller cavities: the cranial cavity and the spinal cavity. The cranial cavity contains the brain, eyes, and ears, while the spinal cavity holds the spinal cord. The brain and spinal cord are covered by three layers of connective tissue called the meninges. The outermost layer is the dura mater; the middle layer is the arachnoid mater; and the innermost layer is the pia mater. The space between the arachnoid mater and the pia mater is filled with cerebrospinal fluid (CSF), which flows throughout the CNS. If an injured patient has clear yellow fluid leaking from the ears, nose, eyes, or mouth, it is probably CSF and indicates a skull fracture.

NEURONS

Neurons are nerve cells that transmit nerve impulses throughout the CNS and PNS. The basic structure of a neuron is a cell body with multiple dendrites and a single axon. The **cell body**, also called the soma, contains the nucleus. The nucleus contains the chromosomes. The **dendrites** of the neuron extend from the cell body and resemble the branches of a tree. The dendrite receives chemical messages from other cells across the

Functional Health Patterns

synapse, a small gap. The **axon** is a thread-like extension of the cell body that varies in length, up to 3 feet in the case of spinal nerves. The axon transmits an electrochemical message along its length to another cell. PNS neurons that deal with muscles are myelinated with fatty Schwann cell insulation to speed up the transmission of messages. Gaps between the Schwann cells that expose the axon, called **nodes of Ranvier**, increase the speed of the transmission of nerve impulses along the axon. Neurons in the PNS that deal with pain are unmyelinated because transmission does not have to be as fast. Some neurons in the CNS are myelinated by oligodendrocytes. If the myelin in the CNS oligodendrocytes breaks down, the patient develops multiple sclerosis (MS).

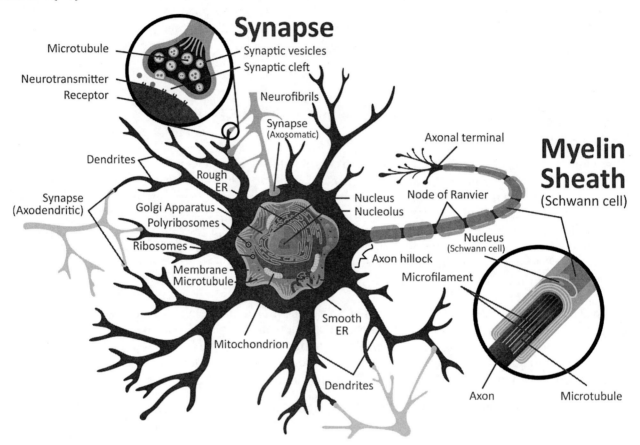

The three **categories of neurons** are as follows:

- **Afferent neurons** carry sensory impulses from the environment to the brain and spinal cord. They are also called sensory neurons or receptor neurons. Afferent neurons are found in the skin, muscles, joints, and sensory organs. They permit the perception of pressure, pain, temperature, taste, odor, sound, and visual stimuli.
- **Efferent neurons** transmit motor impulses from the brain and spinal cord to effectors, such as muscles and glands. Efferent neurons are involved in motor control and stimulate movement throughout the body.
- **Interneurons** connect sensory and motor neurons. Also called connection neurons or relay neurons, interneurons are located in the CNS; sensory and motor neurons are found in both the CNS and PNS.

NEUROTRANSMITTERS AND NEUROMODULATORS

Acetylcholine is a neurotransmitter that transmits nerve impulses at various sites in the brain, brain stem, and autonomic nervous system to muscles. Its mode of action is primarily excitatory. **Serotonin** is another neurotransmitter released from the brain stem, hypothalamus, or dorsal horn of the spinal cord. It acts in an inhibitory manner to suppress spinal cord pain and emotional responses. There are two neurotransmitters of the catecholamine variety: dopamine and norepinephrine. **Dopamine** is released mainly at the base of the brain and usually acts by inhibiting movements and responses, while **norepinephrine** is present at many junctions and is primarily stimulatory. Various **amino acids** such as aspartate, glutamate, and glycine; certain **peptides** such as endorphins and enkephalins; and various other analgesics or hormones appear to have neuromodulatory properties as well. **Nitric acid** released from neurons can also be stimulatory.

DERMATOMES

Dermatomes are cutaneous areas that are innervated by specific spinal nerves. There are 31 pairs of spinal nerves, most of which control or receive sensations from dermatomes. **C2 through C8** of the cervical spinal nerves are related to dermatomes on the front and back of the top parts of the torso, the arms, and the digits. The 12 **thoracic spinal nerves** control muscles and receive sensations in the torso or arms. **Lumbar nerves L1 to L5** innervate regions in the lower torso, legs, and feet. The five **sacral nerves** function in similar areas, in particular the genital and anal regions. There is also one **coccygeal spinal nerve**. Impairment of spinal nerves results in reduced sensations in the corresponding dermatome.

REFLEX ARCS

A reflex arc is a nerve pathway that triggers a reflex action in response to sensory information. If a muscle is stimulated, a reflex arc is triggered in either the brain or spinal cord. The affected muscle releases a signal to the surrounding **sensory neuron**, which in turn transmits a signal to the appropriate area of the spinal cord or brain, where an **interneuron** carries the information. A reflex action is then stimulated by a **motor neuron axon** carrying the information to other muscle fibers. Some sensory information is fed into and emerges from the CNS to affect the same side of the body, as in the **three-neuron ipsilateral reflex arc**, while other times the entry and exit points are on opposite sides, as in a **three-neuron contralateral reflex arc**. Sensory neurons can also diverge and transmit information to several parts of the CNS, resulting in more than one motor neuron response or an **intersegmental reflex arc**.

CONTROL OF LENGTH AND STRENGTH OF MUSCLE CONTRACTION

The **Golgi tendon** receptors and muscle spindles are **stretch receptors**. A muscle is made up primarily of a bundle of **muscle fibers**. At the end, a muscle is connected to a tendon as well as the Golgi tendon organs, which are basically composed of sensory dendrites and collagen. When muscles are contracted, the Golgi tendon receptors are activated and send signals to **inhibitory interneurons** in the CNS that trigger relaxation of the muscle. Conversely, muscle spindles contain specialized muscle fibers called **intrafusal fibers**, which send messages to the CNS when a muscle is stretched, which in turn elicits shortening or contracting muscle reflexes.

ASSESSMENT OF THE NEUROLOGICAL SYSTEM

Assessment of the neurological system includes:

- Assess the **health history** for any trauma, falls, alcoholism, drug abuse, medications taken, and family history of neurological problems.
- Ask about any presenting **neurological symptoms**, the circumstances in which they occur, whether they fluctuate, and any associated factors, such as seizures, pain, vertigo, weakness, abnormal sensations, visual problems, loss of consciousness, changes in cognition, and motor problems.

Assessment includes determining the level of consciousness and cognition. Posture and movements are assessed for abnormalities. Facial expression and movement are noted. Cranial nerve assessment is done. The patient is assessed for strength, coordination, and balance and the ability to perform ADLs. One should assess for clonus and test all reflexes, including Babinski, gag, blink, swallow, upper and lower abdominal, cremasteric in males, plantar, perianal, biceps, triceps, brachioradialis, patellar and ankle. Peripheral sensation is tested by touching the patient with cotton balls and the sharp and dull ends of a broken tongue blade.

CRANIAL NERVE ASSESSMENT

	Name	Function	PE Test
I	Olfactory	Smell	Test olfaction
II	Optic	Visual acuity	Snellen eye chart; Accommodation
III	Oculomotor	Eye movement/ pupil	Pupillary reflex; Eye/eyelid motion
IV	Trochlear	Eye movement	Eye moves down & out
V	Trigeminal	Facial motor/ sensory	Corneal reflex; Facial sensation; Mastication
VI	Abducens	Eye movement	Lateral eye motion
VII	Facial	Facial expression; Taste	Moves forehead, closes eyes, smile/frown, puffs cheeks; Taste
VIII	Vestibulo-cochlear (Acoustic)	Hearing; Balance	Hearing (Weber/Rinne tests); Nystagmus
IX	Glosso-pharyngeal	Pharynx motor/sensory	Gag reflex; Soft palate elevation
X	Vagus	Visceral sensory, motor	Gag, swallow, cough
XI	Accessory	Sternocleidomastoid and trapezius (motor)	Turns head & shrugs shoulders against resistance
XII	Hypoglossal	Tongue movement	Push out tongue; move tongue from side to side

NEUROLOGICAL ASSESSMENT TOOLS

GLASGOW COMA SCALE

The Glasgow coma scale (GCS) measures the depth and duration of coma or impaired level of consciousness and is used for post-operative assessment. The GCS measures three parameters: best eye response, best verbal response, and best motor response, with a total possible score that ranges from 3-15:

Eye opening	4: Spontaneous 3: To verbal stimuli 2: To pain (not of face) 1: No response
Verbal	5: Oriented 4: Conversation confused, but can answer questions 3: Uses inappropriate words 2: Speech incomprehensible 1: No response
Motor	6: Moves on command 5: Moves purposefully respond pain 4: Withdraws in response to pain 3: Decorticate posturing (flexion) in response to pain 2: Decerebrate posturing (extension) in response to pain 1: No response

Injuries/conditions are classified according to the total score: 3-8 Coma; ≤8 Severe head injury likely requiring intubation; 9-12 Moderate head injury; 13-15 Mild head injury.

Review Video: <u>Glasgow Coma Scale</u>
Visit mometrix.com/academy and enter code: 133399

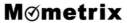

RANCHO LOS AMIGOS LEVELS OF COGNITIVE FUNCTION SCALE

The Rancho Los Amigos Levels of Cognitive Function Scale assesses functional responses after brain injury. The full scale has 10 levels, but usually only the first 8 are used since levels IX and X relate to advanced cognitive skills. The levels are as follows:

Level	Response	Assistance Required for ADLs
Level I	No response: No acknowledgement of pain, touch, sound, or sight	Total assistance
Level II	Generalized reflex response: Unpredictable nonspecific responses	Total assistance
Level III	Localized response: Can blink or move in response to sounds or pain but unpredictable actions upon command	Total assistance
Level IV	Confused-agitated: Alert but agitated with undirected activities and low attention span	Maximal assistance
Level V	Confused-nonagitated: Aware of immediate environment but easily distracted and unable to focus on new tasks	Maximal assistance
Level VI	Confused-appropriate: Awareness of time and place distorted, with some prior (but not good) recall of a recent memory, can follow easy directions	Maximal assistance
Level VII	Automatic-appropriate: Able to cope well in familiar but not strange surroundings in a mechanical fashion, cannot problem-solve	Moderate assistance
Level VIII	Purposeful-appropriate: More self-aware and able to learn new tasks and deal with unfamiliar situations	Minimal assistance
Level IX	Purposeful-appropriate	Standby assistance (if requested)
Level X	Purposeful-appropriate	Modified independent

ABS

The **Agitated Behavior Scale** (ABS) is a tool for behavioral management. It rates 14 different possible **behavioral excesses** that can impair day-to-day functioning and impede treatment. Each behavior is given a numerical value of **1** (absent), **2** (present to a slight degree), **3** (present to a moderate degree), or **4** (found in an extreme fashion). The types of behaviors rated are attention span, patience, cooperativeness, presence of violent actions, volatile anger, self-stimulatory activities, grasping of needed equipment, straying outside the treatment area, too much movement, repetitive actions, talking excessively or loudly, abrupt mood changes, spontaneous crying or laughter, and verbal or physical abuse of self. All scores are added for a total score, or they may be grouped into behavior that is aggressive, labile, or indicates a lack of inhibition. The ABS can be used to look at changes that may be dependent on time of day or that change over the course of recovery.

TOOLS TO ASSESS BRAIN INJURIES

The **Galveston Orientation and Amnesia Test (GOAT)** is often utilized to assess the patient's cognitive and orientation abilities to see whether they have emerged from the post-traumatic amnesia (PTA) period. GOAT is a fast observation that looks at 10 components and assigns a total score ranging from 1 to 100 with a cutoff of 75. The test is administered on consecutive days, indicating PTA clearing.

Functional Health Patterns

Other similar scales include the **Disability Rating Scale (DRS)**, the **Neurobehavioral Rating Scale (NRS)**, and the **Overt Aggression Scale–Modified for Neurorehabilitation (OAS-MNR)**. Katz and Alexander have described 6 stages of recovery from diffuse axonal injury as well; according to their classification, these stages progress through coma, a vegetative state, a condition of minimal consciousness, a confusional state during PTA, increasing independence after PTA resolves, and finally restoration of social abilities and re-entry into the community.

DEFICITS ASSOCIATED WITH UPPER AND LOWER MOTOR NEURON SYNDROMES

Upper motor neuron syndrome (UMN) is CNS damage resulting in the disruption of any motor systems controlled at the point of disturbance. Functional deficits can include loss of muscle tone (hypotonic muscle) and strength, partial inability to move, weakness, fatigue, and a reduction in motor skills. In other instances, UMN can result in increased muscle tone (hypertonic muscle) and magnified reflex reactions or malfunctions such as spasticity. UMN syndromes can occur when damage occurs in the brain areas of the motor cortex, internal capsule or brain stem, and spinal cord. Similar pathological conditions may result from different areas of damage. Examples include childhood cerebral palsies and multiple sclerosis.

Lower motor neuron syndrome (LMN) usually occurs when peripheral nerves, junctions, and associated muscles are damaged, resulting in either paralysis or deficits in reflexes and voluntary movements. Muscular dystrophies, polio, and bulbar palsies are considered LMNs.

ALTERED MUSCLE REFLEXES

Altered muscle reflexes are called either **dyspraxias** or **apraxias**. They can hinder the ability to perform complex movements. The term *reflex* refers to any involuntary or automatic response to provocation. If there is a reduction in the reflex quality or amount of reaction, **hyporeflexia** is occurring. Hyporeflexia is often observed with LMN syndromes. Conversely, a response that is magnified in terms of quality and amount is said to be **hyperreflexia**. This usually happens because the brain's ability to inhibit lower neuronal responses has been compromised, as with spinal cord injuries.

SPINAL CORD INJURY

SPINAL CORD SYNDROMES

The American Spinal Injury Association (ASIA) has characterized 6 major spinal cord injury syndromes.

- **Central cord syndrome** is generally caused by neck hyperextension resulting in a C-region injury; clinically, the patient's upper extremities are weaker than the lower limbs, the sacrum is not affected, and they may have bowel or bladder problems.
- If the front of the spinal cord is compressed (usually through flexion or bone fragments), **anterior cord syndrome** can result, in which sensitivity to pain and temperature is accompanied by motor function loss.
- If penetration or some other trauma occurs on one side of the spinal cord, **Brown-Sequard syndrome** occurs; in this syndrome, nerve endings on the injured side are damaged, resulting in loss of motor function and an inability to feel deep pain on the injured side, plus loss of sensitivity to light touch, pain, and temperature on the opposite side.
- **Conus medullaris syndrome** and **cauda equina syndrome** result from trauma to the sacral and lumbar nerve roots, resulting in involuntary bowel, bladder, and lower limb motions. The basic difference between the two is the area of sensory preservation.
- **Posterior cord syndrome** is the lack of all dorsal column function. This is rare.

TYPES OF SPINAL CORD INJURY

Spinal cord injury (SCI) can be the result of either direct or indirect damage to the structure. In the United States, nearly 80% of spinal cord injuries occur in males. The most common types of **direct trauma** are: violent forward flexion of the neck or forceful backward hyperextension of the head during a motor vehicle accident; twisting (flexion-rotation) of the head; compression of vertebral bodies during a fall; and direct

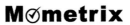

penetration of the cord during incidents such as stabbing or gunshot wounds. **Indirect trauma** can occur through lack of blood to the cord, inflammatory processes, cell destruction and electrolyte imbalances, programmed cell death (apoptosis), and tumors pressing on the spinal cord. The vast majority of SCI victims develop some degree of either **paraplegia** or **tetraplegia**; the latter occurs with damage in higher vertebral areas (about C1 to C8). Many of these people are ventilator dependent.

PROCEDURES FOR CLASSIFICATION

The rehabilitation nurse should follow ASIA's **Impairment Scale** when classifying a patient with spinal cord injury at the time of admittance. The essence of the classification is identification of the sensory and motor levels of impairment, the neurological level of impairment (NLI), whether the injury is complete or incomplete, and whether there are zones of partial preservation (ZPPs). Spinal cord injuries do not affect sensation in the face; therefore, ratings are done relative to facial sensation. Twenty-eight areas (dermatomes) on each side of the body are checked by pinprick and light touch and graded as 0 (incapable of distinguishing sharp from dull), 1 (differentiates sharp from dull but not like on the face), or 2 (a normal response). Impairment at the top cervical (C2 to C8) or first thoracic (T1) level usually indicates tetraplegia, while lower thoracic (T2 to T12), lumbar (L1 to L5), or sacral (S1 to S5) damage generally means only lower extremity paralysis. Ten important flexor or extensor muscles on each side are also tested for strength on a scale from 0 to 5.

MOTOR AND SENSORY EFFECTS OF INJURIES AT THE CERVICAL LEVELS

Upper motor neuron injuries encompass damage to the 8 cervical spinal levels **C1 to C8** as well as thoracic levels **T1 to T10**. For the most part, patients cannot feel sensations or perform voluntary movements below the level of injury. Therefore, if damage occurs at the upper levels **C1 to C3**, patients will be ventilator dependent and have very limited capabilities and mobility; they may have some head movement, but there will be sensory loss in certain areas and their diaphragm and intercostal muscles will be paralyzed. If the **C4 segment** is injured, patients may have some diaphragm function and shoulder movement, and they may be able to breathe without a ventilator or feed themselves at times. As the highest level of damage to the spinal cord moves lower (**C5 and C6**), certain muscle groups in the upper extremities become functional; sensations in the upper extremities are present in individuals with these injuries, and the possibility of independent living increases. People with **C7 injuries** can support normal breathing patterns, have most upper extremity sensations, and can usually function independently. Those with **C8 damage** have full sensation in their hands, can flex their fingers, have normal arm and shoulder positions, and can function independently.

MOTOR AND SENSORY EFFECTS OF INJURIES AT THE THORACIC, LUMBAR, AND SACRAL LEVELS

Damage to the upper thoracic spinal segments is still considered an upper motor neuron injury. If the **T1 through T5 sections** are involved, the patient has full control over their upper extremities. The patient can feel down to the middle chest and back area and has some functionality of the intercostal and thoracic muscles. This means that the patient also has normal pulmonary function and fairly good balance, and can function using just a manual wheelchair. If damage is lower, at the **T6 to T10 levels**, these parameters improve further. When the lower thoracic, lumbar, or sacral levels are the highest levels affected, the SCI is a lower motor neuron injury. From **T11 to L5**, motor functions in the hips, knee, and foot progressively return, and sensations are present in the abdomen, hips, and certain areas of the leg; however, sensation is not present in the genital or buttock regions. People with **S1 through S5 injuries** can eventually gain complete control of the lower extremities, manage their elimination and sexual functions, and feel sensations in all areas, including the groin. Therefore, people with LMN injuries can eventually perform self-care and ambulate with leg braces or independently.

POSSIBLE CHANGES DURING SPINAL SHOCK

A patient with an SCI initially goes through **spinal shock** from shutdown of the sympathetic nervous system. During this period, the patient may experience changes in thermoregulation and orthostasis, cardiac arrhythmias, thrombophlebitis, or a phenomenon called autonomic dysreflexia. The ability of the hypothalamus to regulate **core body temperature** can be affected, resulting in a temperature closer to the external environment, which may be mistaken for infection or other problems. Many people develop

orthostatic hypotension or light-headedness when adjusting from a prone to upright position due to a lessened sympathetic response and blood pooling in the lower extremities. Therefore, the patient's blood pressure needs to be monitored, and their abdomen may be wrapped to establish tissue perfusion. The patient may experience **bradycardia** (a slow heart rate). These changes are most common with injuries at the T6 level or above. **Deep venous thrombosis (DVT)** or **pulmonary embolisms** can potentially occur, indicating interventions such as compression hose or pneumatic devices. When spinal shock is over, the potentially grave phenomenon of **autonomic dysreflexia**, or a rapid increase in blood pressure, can occur.

GOALS FOR URINARY AND BOWEL ELIMINATION FUNCTION RECOVERY

During spinal shock and afterward, any SCI patient may have **altered bladder and/or bowel function**. The goal for urinary elimination is the establishment of a **containment system**, which—depending on individual circumstances—is usually an indwelling, self-intermittent, or external catheter with a drainage system. During acute rehabilitation, a **routine** is established, and long-term, the patient is taught to self-manage the system. The main goal for bowel elimination during spinal shock is the establishment and maintenance of a **clean bowel**. Patients with upper motor neuron damage are prone to develop a reflex bowel when the shock resolves. Patients with lower motor neuron damage lose motor tone and develop a limp rectal sphincter. During the acute rehabilitation period, a **daily bowel program** needs to be started and then continued later at home to prevent incontinence. Program components include hydration and dietary changes. UMN patients are usually given suppositories or other stimulants to encourage reflex emptying, while individuals with LMN damage take medications for motility.

SPASTICITY AND SKIN INTEGRITY RECOVERY GOALS FOR A PERSON WITH UPPER MOTOR NEURON SCI

Spasticity and skin integrity are two major areas of concern in a treatment plan for patients with upper motor neuron SCI. **Spasticity** occurs in the majority of these patients in the acute rehabilitation timeframe after resolution of spinal shock. It is the nurse's responsibility to help identify what stimulates this behavior (often certain body alignments), minimize the activator at that time, and develop a plan for its management after discharge. Range-of-motion and stretching exercises are generally recommended; pain may be managed with various anti-spasmodic drugs, and other measures, including surgery, may be required. Maintenance of **skin integrity** is an issue for all SCI patients because they lose mobility, sensitivity, and automatic functions, resulting in increased risk for pressure ulcers. Skin integrity is addressed through use of specialized sleeping surfaces, frequent repositioning, and weight-shifting changes.

RESPIRATORY FUNCTION GOALS FOR A PATIENT WITH UMN SCI

Respiratory capacity is affected by muscles stimulated by a range of spinal cord nerves at levels from C2 all the way down to T12. If the injury is at the C4 level or above, mechanical ventilation is usually necessary due to respiratory paralysis. Lower-level SCIs generally also require hard-hitting pulmonary management initially, but the goal is later removal of the ventilator. Complications such as pneumonia or respiratory failure can also occur. Interventions such as deep breathing exercises, drugs to control secretions, suctioning devices, or chest physiotherapy may be needed to establish a clear airway, which is the goal. Ultimately, the patient needs to be taught exercises for lung expansion and good pulmonary grooming.

OTHER POSSIBLE PROBLEMS AND GOALS FOR TREATMENT

Patients with SCI often develop **neurogenic pain** within the first half-year after injury. The nurse should stress proper posture and alignment (to decrease the likelihood of muscle spasms and pain), and they should develop a long-term pain management plan (usually incorporating medications). Within the same time frame, many patients experience heterotopic ossification, or the excessive growth of bone into the soft tissue in a joint, resulting in decreased range of motion, pain, spasticity, and other symptoms. ROM exercises and pharmacologic interventions are indicated in this case.

Osteoporosis, or the excessive reabsorption of bone relative to formation, occurs particularly in the initial year after injury due to decreased mobility predisposing the patient to fractures; weight-bearing exercises are indicated.

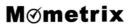

Social and emotional adjustments are difficult for many individuals, and depression is prevalent in the group; the nurse can help by being observant, planning self-care programs, and identifying community resources.

TRAUMATIC BRAIN INJURY
CAUSES

Traumatic brain injury (TBI) is an insult to the brain caused by an external influence that triggers a deterioration or alteration of consciousness, such that cognition or physical functioning is impaired either permanently or temporarily. The main cause of TBI in the United States is **motor vehicle accidents**, particularly motorcycle crashes. In the elderly and young children, the chief cause of TBI is a **fall**. Participation in team or individual **sports** or certain recreational activities is another source of TBI. **Violence**, ranging from use of firearms (including combat-related) to shaken baby syndrome, is another leading cause of TBI and—in many cases—death. **Collisions** in sports such as football or soccer, boxing, and bicycle falls (when helmets are not worn) are among the activities that can result in TBI. Repeated **concussions** (mild blows to the head often causing disorientation or temporary unconsciousness) can eventually lead to cognitive dysfunction. **Alcohol or substance abuse** can accentuate the effects of TBI.

TYPES

TBI can occur at the time of impact (primary) or sometime after the incident (secondary). **Primary injuries** are either open head injuries, in which the brain matter is actually exposed to outside elements through piercing via fracture or a missile, or closed head injuries, where the head collides with an outside surface but no brain matter is exposed directly to the environment. There are four main types of **closed head injuries**:

- **Concussions:** minor transient synaptic disruptions possibly accompanied by brief loss of consciousness
- **Diffuse axonal injuries:** more dispersed and potentially permanent synaptic damage caused by tearing and pulling
- **Contusions:** bruising of brain tissue caused by internal collisions between it and the skull
- **Hematomas:** internal pools of blood caused by hemorrhage or measured leakage from blood vessels

Common late or **secondary complications** of TBI are seizures, abscesses, or hydrocephalus (the buildup of cerebrospinal fluid). Seizures can occur at any time from immediately following an injury to weeks later, with the possibility of development of post-traumatic epilepsy greatest in the latter.

NURSING DIAGNOSES, INTERVENTIONS, AND DESIRED OUTCOMES FOR CHILDREN

TBI can impair many types of **motor and sensory functions**. The type and seriousness of the resulting disability is dependent on the location and nature of the **brain lesion**. Children with TBI can experience disturbed thought processes, urinary and bowel incontinence, various types of sensory deficits, impaired swallowing, speech defects, impaired physical mobility, and possibly delayed growth and development, all of which need to be addressed. **Level of cognitive functioning** is usually assessed by a scale such as the Rancho Los Amigos Levels of Cognitive Function Scale, which can indicate the types of interventions needed. For example, at levels I to III, activities that stimulate the patient and aid simple functions such as elimination and feeding are important, while for the child with level VI or higher functioning, the focus is on neurological and psychological testing and management to promote school and community reintegration.

DIFFUSE BRAIN INJURIES

Diffuse brain injuries involve extensive and scattered damage within the brain. They are primarily **diffuse axonal injuries** in which the forces of the injury (acceleration, deceleration, and shearing) cause widespread damage. The damage can be **transient impairment** or **scattered axonal disruption and loss**. These patients are usually comatose initially followed by increasing arousal and then confusion, or they have a period of post-traumatic amnesia, and then they overcome the confusion. Many **neuronal defects** can be associated. If there is a considerable increase in intracranial pressure or compromise of the cardiovascular and/or respiratory tract, another diffuse type of injury called **diffuse hypoxic-ischemic injury** can occur. Here, the lack of oxygen to the brain—particularly the hippocampus, basal ganglia, or cerebellum—results in diffuse neuronal loss, a phenomenon known as **watershed infarction** (stroke from lack of oxygen perfusion), and/or memory problems.

FOCAL BRAIN INJURIES

Focal brain injuries are those involving distinct localized damage. **Focal cortical contusions** commonly occur in the frontal or temporal lobes because of the associated bony structures. Associated hemorrhaging, swelling, and tissue disruptions (including lacerations or tearing of the meninges layer) are prevalent as well. **Frontal lobe contusions** manifest as emotional or social problems in the patient, whereas **temporal lobe injuries** usually show up as language or cognitive issues. Another type of focal damage, called **focal hypoxic-ischemic injury**, is secondary brain blood vessel blockage or necrosis. This occurs due to swelling, pressure, or herniation within the brain. **Herniation** is the abnormal projection of areas of the brain due to shifting of tissue following injury, resulting in compression and damage of nerves and blood vessels. Amnesia, aphasias, disorientation, or other problems can result. **Deep hemorrhages in the basal ganglia** area are rare examples of focal lesions usually manifesting as opposite-side motor weakness.

EXTRACEREBRAL HEMATOMAS

Extracerebral hematomas are areas of bleeding external to the actual brain, occurring between layers of the meninges. They create pressure on the cranial space. Types include epidural and subdural hematomas.

- **Epidural hematomas** occur on the outside of the dural layer of the meninges, usually subsequent to a skull bone fracture and cutting of the middle meningeal artery.
- **Subdural hematomas** occur in the area between the dural and arachnoid layers of the meninges. Typically caused by a tear to bridge veins or pial arteries or by lacerations to the brain, they may occur rapidly or develop over time. The latter slow-growing versions are known as hygromas. If subdural hematomas are not addressed rapidly, inadequate oxygen supply and hypoxic damage can result.

ANOXIC BRAIN INJURY

Anoxic brain injury (ABI) is any brain damage that results from **inadequate blood flow and oxygen perfusion** to the area. It often occurs after cardiac arrest, choking, drug overdosing, or near drowning; during surgery; or after a traumatic injury. The person can develop speech or movement problems and loss of recognition. Mild cases are typically characterized by amnesia, lack of attention, poor balance, and agitation. With severe anoxic brain injuries, the individual can also develop seizures, spasticity, and language problems. In the most severe cases, the patient is not able to communicate reliably and responds inconsistently to the environment. ABI patients generally are not completely comatose, and they can open their eyes.

BEHAVIORS ASSOCIATED WITH COGNITIVE DEFECTS

Some behaviors that can occur with brain damage include the following:

- **Disorientation/confusion**: Bewilderment and loss of direction, position, or time resulting from altered attention span and memory.
- **Depression**: A state of unhappiness and hopelessness manifesting as withdrawal, weeping, apprehension, and petulance.
- **Impaired judgment**: Incapacity to assess the consequences of actions and respond appropriately.
- **Impaired problem solving**: Incapacity to describe and analyze a problem, come up with a strategy to deal with the problem, and analyze the results.
- **Impulsivity**: Inclination to act in response to sudden urges or desires without considering the consequences.
- **Disinhibition**: Loss of inhibition and the incapacity to verbalize and behave within societal and cultural standards.

- **Agitation**: Highly unrestrained behavior characterized by nervous anxiety, irritability, and lack of attention span.
- **Apathy**: Lack of motivation and energy, and emotional emptiness.
- **Lack of initiation**: Failure to independently instigate and follow through on actions.
- **Lack of insight**: Lack of self-awareness and inability to see situations clearly, often leading to denial.
- **Emotional lability**: Quickly changeable and inexplicable shows of emotion such as crying or laughing.
- **Perseveration**: Reflexive repetitive responses in inappropriate situations; responses can be either spoken phrases or repeated actions.
- **Confabulation**: Fictitious creation of details about past events to compensate for memory loss and to alleviate anxiety, often seen in patients with dementia.

The nurse should not merely tolerate any of these behaviors, but should instead strive to provide an environment that will enable the patient to gain some control over the behaviors.

STROKES
HEMORRHAGIC STROKES

Hemorrhagic strokes account for about 20% of all strokes and result from a ruptured cerebral artery, causing not only a lack of oxygen and nutrients but also edema that causes widespread pressure and damage:

- **Intracerebral** is bleeding into the substance of the brain from an artery in the central lobes, basal ganglia, pons, or cerebellum. Intracerebral hemorrhage usually results from atherosclerotic degenerative changes, hypertension, brain tumors, anticoagulation therapy, or use of illicit drugs, such as cocaine.
- **Intracranial aneurysm** occurs with ballooning cerebral artery ruptures, most commonly at the Circle of Willis.
- **Arteriovenous malformation**. Rupture of AVMs can cause brain attack in young adults.
- **Subarachnoid hemorrhage** is bleeding in the space between the meninges and brain, resulting from aneurysm, AVM, or trauma. This type of hemorrhage compresses brain tissue.

Treatment includes: The patient may need airway protection/artificial ventilation if neurologic compromise is severe. Blood pressure is lowered to control rate of bleeding but with caution to avoid hypotension and resulting cerebral ischemia (Goal – CPP >70). Sedation can lower ICP and blood pressure, and seizure prophylaxis will be indicated as blood irritates the cerebral cells. An intraventricular catheter may be used in ICP management; correct any clotting disorders if identified.

> **Review Video: Stroke**
> Visit mometrix.com/academy and enter code: 310572

ISCHEMIA STROKES

Strokes (brain attacks, cerebrovascular accidents) result when there is interruption of the blood flow to an area of the brain. The two basic types are ischemic and hemorrhagic. About 80% are **ischemic**, resulting from blockage of an artery supplying the brain:

- **Thrombosis** in a large artery, usually resulting from atherosclerosis, may block circulation to a large area of the brain. It is most common in the elderly and may occur suddenly or after episodes of transient ischemic attacks.
- **Lacunar infarct** (a penetrating thrombosis in a small artery) is most common in those with diabetes mellitus and/or hypertension.
- **Embolism** travels through the arterial system and lodges in the brain, most commonly in the left middle cerebral artery. An embolism may be cardiogenic, resulting from cardiac arrhythmia or surgery. An embolism usually occurs rapidly with no warning signs.
- **Cryptogenic** has no identifiable cause.

Functional Health Patterns

Medical management of ischemic strokes with tissue plasminogen activator (tPA) (Activase), the primary treatment, should be initiated within 3 hours (or up to 4.5 hours if inclusion criteria are met):

- **Thrombolytic,** such as tPA, which is produced by recombinant DNA and is used to dissolve fibrin clots. It is given intravenously (0.9 mg/kg up to 90 mg) with 10% injected as an initial bolus and the rest over the next hour.
- **Antihypertensives** if MAP >130 mmHg or systolic BP >220
- **Cooling** to reduce hyperthermia
- **Osmotic diuretics** (mannitol), hypertonic saline, loop diuretics (Lasix), and/or corticosteroids (dexamethasone) to decrease cerebral edema and intracranial pressure
- **Aspirin/anticoagulation** may be used with embolism
- Monitor and treat hyperglycemia
- **Surgical Intervention:** Used when other treatment fails, may go in through artery and manually remove the clot

SYMPTOMS OF BRAIN ATTACKS IN RELATION TO AREA OF BRAIN AFFECTED

Brain attacks most commonly occur in the right or left hemisphere, but the exact location and the extent of brain damage from a brain attack affects the type of presenting symptoms. If the frontal area of either side is involved, there tends to be memory and learning deficits. Some symptoms are common to specific areas and help to identify the area involved:

- **Right hemisphere**: This results in left paralysis or paresis and a left visual field deficit that may cause spatial and perceptual disturbances, so people may have difficulty judging distance. Fine motor skills may be impacted, resulting in trouble dressing or handling tools. People may become impulsive and exhibit poor judgment, often denying impairment. Left-sided neglect (lack of perception of things on the left side) may occur. Difficulty following directions, short-term memory loss, and depression are also common. Language skills usually remain intact.
- **Left hemisphere**: Results in right paralysis or paresis and a right visual field defect. Depression is common and people often exhibit slow, cautious behavior, requiring repeated instruction and reinforcement for simple tasks. Short-term memory loss and difficulty learning new material or understanding generalizations is common. Difficulty with mathematics, reading, writing, and reasoning may occur. Aphasia (expressive, receptive, or global) is common.
- **Brain stem**: Because the brain stem controls respiration and cardiac function, a brain attack in the brain stem frequently causes death, but those who survive may have a number of problems, including respiratory and cardiac abnormalities. Strokes may involve motor or sensory impairment or both.
- **Cerebellum**: This area controls balance and coordination. Brain attacks in the cerebellum are rare but may result in ataxia, nausea and vomiting, and headaches and dizziness or vertigo.

REHABILITATION GOALS

Rehabilitation of a patient who has undergone a cerebrovascular accident should be directed toward improving their **functional abilities** based on the identified impairments. These patients can have a range of physical, cognitive, and behavioral issues. The most common areas affected are attention span, memory, decision-making, perception, ability to choose, communication, mood, and emotional lability. People who have had a stroke are often **dependent** on others and may undergo a period of **depression**. They can lose **flexibility** or have problems with **mobility**; thus, correct positioning and passive stretching are important rehabilitative interventions. A rehabilitation program should address cognitive, physical, and language defects. There are a number of nursing approaches based on the theory that the brain can be retrained and some functionality restored through reprogramming; these include the **Motor Relearning Program** and the **Bobath approach**.

DEMENTIA

ALZHEIMER'S DISEASE

Alzheimer's disease (AD) is a slowly and subtly destructive form of dementia. It involves cognitive and intellectual deterioration due to the destruction of brain cells. Another type of dementia, called **vascular dementia**, can result from diminished blood flow to nerve cells in the brain, and the term **mild cognitive impairment (MCI)** is used to describe the transition to dementia. AD's primary risk factor is aging; the presence of AD in a close relative also increases the probability of its development. While the exact etiology of AD is undetermined, pathological alterations include development of **neuritic plaques** containing the protein β-amyloid, **neurofibrillary tangles** enclosing abnormal proteins, and a **deficit of cholinergic neurons** related to memory and cognition. The **initial stage** of AD, called mild AD, can last up to 3 years. The typical presentation is primarily mild memory loss. In a person with **stage II** moderate AD (lasting up to 10 years after onset), the memory impairment is more pronounced. Other symptoms at this stage include spatial disorientation, restlessness, indifference, irritability, delusions, speech deficits, and self-care issues. By **stage III** (usually at 11 years or more) severe AD, an individual with AD is grossly impaired cognitively, has rigid limbs, and is incontinent.

MANAGEMENT

AD is currently managed **pharmacologically** and through other types of interventions. Most of the currently approved drugs for AD fall into the category of **cholinesterase inhibitors**. These include galantamine, rivastigmine tartrate, and donepezil, all of which employ different mechanisms to stabilize the neurotransmitter acetylcholine, which is diminished in AD. There is also a drug called **memantine**, which works by depressing levels of another neurotransmitter, glutamate. **Glutamate** can kill brain cells if present in excess. Unfortunately, only about half of AD patients benefit from these drugs, and other drugs are being investigated. **Nonpharmacological interventions** primarily address the behavioral abnormalities associated with AD and include things such as music therapy, movement therapy, and auditory or tactile stimulation techniques.

NON-ALZHEIMER'S DEMENTIA

Dementia is a chronic condition in which there is progressive and irreversible loss of memory and function. There are many types of dementia a nurse may encounter:

- **Creutzfeldt-Jakob disease**: Rapidly progressive dementia with impaired memory, behavioral changes, and incoordination
- **Dementia with Lewy Bodies**: Similar to Alzheimer's, but symptoms may fluctuate frequently; may also include visual hallucinations, muscle rigidity, and tremors
- **Frontotemporal dementia**: Causes marked changes in personality and behavior; characterized by difficulty using and understanding language
- **Mixed dementia**: Combination of different types of dementia
- **Normal pressure hydrocephalus**: Characterized by ataxia, memory loss, and urinary incontinence
- **Parkinson's dementia**: Involves impaired decision making and difficulty concentrating, learning new material, understanding complex language, and sequencing
- **Vascular dementia**: Memory loss less pronounced than that common to Alzheimer's, but symptoms are similar

Nursing considerations: Distraction is usually the best course of action to deter the patient with dementia. Reorient frequently, but do not argue with the patient. Avoid restraints or sedatives, which worsen confusion.

DELIRIUM

Delirium is an acute, sudden, and fluctuating change in consciousness. Delirium occurs in 10-40% of hospitalized older adults and about 80% of patients who are terminally ill. Delirium may result from drugs, infections, hypoxia, trauma, dementia, depression, vision and hearing loss, surgery, alcoholism, untreated pain,

Functional Health Patterns

fluid/electrolyte imbalance, and malnutrition. If left untreated, delirium greatly increases the risk of morbidity and death.

Signs/Symptoms: Reduced ability to focus/sustain attention, language and memory disturbances, disorientation, confusion, audiovisual hallucinations, sleep disturbance, and psychomotor activity disorder.

Diagnosis: Patient interview, history/chart/medication review, and possible blood tests to identify electrolyte imbalance/abnormalities.

Treatment includes:

- **Medications**: Trazodone, lorazepam, haloperidol—though these may make confusion worse in elderly patients
- **Procedures**: Provide a sitter to ensure safety, decreasing dosage of hypnotics and psychotropics, correct underlying cause

Prevention: Reorient patient frequently, ensure adequate rest/nutrition, monitor response to medications, and treat infections and dehydration/malnutrition early.

AGITATION

Agitation is a common occurrence in the critically ill patient. Factors contributing to the development of agitation include drug or alcohol withdrawal, sleep deprivation, hypoxemia, electrolyte or metabolic imbalance, anxiety, pain, and adverse drug reactions. Delirium may also include agitation as a manifestation.

Diagnosis: The physiologic effects of agitation may include increases in heart rate, respiratory rate, blood pressure, intracranial pressure, and oxygen consumption. In addition, agitation can contribute to the self-removal of lines or tubes and combative behavior that may result in patient harm.

Treatment: Treatment of agitation involves the identification and correction of causative factors. The use of pharmacologic agents to manage pain, anxiety, and agitation are often utilized. Non-pharmacologic interventions including verbal de-escalation (when possible). The promotion of normal sleep patterns and relaxation techniques may also be effective. Early identification of signs and symptoms is also critical in the successful management of agitation.

SITTERS AND RESTRAINTS FOR SAFETY DURING DELIRIUM AND CONFUSION

For patients with delirium or confusion, safety is the priority, but returning patients to their baseline neurologic levels is critical as well. Interventions such as orientation protocols, medication review (benzodiazepines should usually be avoided in this population), early mobilization, and mental stimulation are key. At times, these interventions will not be sufficient for keeping the patient safe and managing agitation that can turn combative. While it is usually most beneficial to use a familiar person for the patient, at times **professional sitters** may be needed and can be a valuable resource. Family or professional sitters should be educated about effective calming strategies, including diversion, reorientation, frequently reassuring the patient, and not challenging the patient. They shouldn't affirm delusional thinking and should be educated on when to call for help from staff if the patient's condition becomes more severe or unsafe. **Restraints** should be used only as a last resort, as they have been shown to increase time of delirium. When restraints are used, state laws must be followed. This includes safety checks, ensuring basic needs are being met, and periodic reevaluation for removal of restraints.

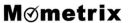

COGNITIVE DEFICITS

POSSIBLE NURSING DIAGNOSES FOR COGNITIVE DEFECTS

There are four main nursing diagnoses indicating cognitive defects:

- **Disturbed thought process**: A disturbance of cognitive function relative to age expectations. It is characterized by memory issues, lack of decision-making abilities, and inattention, and it can be caused by a variety of neurological problems as well as electrolyte imbalances or infection.
- **Chronic confusion**: The progressive worsening of intellectual processes and behavior. This is generally a sign of dementia, stroke, or other injuries and is characterized by disorientation, altered personality, and memory problems.
- **Impaired memory without other symptoms**: This may be caused by a number of factors, such as stress, congestive heart failure, and neurological disorders; these patients are forgetful, particularly in terms of recent events.
- **Impaired environmental interpretation syndrome:** Describes people who have been unable to orient themselves to their environment over a period of at least three months and are chronically confused and unable to concentrate or reason. This syndrome often occurs in Alzheimer's, Parkinson's, and Huntington's diseases.

NURSING INTERVENTIONS AND OUTCOMES IN ACUTE REHABILITATION UNITS

Appropriate nursing outcomes and interventions for patients with cognitive deficits in **acute rehabilitation** units include the following:

Intervention	Desired Outcome
Promotion of cognitive function through use of testing, aids, and stimulating activities	Execution of complex mental processes
Encouragement of appropriate decision making by identifying choices, providing support, and introducing increasingly difficult tasks	Ability to make decisions between alternatives
Establishment of appropriate thought control by reinforcing appropriate behavior and discouraging unsuitable behavior	Establishment of appropriate thought processes and subject matter and perception thereof
Promotion of correct information processing through conversation and discussion	Demonstration of ability to acquire, organize, and use information
Stimulation of memory through use of repetition, memory games, group training programs, etc.	Recovery and report of previously gathered information
Safety promotion by identification of risk factors and providing safe environment	No falls
Control of aggressive behavior through identification of precipitating factors and development of behavioral management plan	Practice of self-restraint

APPROPRIATE NURSING INTERVENTIONS AND OUTCOMES IN SUBACUTE REHABILITATION UNIT

Potential rehabilitation nursing interventions and outcomes in smaller **subacute rehabilitation** units include the following:

Intervention	Desired Outcome
Establishment of a comfortable, safe, and consistent environment and an orientation to reality for the patient	Cognitive recognition of people, places, and times

Functional Health Patterns

Intervention	Desired Outcome
Promotion of attention span and focus by keeping outside stimuli at a minimum and making sure the patient has enough rest	Increased concentration needed for tasks
Use of smells, sounds, touch, and/or visual aids to aid return to consciousness	To demonstrate the ability to be stimulated and adjust to their environment
Elevation of activity level in terms of both frequency and length through development of individualized program	To increase activity tolerance to the point of participation in daily activities
Promotion of family participation in care and understanding of the patient's needs and cognitive deficits via support and education	To keep the family informed enough to assist in decision making and care and understand underlying processes
Provision of available resources for family and patient	To inform the decision on the next level of care

APPROPRIATE NURSING INTERVENTIONS AND OUTCOMES IN OUTPATIENT REHABILITATION SETTING

Interventional and outcome goals for the rehabilitation nurse for **outpatient rehabilitation** in day care centers or at home include:

Intervention	Desired Outcome
Promotion of safety in the patient's home through use of aids, adaptive equipment, grab bars, etc.	Lack of evidence of any physical harm
Establishment of readiness of the caregiver by evaluating their abilities and working with the caregiver on planning and resources	Capability of assuming full responsibility in the home setting
Encouragement of good care by the caregiver by helping them to set up a plan, supporting the caregiver, and anticipating their needs	Recognition of behavioral changes and needed services
Monitoring of the caregiver's health and directing the caregiver to support services if needed	Ensuring that the caregiver can deal with the stress involved
Promotion of normalization and the integrity of the family through any strategies	Optimizing family interactions and supporting the family during crises
Provision of resources	To enhance and promote the wellness, recuperation, and rehabilitation of the patient, including stress reduction, exercise, and education
Techniques such as group therapy, role-playing, and positive feedback	Enhancement of social skills in the patient

APPROPRIATE NURSING INTERVENTIONS AND OUTCOMES IN OTHER REHABILITATION SETTINGS

Other rehabilitation settings are primarily residential facilities. In those environments, the following are generally the potential rehabilitation nursing interventions and outcomes:

Intervention	Desired Outcome
Promotion of personal safety of the patient by controlling their environment, establishing a routine, and monitoring behavior	Successful control of any behaviors that could lead to injury

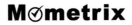

Intervention	Desired Outcome
Control of the individual's tendency toward aggressive behavior through diet, removing the individual from any situation that can provoke aggression, identifying triggers and solutions, and education	Self-restraint of the patient
Inclusion of the caregiver in as many aspects as possible and establishing lines of communication	Assisting the caregiver in adapting to the patient's transfer to an institution
Promotion of the patient's quality of life, including aspects such as medication administration, psychosocial support, and encouragement of self-care activities	Patient and family satisfaction

NEUROMUSCULAR DISORDERS

MULTIPLE SCLEROSIS

Multiple sclerosis is an autoimmune disorder of the CNS in which the myelin sheath around the nerves is damaged and replaced by scar tissue that prevents conduction of nerve impulses.

Symptoms vary widely and can include problems with balance and coordination, tremors, slurring of speech, cognitive impairment, vision impairment, nystagmus, pain, and bladder and bowel dysfunction. Symptoms may be relapsing-remitting, progressive, or a combination. Onset is usually at 20-30 years of age, with incidence higher in females. Patient may initially present with problems walking or falling or optic neuritis (30%) causing loss of central vision. Males may complain of sexual dysfunction as an early symptom. Others have dysuria with urinary retention.

Diagnosis is based on clinical and neurological examination and MRI. **Treatment** is symptomatic and includes treatment to shorten duration of episodes and slow progress.

- **Glucocorticoids**: Methylprednisolone
- **Immunomodulator**: Interferon beta, glatiramer acetate, natalizumab
- **Immunosuppressant**: Mitoxantrone
- **Hormone**: Estriol (for females)

> **Review Video: Multiple Sclerosis**
> Visit mometrix.com/academy and enter code: 417355

ALS

Amyotrophic lateral sclerosis (ALS) is a progressive degenerative disease of the upper and lower motor neurons, resulting in progressively severe symptoms such as spasticity, hyperreflexia, muscle weakness, and paralysis that can cause dysphagia, cramping, muscular atrophy, and respiratory dysfunction. ALS may be sporadic or familial (rare). Speech may become monotone; however, cognitive functioning usually remains intact. Eventually, patients become immobile and cannot breathe independently.

Diagnosis is based on history, electromyography, nerve conduction studies, and MRI. Treatment includes riluzole to delay progression of the disease. Patients in the ED usually have been diagnosed and have developed an acute complication, such as acute respiratory failure, aspiration pneumonia, or other trauma.

Functional Health Patterns

123

Treatment includes:

- Nebulizer treatments with bronchodilators and steroids
- Antibiotics for infection
- Mechanical ventilation

If **ventilatory assistance** is needed, it is important to determine if the patient has a living will expressing the wish to be ventilated or not or has assigned power of attorney for health matters to someone to make this decision.

PARKINSON'S DISEASE

Parkinson's disease (PD) is an extrapyramidal movement motor system disorder caused by loss of brain cells that produce dopamine. Typical symptoms include tremor of face and extremities, rigidity, bradykinesia, akinesia, poor posture, and a lack of balance and coordination causing increasing problems with mobility, talking, and swallowing. Some may suffer depression and mood changes. Tremors usually present unilaterally in an upper extremity.

Diagnosis includes:

- **Cogwheel rigidity test**: The extremity is put through passive range of motion, which causes increased muscle tone and ratchet-like movements.
- Physical and neurological exam
- Complete history to rule out drug-induced Parkinson akinesia

Treatment includes:

- Symptomatic support
- Dopaminergic therapy: Levodopa, amantadine, and carbidopa
- Anticholinergics: Trihexyphenidyl, benztropine
- For drug-induced Parkinson's, terminate drugs

Drug therapy tends to decrease in effectiveness over time, and patients may present with a marked increase in symptoms. Discontinuing the drugs for 1 week may exacerbate symptoms initially, but functioning may improve when drugs are reintroduced.

GUILLAIN-BARRÉ SYNDROME

Guillain-Barré syndrome (GBS) is an autoimmune disorder of the myelinated motor peripheral nervous system, causing ascending and descending paralysis. GBS is often triggered by a viral infection, but may be idiopathic in origin. Diagnosis is by history, clinical symptoms, and lumbar puncture, which often show increased protein with normal glucose and cell count although protein may not increase for a week or more.

> **Review Video: Guillain-Barre Syndrome**
> Visit mometrix.com/academy and enter code: 742900

Symptoms include:

- Numbness and tingling with increasing weakness of lower extremities that may become generalized, sometimes resulting in complete paralysis and inability to breathe without ventilatory support.
- Deep tendon reflexes are typically absent and some people experience facial weakness and ophthalmoplegia (paralysis of muscles controlling movement of eyes).

Treatment includes:

- Supportive: Fluids, physical therapy, and antibiotics for infections
- Patients should be hospitalized for observation and placed on ventilator support if forced vital capacity is reduced.
- While there is no definitive treatment, plasma exchange or IV immunoglobulin may shorten the duration of symptoms.

CEREBRAL PALSY

Cerebral palsy (CP) is a non-progressive motor dysfunction related to CNS damage associated with congenital, hypoxic, or traumatic injury before, during, or ≤2 years after birth. It may include visual defects, speech impairment, seizures, and intellectual disability. There are four **types of motor dysfunction:**

- **Spastic**: Damage to the cerebral cortex or pyramidal tract. Constant hypertonia and rigidity lead to contractures and curvature of the spine.
- **Dyskinetic**: Damage to the extrapyramidal, basal ganglia. Tremors and twisting with exaggerated posturing and impairment of voluntary muscle control.
- **Ataxic**: Damage to the extrapyramidal cerebellum. Atonic muscles in infancy with lack of balance, instability of muscles, and poor gait.
- **Mixed**: Combinations of all three types with multiple areas of damage.

Characteristics of CP include:

- Hypotonia or hypertonia with rigidity and spasticity
- Athetosis (constant writhing motions)
- Ataxia
- Hemiplegia (one-sided involvement, more severe in upper extremities)
- Diplegia (all extremities involved, but more severe in lower extremities)
- Quadriplegia (all extremities involved with arms flexed and legs extended)

MYASTHENIA GRAVIS

Myasthenia gravis is an autoimmune disorder that results in sporadic, progressive weakness of striated (skeletal) muscles because of impaired transmission of nerve impulses. Myasthenia gravis usually affects muscles controlled by the cranial nerves although any muscle group may be affected. Many patients also have thymomas.

Signs and symptoms include weakness and fatigue that worsens throughout the day. Patients often exhibit ptosis and diplopia. They may have trouble chewing and swallowing and often appear to have masklike facies. If respiratory muscles are involved, patients may exhibit signs of respiratory failure. Myasthenic crisis occurs when patients can no longer breathe independently.

Diagnosis includes electromyography and the Tensilon test (an IV injection of edrophonium or neostigmine, which improves function if the patient has myasthenia gravis, but does not improve function if the symptoms are from a different cause). CT or MRI to diagnose thymoma.

Treatment includes anticholinesterase drugs (neostigmine, pyridostigmine) to relieve some muscle weakness, but these drugs lose effectiveness as the disease progresses. Corticosteroids may be used. Thymectomy is performed if thymoma is present. Tracheotomy and mechanical ventilation may be needed for myasthenic crisis.

> **Review Video: <u>Myasthenia Gravis</u>**
> Visit mometrix.com/academy and enter code: 162510

Functional Health Patterns

HUNTINGTON'S DISEASE

Huntington's disease (HD) is a hereditary degenerative neuromuscular disorder that usually presents in middle age. It is caused by accumulation of the amino acid **glutamine** in the brain, where it kills cells. Brain centers related to movement, perception and memory, and balance and coordination are affected. Individuals with HD develop involuntary, unusual movements due to increased levels of the inhibitory neurotransmitter **dopamine** and diminished amounts of **acetylcholine**. All of their muscle actions eventually become uncontrolled, and they develop dementia. Besides the aforementioned clinical symptoms, diagnostic tests for this disease should include a neurological examination, imaging procedures (including an MRI and a CT scan to look for brain shrinkage), and a search for genetic predisposition—through family history and genetic studies—to look for the associated abnormal gene on chromosome 4.

SPINA BIFIDA

Spina bifida is a blanket term for conditions present at birth in which the neural tubes in the spinal column or meninges protrude through a cleft in the column, resulting in loss of neuromuscular function below the level of injury. Its genesis is not completely understood, but insufficient folic acid intake by the mother during pregnancy appears to contribute to the condition. The major diagnostic components include lower extremity paralysis and impaired physical mobility, elimination problems, and sexual dysfunction. These can be addressed through use of a wheelchair and exercise therapies, urinary elimination management and bowel training, and enhancement of self-esteem. Individuals with spina bifida may have delayed growth and development as well. Patients with spina bifida also have increased risk for obesity, injuries, latex allergies, poor skin integrity, and hydrocephalus. Hydrocephalus—increased cerebrospinal fluid around the brain, resulting in head enlargement and intracranial pressure—must be controlled if present through use of shunts.

TEAM MEMBERS IN THE MANAGEMENT OF PATIENTS WITH NEUROMUSCULAR DISORDERS

All degenerative neuromuscular disorders share some common characteristics, such as the functions generally compromised (respiration, speech, swallowing, ambulation, etc.) and typical palliative measures (maintenance of function, self-care education, and more). Care for people with these disorders also requires considerable planning because the disease is debilitating and usually progressive. Additional team members usually have to be called upon at some point. Team members may include the following:

- The **physician** and **nurse** as the primary professionals involved
- A **respiratory therapist** for ventilatory support
- A **speech pathologist** to address speech difficulties
- A **dietitian** as a nutrition consultant
- A **urologist** and **enterostomal nurse** for elimination problems
- **Psychosocial professionals** (including help for caregivers under strain if needed)
- A **physical therapist** and possibly an **occupational therapist** to help address muscular weakness and mobility issues
- A **sexual therapist** if appropriate

DRUG CLASSES TO MANAGE NEUROMUSCULAR DISEASES

Medications used to manage neuromuscular diseases are specific to the causes and symptoms of the disease:

- **Antidepressants** and **stool softeners** are routinely used in patients with spinal cord injuries or any of the specific disorders discussed, namely ALS, Guillain-Barré, Huntington's, myasthenia gravis, multiple sclerosis, and Parkinson's.
- **Corticosteroids**, **immunomodulators**, **methotrexate**, **T-cell receptor peptides**, and **monoclonal antibodies** are used to suppress immune and inflammatory responses, particularly in multiple sclerosis or myasthenia gravis patients.
- **Methylprednisolone** is often administered to spinal cord injury patients to reduce swelling and improve blood flow.

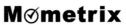

- **Drugs that impact neurotransmission and/or muscle properties** are used to manage symptoms such as urinary retention or frequency, spasticity, bradykinesia, tremor, and rigidity primarily in individuals with multiple sclerosis, Parkinson's, or spinal cord injury; these include cholinergics, anticholinergics, muscle relaxants, antispasmodics, dopaminergic drugs, MAO inhibitors, antihistamines, and COMT and GABA antagonists.
- **Antioxidants** are given to patients with Parkinson's disease to slow disease progression.

GOALS AND ADLS FOR PATIENTS WITH NEUROLOGICAL DEFECTS

PATIENTS WITH LOW VISION OR COGNITIVE DEFECTS

For individuals with low vision, safety is the main issue. Personal care, food-related items, furniture, and medications should be presented in a **consistent environment or pattern**. **Direct lighting** should be selected to reduce glare and maximize contrast. If the person is blind, there are services available to assist with most activities of daily life.

For individuals with cognitive defects, again, providing a safe environment is paramount while preserving their dignity. These types of patients may have problems with memory, lack of attention, problem-solving ability, and the like. Thus, **consistency** is important in the rehabilitation plan of these patients. **Rehabilitation plans** should include such things as incorporation of cues or memory aids, close management of the patient's environment, reinforcement of behavioral patterns, and consideration of familial and cultural values.

PATIENTS WITH HEMIPLEGIA

Patients with hemiplegia have partial or total inability to move one side, usually due to CNS damage. The primary goal is for the patient to make **best use of the affected side** without causing frustration or engaging in unsafe maneuvers. The plan should include **exercises**, such as massed practice exercises, which have frequent repetition and assistance to carry out tasks, and are based on the concept of **neuroplasticity**, the ability of the CNS to form new neural connections or repair damaged connections. Different techniques include constraint-induced movement therapy, adaptive task practice (shaping), active assist, body-weight-supported treadmill training, and robot-assisted movement. The patient can basically follow the dressing procedures with assistance from the nurse or other helper. If the patient has **balance issues**, they can dress while seated or braced against a door or wall frame. Recommendations for eating include anything that will prevent accidents and add to the patient's goals for improvement. It is especially important to provide a safe environment in the **bathroom** with devices such as shower seats, grab bars, and ramps. Good **lighting** is important. Personal care items that can be used with **one hand** should be made available.

PATHOPHYSIOLOGY OF PAIN

NOCICEPTORS

Nociceptors are the primary neurons, or **sensory receptors**, responding to stimuli in the skin, muscle, and joints, as well as the stomach, bladder, and uterus. These neurons have specialized responses for mechanical, thermal, or chemical stimuli. The **neuron stimulation** is a direct result of tissue injury and follows four stages: **transduction** where a change occurs, **transmission** where the impulse is transferred along the neural path, **modulation** or translation of the signal, and **perception** by the patient. When injury occurs, the nociceptors initiate the process that begins **depolarization of the peripheral nerve**. Nociceptors may consist of either A-fiber axons or C-fiber axons. The message travels along the neural pathway and creates a perception of pain. A-fiber axons carry these pain messages at a much faster rate than C-fiber axons.

Functional Health Patterns

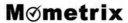

NOCICEPTIVE PAIN

Nociceptive pain is an umbrella term for pain caused by **stimulation of the neuroreceptor**. This stimulation is a direct result of tissue injury. The severity of pain is proportionate to the extent of the injury. Nociceptive pain can be subdivided into two classifications: somatic and visceral pain. **Somatic pain** is located in the cutaneous tissues, bone joints, and muscle tissues. **Visceral pain** is specific to internal organs protected by a layer of viscera, such as the cardiovascular, respiratory, gastrointestinal, or genitourinary systems. Both types are treatable with opioids.

VISCERAL PAIN

Visceral pain is associated with the internal organs. It can be very different depending on the affected organ. Not all internal organs are sensitive to pain (some lack **nociceptors**, such as the spleen, kidney, and pancreas), and may withstand a great deal of damage without causing pain. Other internal organs, such as the stomach, bladder, and ureters, can create significant pain from even the slightest damage. Visceral pain generally has a **poorly defined area**. It is also capable of referring pain to other remote locations away from the area of injury. It is described as a squeezing or cramping: a deep ache within the internal organs. The patient may complain of a generalized sick feeling or have nausea and vomiting. Visceral pain generally responds well to treatment with **opioids**.

> **Review Video: <u>Visceral Pain</u>**
> Visit mometrix.com/academy and enter code: 430402

SOMATIC PAIN

Somatic pain refers to messages from pain receptors located in the **cutaneous or musculoskeletal tissues**. When the pain occurs within the musculoskeletal tissue, it is referred to as **deep somatic pain**. Metastasizing cancers commonly cause deep somatic pain. **Surface pain** refers to pain concentrated in the **dermis and cutaneous layers** such as that caused by a surgical incision. Deep somatic pain is generally described as a dull, throbbing ache that is well focused on the area of trauma. It responds well to **opioids**. Surface somatic pain is also directly focused on the injury. It is frequently described as sharper than deep somatic pain. It may also present as a burning or pricking sensation.

> **Review Video: <u>Somatic Pain</u>**
> Visit mometrix.com/academy and enter code: 982772

NEUROPATHIC PAIN

Neuropathic pain results from injury to the **nervous system**. This can result from cancer cells compressing the nerves or spinal cord, from actual cancerous invasion into the nerves or spinal cord, or from chemical damage to the nerves caused by chemotherapy and radiation. Other causes include diabetes- and alcohol-related damage, trauma, neuralgias, or other illnesses affecting the neural path either centrally or peripherally. When the nerves become damaged, they are unable to carry accurate information. This results in more severe, distinct **pain messages**. The nerves may also relay pain messages long after the original cause of the pain is resolved. It can be described as sharp, burning, shooting, shocking, tingling, or electrical in nature. It may travel the length of the nerve path from the spine to a distal body part such as a hand, or down the buttocks to a foot. NSAIDs and opioids are generally ineffective against neuropathic pain, though adjuvants may enhance the therapeutic effect of opioids. Nerve blocks may also be used.

> **Review Video: <u>Neuropathic Pain</u>**
> Visit mometrix.com/academy and enter code: 780523

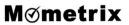

ADVERSE SYSTEMIC EFFECTS OF PAIN

Acute pain causes adverse systemic effects that can negatively affect many body systems.

- **Cardiovascular**: Tachycardia and increased blood pressure is a common response to pain, causing increased cardiac output and systemic vascular resistance. In those with pre-existing cardiovascular disease, such as compromised ventricular function, cardiac output may decrease. The increased myocardial need for oxygen may cause or worsen myocardial ischemia.
- **Respiratory**: Increased need for oxygen causes an increase in minute ventilation and splinting due to pain, which may compromise pulmonary function. If the chest wall movement is constrained, tidal volume falls, impairing the ability to cough and clear secretions. Bed rest further compromises ventilation.
- **Gastrointestinal**: Sphincter tone increases and motility decreases, sometimes resulting in ileus. There may be an increased secretion of gastric acids, which irritates the gastric lining and can cause ulcerations. Nausea, vomiting, and constipation may occur. Reflux may result in aspiration pneumonia. Abdominal distension may occur.
- **Urinary**: Increased sphincter tone and decreased motility result in urinary retention.
- **Endocrine**: Hormone levels are affected by pain. Catabolic hormones such as catecholamine, cortisol, and glucagon increase, and anabolic hormones such as insulin and testosterone decrease. Lipolysis increases along with carbohydrate intolerance. Sodium retention can occur because of increased ADH, aldosterone, angiotensin, and cortisol. This in turn causes fluid retention and a shift to extracellular space.
- **Hematologic**: There may be reduced fibrinolysis, increased adhesiveness of platelets, and increased coagulation.
- **Immune**: Leukocytosis and lymphopenia may occur, increasing risk of infection.
- **Emotional**: Patients may experience depression, anxiety, anger, decreased appetite, and sleep deprivation. This type of response is most common in those with chronic pain, who usually have different systemic responses from those with acute pain.

CORE PRINCIPLES OF PAIN ASSESSMENT AND MANAGEMENT

According to the Joint Commission, assessing pain should be a priority in patient care, and organizations must establish **policies** for assessment and treatment of pain and must educate staff members about these policies. The Joint Commission considers a **plan of care** regarding pain control an essential patient right. Hospitals should be consistent in the use of the same assessment tools throughout the organization, specific to different patient populations (for example, pediatrics and geriatrics). The latest standards (2018) of evidence-based practice include the following:

- Organizations must establish a clinical leadership team to oversee pain management and safe prescription of opioids.
- Patients must be involved in planning and setting goals and should receive education regarding safe use of opioid and non-opioid medications.
- Patients should be screened for pain in all assessments, including visits to the emergency department.
- Patients at high risk for opioid misuse or adverse effects must be identified and monitored.
- Healthcare providers should have access to prescription drug monitoring safety databases, such as the prescription databases provided by most states.
- Organizations must provide performance improvement educational programs regarding pain assessment and management and must collect and analyze data on its pain assessment and management.

AREAS ADDRESSED WHEN ASSESSING PAIN

Information concerning a patient's pain can be gathered from a variety of sources, including observations, interviews with the patient and family, medical records, and observations of other health care providers.

Functional Health Patterns

129

However, it is important to remember that each patient's pain is **subjective** and **personal**. Pain is defined as whatever the patient says it is. Having the patient give parameters of quality, location, duration, speed of onset, and intensity can all be beneficial in forming a treatment plan based on the patient's needs. Pain is also influenced by psychological, social, and spiritual factors. Behavioral, psychological, and subjective assessment information such as physical demeanor and vital signs can be helpful in further defining a patient's pain parameters.

PHYSICAL SIGNS OF PAIN

The best assessment of the patient's pain is **the patient's own report**. All other information is assessed as supporting this report. However, when this method is restricted or unavailable, **physical signs and symptoms** can help the nurse's assessment capabilities. It is important to be familiar with the patient's **baseline** or resting information to give a clear picture of the changes the body may go through when experiencing significant pain. Systolic blood pressure, heart rate, and respirations may all increase above the patient's normal parameters. Tightness or tension may be felt in major muscle groups. Posturing can also occur: the patient may guard areas of the body, curl themselves up into a fetal position, or hold only certain body portions rigid. Calling out, increased volume in speech, and moaning can also be indicators. Facial expressions, such as flat affect or grimacing, and distraction from their surroundings also indicate a significant increase in stressful stimuli.

PAIN ASSESSMENT TOOLS
ABCDE MNEMONIC APPROACH TO PAIN ASSESSMENT

The Agency for Healthcare Policy and Research recommends use of the **ABCDE method** for assessing and managing pain:

- **A**sking the patient about the extent of pain and assessing systematically.
- **B**elieving that the degree of pain the patient reports is accurate.
- **C**hoosing the appropriate method of pain control for the patient and circumstances.
- **D**elivering pain interventions appropriately and in a timely, logical manner.
- **E**mpowering patients and family by helping them to have control of the course of treatment.

The **5 key elements of pain assessment** include:

- **Quality**: Words are used to describe pain, such as *burning*, *stabbing*, *deep*, *shooting*, and *sharp*. Some may complain of pressure, squeezing, and discomfort rather than pain.
- **Intensity**: Use of a 0-10 scale or other appropriate scale to quantify the degree of pain.
- **Location**: Where does the patient indicate pain?
- **Duration**: Is it constant; does it come and go; is there breakthrough pain?
- **Aggravating/alleviating factors**: What increases the intensity of pain and what relieves the pain?

UNIDIMENSIONAL TOOLS FOR PAIN ASSESSMENT

Unidimensional tools for pain assessment focus on one aspect only: the patient's level of pain. Tools include:

- **Visual analog/numeric rating scale**: A 1-10 rating scale presented visually or verbally from which the patient chooses a number to describe the degree of pain the patient is experiencing. Zero represents no pain, 1 very mild pain, and 10 the most severe pain the patient can imagine.
- **Descriptive**: Pain is described in simple terms that a patient can choose from: mild, moderate, or severe. This may be especially helpful for patients from other countries or cultures where the 1-10 scale is not generally used.

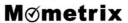

- **FACES**: A chart shows a facial expression scale of simple drawings showing faces with different emotions, such as happiness, fear, and pain. Used primarily for children over age 3 and for nonverbal adults, although both a child's and an adult's version are available. A revised version applies numeric values to expressions so that pain can be assessed according to a numeric rating scale as well.

> **Review Video: How to Accurately Assess Pain**
> Visit mometrix.com/academy and enter code: 693250
>
> **Review Video: Assessment Tools for Pain**
> Visit mometrix.com/academy and enter code: 634001

MULTIDIMENSIONAL TOOLS FOR PAIN ASSESSMENT

Multidimensional tools used for pain assessment include:

- **Multidimensional pain inventory**: The patient begins by identifying a significant other and then answering 20 questions (rating scale 0-6) about the current rate of pain, the degree of interference in daily life, the ability to work, satisfaction from social/recreational activities, support level of the significant other, mood, pain during the previous week, changes brought about by pain, concerns of the significant other, ability to deal with pain, irritability, and anxiety.
- **Brief pain inventory**: Patients are assessed on the severity of pain (on a 1-10 scale), location of pain, impact of pain on daily function, pain medication, and amount of pain relief in the past 24 hours or the past week. They are asked if the pain interferes with general activity, walking, normal work, mood, interpersonal relations, sleep, or enjoyment of life.
- **McGill pain questionnaire**: The patient marks areas of internal and external pain on body diagrams and selects appropriate adjectives for 20 different sections regarding sensory, affective, and evaluative perceptions. For example, the questionnaire allows the patient to indicate if the pain is "flickering, quivering, pulsing, throbbing, beating, or pounding." The patient also rates present pain intensity (PPI) from 0 (none) to 5 (excruciating).

ASSESSMENT TOOLS FOR COGNITIVELY IMPAIRED OR NONVERBAL PATIENTS

The following are types of assessment tools available for use with cognitively impaired or nonverbal patients:

- **Discomfort Scale for Dementia of the Alzheimer Type (DS-DAT)**: For use with elderly persons experiencing dementia, decreased cognition, and decreased verbalization
- **Assessment of Discomfort in Dementia Protocol (ADD)**: Particularly designed for use with patients exhibiting difficult behaviors
- **Checklist of Nonverbal Pain Indicators (CNPI)**: Pain measurement with cognitive impairment
- **Noncommunicative Patient's Pain Assessment Instrument (NOPPAIN)**: Specifically for use by nursing assistants
- **Pain Assessment for the Dementing Elderly (PADE)**: Assessing physical pain behaviors
- **Pain Assessment Tool in Confused Older Adults (PATCOA)**: Focuses on the observation of nonverbal cues
- **Pain Assessment in Advanced Dementia (PAINAD)**: Adapted from the DS-DAT
- **Pain Assessment Checklist for Seniors with Limited Ability to Communicate (PACSLAC)**: To assess common and subtle symptoms
- **Abbey Pain Scale**: For late-stage dementia in nursing home environments

Functional Health Patterns

131

NEUROPATHIC PAIN SCALE

The **neuropathic pain scale** (**NPS**) is the first tool designed specifically to assess the types of pain associated with neuropathy. The NPS comprises 10 sections with 9 assessed with a 0-10 (not unpleasant to intolerable) scale:

- Intensity of pain
- Sharpness of pain
- Heat of pain
- Dullness of pain
- Coldness of pain
- Skin sensitivity to touch, clothing
- Itchiness
- Overall unpleasantness of pain
- Intensity of deep and surface pain

The 10th section asks for narrative descriptions of the **time quality** of pain. The patient chooses from three options:

- Feeling background pain all of the time with occasional flare-ups
- Feeling a single type of pain all the time
- Feeling a single type of pain sometimes while having some pain-free periods. The patient then is asked to describe the pain experienced

ASSESSING PAIN IN PEDIATRIC PATIENTS

When assessing the pediatric patient, the nurse must take into consideration the **chronological and developmental age** of the child. These factors help determine which measure the child might use to express pain, as well as treatments that might prove most successful. Assessment parameters must also include the presence of and parameters surrounding chronic illness, as well as neurological impairment. The nurse must identify the underlying cause of the pain, what nonpharmacological measures have been tried for pain control, and what methods can be used to deliver pharmacological interventions. The weight of the child in kilograms determines the appropriate dosages of medications. If the child is able to speak, do the child and the parents speak the same language as the health care provider, and are there any other obvious barriers to communication or pain relief measures?

> **Review Video: <u>Pediatric Pain Assessment</u>**
> Visit mometrix.com/academy and enter code: 264352

PRETEEN/ADOLESCENT PAIN SCALE

Pain is subjective and may be influenced by the individual's pain sensation threshold (the smallest stimulus that produces the sensation of pain) and tolerance threshold (the maximum degree of pain that a person can tolerate). The most common current pain assessment tool for preteens and adolescents is the 1-10 pain scale:

- 0 = no pain
- 1-2 = mild pain
- 3-5 = moderate pain
- 6-7 = severe pain
- 8-9 = very severe pain
- 10 = excruciating pain

However, assessment also includes information about onset, duration, and intensity. Identifying pain triggers and what relieves the pain is essential when developing a pain management plan. Children may show very different behaviors when they are in pain. Some may cry and moan with minor pain, and others may seem

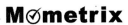

indifferent even when they are truly suffering. Thus, judging pain by behavior alone can lead to the wrong conclusions.

Numeric Pain Rating Scale

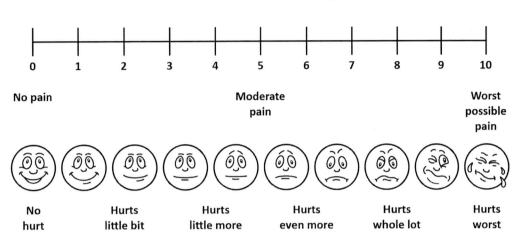

Non-Communicating Children's Pain Checklist

The **Non-Communicating Children's Pain Checklist** (NCCPC) is designed for children ages 3-8 who are cognitively impaired, but a modified version may be used for children recovering from anesthesia. The checklist contains 7 categories with sub-listings that are each scored: 0 (not occurring), 1 (occurring occasionally), 2 (occurring fairly often), 3 (occurring frequently), and NA (not applicable).

- **Vocal**: Moaning, whining, crying, screaming, yelling, or using a specific word for pain
- **Social**: Uncooperative, unhappy, withdrawn, seeking closeness, or can't be distracted
- **Facial**: Furrowed brow, eye changes, not smiling, lips tight or quivering, or clenching or grinding teeth.
- **Activity**: Not moving and quiet or agitated and fidgety.
- **Body and limbs**: Floppy, tense, rigid, spastic, pointing to a part of body that hurts, guarding part of the body, flinching, or positioning body to show pain.
- **Physiological**: Shivering, pallor, increased perspiration, tears, gasping, or holding breath
- **Eating and sleeping**: Eating less or sleeping significantly more or less than usual

The child is usually observed for 2 hours and then scored. All scores are then added together. A score of ≥7 indicates pain.

QUESTT Pediatric Pain Assessment Tool

QUESTT is designed to focus on assessment, action, and consequent reassessment for results.

- **Question** both the child and parent about the pain experience.
- **Use** assessment tools and rating scales that are appropriate to the developmental stage and situation and understanding of the child.
- **Evaluate** the patient for both behavioral and physiological changes.
- **Secure** the parent's participation in all stages of the pain evaluation and treatment process.
- **Take the cause of the pain into consideration** during the evaluation and choice of treatment methods.
- **Take action** to treat the pain appropriately, and then evaluate the results on a regular basis.

Functional Health Patterns

BARRIERS TO OPTIMAL PAIN ASSESSMENTS

Barriers to optimal pain assessments include:

- **Professional**: Health care providers may lack knowledge about pain assessment and management of different patient populations or may carry out assessments based on personal perceptions rather than validated pain assessment instruments. Some may be concerned about managing adverse effects or the patient's development of tolerance or addiction. In other cases, healthcare providers may lack empathy for patients' suffering. Lack of cultural awareness may affect interpretation of pain. For example, patients in cultures that encourage expression of pain may be assessed as having more pain than patients from cultures that value stoicism.
- **System**: The organization may lack clear policies regarding pain assessment and management, and may not have established clear guidelines for consistent use of pain assessment instruments. Additionally, supervision and accountability may be inadequate, and the organization may be concerned about costs and reimbursement for treatment.
- **Patient**: For personal or cultural reasons, patients may minimize or overstate the degree of pain, interfering with assessment. Some patients may be concerned about addiction or the effects of drugs on cognition (confusion, disorientation, lethargy) or other side effects (constipation, nausea, itching). Some may want to protect family from knowing the extent of pain.
- **Family**: Cultural biases may influence how the family responds to a patient's pain, and this can influence the patient's response as well. Families may lack understanding of the role of pain assessment and management. Some lack understanding about the difference between addiction and pain control at the end of life.
- **Society**: Concerns about drug abuse and addiction often permeate society and influence societal attitudes toward pain control and appropriate drugs to use. Laws and regulations may make access to certain drugs, such as those derived from marijuana, difficult or impossible to obtain.

INFLUENTIAL FACTORS IN PAIN PERCEPTION

Factors that can influence the perception of pain include:

- **Emotional state/Attitude**: Patients who are extremely upset or anxious may be so overwhelmed they don't feel the pain, or they may experience pain as more severe than those who are relaxed and calm. If patients expect to suffer from pain, they are also more likely to report severe pain than patients who expect that their pain will be controlled.
- **Cultural expectations**: Perception may vary according to cultural beliefs about pain. For example, if a patient believes that pain is punishment, the patient may agonize over past sins. If a patient believes that pain is fate and reflects karma, then the patient may feel that bearing pain is necessary.
- **Pain threshold**: Different patients simply perceive and experience pain to different degrees. What may be a minor pain to one individual may be severe to another.

EFFECTS OF GENDER ON PAIN EXPERIENCE

Gender can affect pain sensitivity, tolerance, distress, and exaggeration of pain, and the patient's willingness to report pain, as well as displayed nonverbal cues concerning the pain experience. Studies indicate that women generally have **lower pain thresholds** and **less tolerance** for noxious stimuli or pain factors that hinder them from doing things they enjoy. Women seek help for pain-related problems sooner than men and respond better to therapy. Women also experience more **visceral pain** than men. Men are more prone to experience **somatic pain** and show more stoicism regarding pain experiences than women. **Neuropathic pain** seems to be experienced equally between men and women. Nurses need to be careful that biases concerning gender experiences with pain do not skew their assessments of pain. However, they need to be aware that pain experiences are always individual and may differ between the sexes.

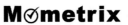

CULTURAL CONSIDERATIONS FOR PAIN MANAGEMENT

The following are cultural considerations for pain management:

- **American Indian** and **Alaskan natives** may be unwilling to show pain or request medications. Pain is a difficulty that must be endured rather than treated.
- **Asian and Pacific Islanders** may not vocalize pain and may have an interest in pursuing nontraditional and nonpharmacological treatments to help relieve pain.
- **Black and African American** cultures may tend to openly express their pain but still believe that it is to be endured. They may avoid medication because of personal fears of addiction or cultural stigmatism.
- **Hispanic cultures** may value the ability to endure pain and suffering as a personal quality of strength. Expression of pain, especially for a male, may be considered a sign of weakness. They may feel that pain is a form of divine punishment or trial.

PSYCHOLOGICAL FACTORS IN EXPERIENCE OF PAIN

Psychological factors that may influence a patient's experience of pain include:

- **Fear**: The fear of pain and the anticipation of having pain are factors in how much pain a person feels, because the fear stimulates areas of the brain that focus attention on the body so that the patient experiences an increased sensation of pain. Fear also causes muscles to tense, blood pressure to increase, and the heart rate to increase, and all of these can exacerbate the perception of pain. While pain medications may be necessary, practicing relaxation and mindfulness exercises may help to reduce anxiety and have a positive effect.
- **Depression**: The same neurotransmitters that transmit sensations of pain are also those that transmit moods, so many people with depression present first with complaints of pain or discomfort, and this can result in chronic pain if the depression is not resolved. In some cases, pain may lead to depression, but then the depression worsens the pain so it becomes a cycle of worsening discomfort. Patients may benefit from cognitive behavioral therapy or medication such as SSRIs.

PAIN DOCUMENTATION IN MEDICAL RECORDS

Recommendations for **pain documentation** in the medical record include:

- Describe the time of onset, the location of pain, the character of the pain, and the degree of pain, using a validated pain assessment instrument (either a self-reporting instrument, such as the visual analog scale, or one based on observation, such as PAINAD).
- Document all interventions, both pharmacological (opioids, adjuvants) and nonpharmacological (positioning, massage, relaxation exercises), including the time, the dosage, and the method of administration.
- Assess and document the initial response to the medication based on the expected response time. For example, an IV medication should take effect almost immediately, but oral medications may take up to 20 minutes to take effect.
- Assess and document the duration of response based on the expected duration of the medication. For example, if a medication response is expected to last for 6 hours, the patient's pain level should be assessed at least every 2 hours and more frequently if the rate of pain increases.
- Describe any adverse effects, such as itching or nausea.

> **Review Video: Pain Assessment Documentation**
> Visit mometrix.com/academy and enter code: 248521

Functional Health Patterns

CLASSES OF DRUGS AFFECTING THE CNS

Most drugs affecting the central nervous system (CNS) are antidepressants, anticonvulsants, or anticholinergics.

- **Antidepressants** are used to prevent or control depression. They are primarily either tricyclic antidepressants (made up of three linked carbon rings), such as doxepin (Silenor) or clomipramine (Anafranil), or selective serotonin reuptake inhibitors, such as paroxetine (Paxil) or fluoxetine (Prozac). There are also some unique antidepressants such as bupropion (Wellbutrin).
- **Anticonvulsants**, used to prevent or reduce seizures, are classified as first or second generation (referring to sequence of development). First-generation drugs include phenytoin (Dilantin), carbamazepine (Tegretol), and valproic acid (Depakote and others). Topiramate (Topamax) is an example of a second-generation drug.
- **Anticholinergics** block nerve impulses controlling the stress response. These drugs include benztropine (Cogentin). Anticholinergics are all primarily used to treat Parkinsonism, which is also responsive to a separate antiparkinsonian drug called carbidopa or levodopa (Sinemet, etc.) and other classes of drugs. Dopamine agonists, ergot derivatives, and other formulations also affect the CNS.

CENTRAL LINES, PORTS, AND CATHETERS
TRIPLE-LUMEN CENTRAL LINES

The CRRN must be familiar with triple-lumen central lines and their management when dealing with particular patients. **Triple-lumen central lines**, such as the Hickman catheter, are most often placed in the internal jugular or subclavian vein, but PICCs (peripherally inserted central catheters) may also have triple lumens. A triple-lumen central line is a catheter with three internal channels so that each channel can be used for a different purpose. For example, one may be used for total parenteral nutrition (TPN), another for medications, and a third for blood draws and monitoring. The exit site must be carefully monitored for signs of infection, and the lumens must be flushed before and after each use, usually with saline, although some may use heparin. Open-ended catheters are typically flushed with heparin because the tip is not smooth and can result in blood turbulence and clotting. These catheters can be identified by the presence of a clamp. Valved, or closed-end, catheters do not require heparin flushes and have no clamp. Some central lines are tunneled, meaning they enter into the skin, but tunnel under the skin prior to entering into the vein, especially if they will be left in place for extended periods of time. Caps should be color coded and/or labeled in some way to ensure that the correct lumen is used for treatments.

HEMODIALYSIS ACCESS CATHETERS

Hemodialysis access catheters may be in place in the CRRN's patient. These catheters are typically tunneled double-lumen catheters placed in the internal jugular vein but may be placed in the femoral vein for temporary acute vascular access. Patients with femoral vein access must remain on bedrest while the catheter is in place. Use of the subclavian vein is generally avoided in those who will have chronic dialysis because of the risk of subclavian vein stenosis, which will prevent use of the ipsilateral arm for fistula placement. Non-tunneled internal jugular vein catheters should be removed within 7 days because of risk of infection. Temporary catheters should be replaced with permanent access if use is likely to exceed 7 days. Catheter access is generally temporary while patients are waiting for a fistula or graft to heal, except for patients who have no fistula or graft sites available. The catheter lumens are color coded, with the red used to withdraw blood into the dialyzer and blue used to return the cleaned blood to the patient.

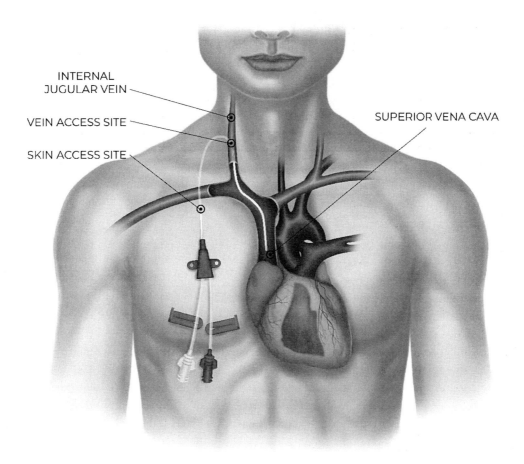

VENOUS ACCESS PORTS

A venous access port is an implanted central line device that can be left in place for extended periods, up to 5 years or longer. The device contains a small reservoir, which is inserted into the upper chest, and a catheter, which is fixed to the port and fed through the internal jugular vein (preferred) or subclavian vein (increased risk of pneumothorax) into the superior vena cava near the right atrium of the heart. This device is implanted for those who require long-term intermittent treatments, such as transfusions or chemotherapy, although a needle can be left in place for up to a week for extended intravenous therapy. Once the port has healed, it can generally be used for up to 2000 treatments. The port can also be used to take blood samples by those trained to do so. A special needle, such as the curved Huber needle, is usually used for access.

MEDICAL EQUIPMENT AND TECHNOLOGY

TENS AND BACLOFEN PUMP

A **transcutaneous electrical nerve stimulation** (TENS) unit is a battery-operated device that delivers low-voltage electrical current through 2 or 4 electrodes for pain management. Generally, the current should be applied at an intensity that is strong, but does not induce pain itself. This interferes with the pain signals being sent to the brain and may stimulate the release of endorphins. TENS is commonly used for back and neck pain, arthritic pain, and sports injuries. Treatments are usually at least 30 minutes, 3 or 4 times daily, although some individuals use the device for hours at a time without harm. Pain relief may persist for a few minutes to up to 18 or more hours after treatment.

A **baclofen pump** is a lithium battery-powered device implanted under the skin of the abdomen. A catheter leading from the pump is inserted into the spinal column to administer baclofen, a muscle relaxer medication that reduces spasticity. The baclofen pump is commonly used for those with cerebral palsy, stroke, or spinal

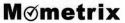

cord or brain injuries that result in tight, stiff muscles. Baclofen is injected through the skin to refill the pump every 2 to 3 months. The device battery usually lasts 4 to 7 years.

LVADs

The **left ventricular assist device** (LVAD) is implanted in the chest; it takes blood from the base of the left ventricle though a cannula to the small LVAD pump, and through an outflow cannula directly into the aorta to allow the left ventricle to rest. The LVAD pump is attached through a percutaneous line to an external controller and battery pack with rechargeable batteries. The LVAD is most commonly used for individuals with end-stage heart failure who are awaiting a heart transplant, or as a destination treatment for those who are not candidates for transplantation. Individuals are sometimes able to stay on the LVAD for years with relief of many of their symptoms because the blood is circulating more effectively. A newer LVAD, the Impella 2.5, is an FDA-approved mini heart pump that is placed in the left ventricle through a catheter and activated by an external console. This device is used for temporary left ventricular assist during procedures such as stenting or angioplasty.

Sensory Function

ANATOMY OF THE EYE

There are three layers in the eye.

- The outer layer is the **protective fibrous tunic,** comprising the membranous *cornea* in the front (covering the iris and pupil) and the *sclera* or tough outer coating of the eyeball.
- The central layer is called the **vascular tunic**. It comprises the following:
  - The *iris*, which is the colored muscular part surrounding the pupil
  - The *ciliary body*, which is also muscular and controls the shape of the lens
  - The *choroid*, which contains blood vessels and pigmented cells and removes waste from the front of the retina
- The inside layer is called the **nervous tunic** because it contains the *retina*, a light-sensitive membrane in the rear of the eye that receives images from the lens and communicates them to the brain via the optic nerve. The retina is composed of **rods**, which are sensitive to dim light and account for peripheral vision, and **cones**, which are sensitive to colors and are responsible for daylight vision.

Other eye structures include the eyelids, the membranous conjunctiva lining the lids, the aqueous lens (which changes shape to accommodate near versus far vision), cavities that primarily control pressure in the eye called the aqueous (anterior) and vitreous humors, and a system of glands and ducts controlling tear production and secretion called the lacrimal apparatus.

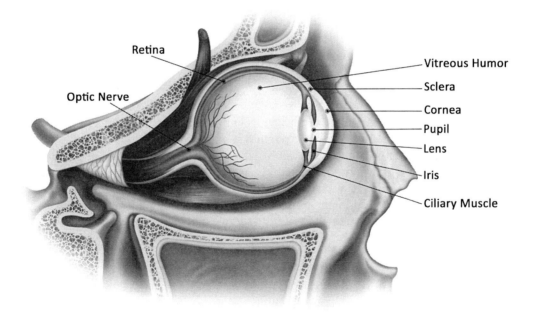

NEURONAL PATHWAYS ASSOCIATED WITH THE EYE

Light rays enter the eye through the **pupil**, which is controlled by the darker adjoining iris, and an image is recorded on the retina in the posterior of the eye. Light passing through the center of the visual field crisscrosses at the **retina**. There are also other visual fields, such as those associated with peripheral vision. At the retina, electrical impulses are generated. These travel along the optic nerves through the **optic chiasma**, or crossing point, into optic tracts and then into the **lateral geniculate nuclei** on the opposite side. These nuclei are located in the geniculate body of the **thalamus**, which is further enclosed by the optic radiations, terminating in the visual cortex of the **occipital lobe** of the brain, where the impulses are deciphered.

TESTS TO EVALUATE VISION

The first step in assessment of vision is a thorough history. Individuals are considered to be visually impaired if they indicate that they are blind in one or both eyes. The most common visual acuity test is the **Snellen reading test**. The individual being tested stands 20 feet away from an eye chart, and glasses may be worn if needed. Each eye is separately tested and rated as $20/x$, with x being the number of feet away a person with normal vision can read what the examinee can see at 20 feet. **Visual fields** should also be checked by bracing the patient's head and having them follow the movement of a pen; restricted eye movement may indicate visual lesions. The eyelids, conjunctiva, sclera, and pupil are visually inspected to look for evidence of **inflammation** and underlying medical problems. The size and shape of the **pupil** is examined (pupil should be 3–5 mm). **Pupillary reaction** is tested by moving a penlight across the visual field from a distance and assessing whether the pupils converge and constrict symmetrically in response. The **lacrimal sacs** and **eyelids** are examined to look for obstructions or inflammation.

VISUAL DISTURBANCES

BLINDNESS

A person is considered **legally blind** when they have a corrected visual acuity of at least 20/200 (meaning the individual can see only 1/10 the amount of a normal person) in the stronger eye. Another term, **functional blindness**, is used to describe people who cannot see light and are totally blind, but without any identifiable cause for the blindness. An individual is considered to have **low vision** if their Snellen reading is a minimum of 20/40. The most prevalent cause of blindness and low vision in Caucasians is **macular degeneration**, the progressive deterioration of the macula lutea, resulting in central vision deficit. The most common causes of blindness and poor vision in African Americans are **cataracts** and **glaucoma**. Diabetic retinopathy can also precipitate visual shortfalls in certain fields.

VISION DISTURBANCES OTHER THAN BLINDNESS

A nurse or other professional may diagnose a number of **visual disturbances** that are not blindness. The most widespread type of visual impairment is a **refractive error**, which is blurriness due to a lack of precise retinal focus; this is completely treatable using corrective lenses. There are several types of **intraocular diseases**, notably cataracts, glaucoma, and retinal detachment. **Cataracts** are an eye disease in which the lens becomes covered with an opaque film that impedes the passage of light and causes blurriness, image distortion, and problems perceiving colors; treatment is generally removal of the cataracts. **Glaucoma** is generally imperceptible high pressure within the eyeball that can eventually damage the optic nerve and cause vision loss if untreated; it is treated with eye drops containing prostaglandins (preferred treatment) or β-blockers, laser therapy, or surgery. A serious variant is **closed-angle glaucoma**, in which displacement of the iris occurs, pressure increases rapidly, and there is acute pain. β-blockers combined with an α2-agonist (iopidine) are administered in acute closed-angle glaucoma to rapidly reduce intraocular pressure. With **retinal detachment**, the rods and cones deteriorate, and a surgical vitrectomy is generally performed.

> **Review Video: <u>Glaucoma and Cataracts</u>**
> Visit mometrix.com/academy and enter code: 279024

HEMIANOPSIA

Hemianopsia is blindness affecting half of the visual field in one or both eyes after brain injuries or other impairments. There are three types of hemianopsia.

- The most common type is **homonymous hemianopsia**, in which vision is lost in different visual fields of each eye. For example, the temporal part (affecting peripheral vision) is lost in one eye, and the nasal field (which is more centrally located) is lost in the other.
- Another type is **bitemporal hemianopsia**, in which peripheral vision in both eyes is affected.

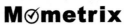

- Another type is **altitudinal**. A person can have anopsia or blindness in one eye or have vision loss in one area of a single eye, such as right nasal hemianopsia, which is visual impairment affecting only the nasal or overlap field.

REHABILITATION APPROACHES FOR PEOPLE WITH LOW VISION

Rehabilitation approaches for people with low vision center around the use of large font or instruments to magnify the images or change the light received in some way. Many large-font books and other documents are currently available, and a person can use a movable reading triangle to focus on small passages of reading material. Depending on the distance of the object(s) being observed, instruments for **magnification** include microscopes for close work, magnifying glasses for reading and writing, and binoculars or field glasses (both of which are really telescopes) for distant observations. The major drawback to all of these is that they all require hand use and coordination. **Eyeglasses** can be modified to reduce glare, either through use of light filters over the glasses or by incorporation of tinted lenses. **Glass prisms** that redirect images in the retina can be utilized as adjuncts to promote vision, but again, these require use of the hands.

HELPING THE VISUALLY IMPAIRED INDIVIDUAL DEAL WITH DAILY LIFE

The nurse's **manner of speaking** to the patient is important. For example, the nurse should speak in a natural tone of voice with very clear instructions that are separated into small, discrete steps. The nurse can help the visually impaired patient cope with daily life by **organizing** the patient's personal space, maintaining the **layout** of personal items and furniture, and using **aids** such as symbols sewn on clothing to help the person identify objects. There are techniques that can be utilized in regard to **meals**, such as describing the location of foods on plates in terms of clock positions, or holding glasses at a certain level to avoid exposure to overly hot or cold liquids. When providing **walking assistance**, the helper should be slightly ahead of the visually impaired patient while the patient clasps the helper's arm above the elbow with their thumb on the outside; if both people keep their arms near their bodies, the patient can feel and respond to movements.

ANATOMY OF THE EAR

The ear is divided into three sections: the external auditory area, the middle ear, and the inner ear. The **external auditory canal** consists of the outer ear, the approximately 1-inch-long auditory canal, and the tympanic membrane, which gathers sound waves. The air-filled **middle ear** is a narrow section that primarily transfers pressure variations; the eustachian tube connects this part to the pharynx as well for pressure equalization. After traveling through the oval window, the pressure waves are received by the **inner ear** and ultimately transferred to a bony portion called the cochlea. The **organ of Corti** is the hearing sensory organ within the cochlea; it contains hair cells that are shifted by the sound waves and converted into neural responses transmitted via the acoustic nerve to the brain. The inner ear also preserves balance and equilibrium. The inner ear also includes bony elements, the vestibule and three semicircular canals, that contain nerve receptors as well as membranous portions called the utricle and saccule.

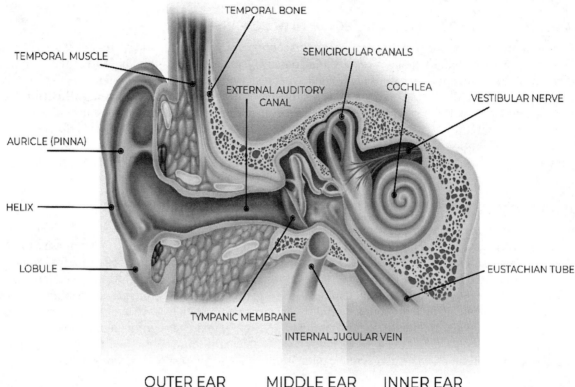

OUTER EAR   MIDDLE EAR   INNER EAR

HEARING ASSESSMENT TECHNIQUES

A hearing assessment should be completed by the rehabilitation nurse upon initial patient contact. The **external ear** should be examined visually and palpated for tenderness, and the **ear canal** should be inspected using an otoscope. In addition, **hearing acuity** should be assessed using one or more of the following tests.

- **Earphones** can be used to test air conduction of sound.
- Several techniques use a **tuning fork** to test bone conduction of sound. The techniques used are direct stimulus of the inner ear, Weber's test (placing the tuning fork at midline to test symmetry of response), or Rinne's test (placing the tuning fork near the mastoid process and pinna to differentiate between bone and air conduction, which is usually greater).
- **Audiometry** uses specific tone frequencies.
- **Speech audiometry** evaluates the percentage of specific two-syllable words understood.
- **Tympanometry** quantifies the energy absorbed by the middle ear when sound is introduced into the canal.
- Other tests include acoustic **reflex testing**, **otoacoustic emissions**, and the **auditory brainstem response** (which examines electric waveforms).

TYPES OF HEARING LOSS

A nurse or other clinician might find one of two types of hearing loss in a hearing-impaired patient. The first is **conductive hearing loss**, indicating a lack of proper sound wave transmission. **Otitis media**, ear infection and associated inflammation, is the greatest cause of conductive hearing loss, and smoking is also a risk factor. **Sensorineural hearing loss** is less common but more critical. About 0.1% of the population is born with sensorineural hearing loss or deafness due to sensory hair cell issues or neural defects of the spiral ganglion cells. This type of hearing loss can also be acquired through certain infections, in conjunction with autoimmune

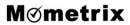

diseases, through use of potentially ototoxic drugs (such as cisplatin and aminoglycosides), exposure to loud sounds, head trauma, spongy bone growth in the inner ear (called otosclerosis), or the presence of a benign tumor (called acoustic neuroma). The latter two conditions can precipitate **balance problems** and possibly other problems in addition to hearing loss.

> **Review Video: What is Otitis Media?**
> Visit mometrix.com/academy and enter code: 328778

INTERVENTIONS FOR HEARING LOSS

There are several available types of **hearing aids** that amplify sound (acoustic aids), utilize skull bones to transmit sound (conduction aids), or functionally replace the cochlea through implantation (cochlear implants). **American Sign Language** is an official language developed and used in the United States and Canada for communication with and among the hearing impaired. Hearing-impaired people can use the **internet** for correspondence. There are also a number of assistive listening devices, computer aids, and telephone configurations that are useful. **Assistive listening devices** include microphones, headphones, pocket talkers, and systems that can be used in group settings such as infrared connections or permanent installations. There are devices that can be connected to **telephones** to amplify sound; and there are TTYs and TDDs (teletypewriters and telecommunications devices for the deaf), and relay services using these TTYs and TDDs. There are also several **automatic speech recognition (ASR) systems** that use microphones to pick up speech and interpret it on a computer screen. **Alarm systems** are available with visual or vibrating indicators for doorbells, telephones, and smoke alarms.

SENSE OF SMELL

In the epithelium of the nose, odors are converted into chemicals that arouse **olfactory receptors** in the cilia of the nasal passages. Sensory responses are then transported through the **olfactory bulb and tract** to portions of the **cerebral cortex** without thalamic involvement. Two separate smell pathways are generated in the brain, one involved with the **perception of odor and smell** and the other related to the **memory of and emotional response to the smell**. Some loss of the sense of smell is often found in geriatric patients, but it can also be observed along with cognitive impairment, strokes, vitamin deficiencies, radiation, certain drugs, respiratory infections, and any untoward stimulus of the nasal cavity. Olfactory sensation can be **assessed** by having the patient shut their eyes and smell ampoules of coffee, peppermint oil, and lemon juice to see if the patient can distinguish them. Olfactory problems can lead to weight issues, which should be monitored, and an inability to sense dangerous situations such as gas leaks or fires.

SENSE OF TASTE

Alterations in the sense of taste are not life-threatening, but they can affect quality of life. Taste can be affected by aging, cigarette use, desquamation of the tongue, radiation of the area, infections, and strokes. **Taste buds** are nerve endings on the surface of the tongue and in the mouth that send signals through the vagus, glossopharyngeal, and facial nerves to the thalamus and then to the **ipsilateral gustatory cortex** in the cerebrum. Taste sensations can be **evaluated** in patients with poor appetites or invariable responses to foods. This is done by saturating cotton swabs with solutions of sugar, salt, lemon juice, or coffee and then placing one swab at a time on the tongue to see if the person can distinguish the category (sweet, salty, sour, and bitter, respectively).

SENSES OF TOUCH AND SENSATION

There are six kinds of sensory receptors.

- The **mechanoreceptors** are situated within the skin and are involved with the sensations of touch, vibration, flutter, and pressure.
- **Proprioceptors** are located in muscles and other soft tissues associated with sense of position.
- **Thermoreceptors** are located in the skin and sense heat and cold.
- **Nociceptors** react to pain or injury.

Functional Health Patterns

- **Chemoreceptors** respond to chemical stimuli.
- **Photic receptors** respond to light.

The latter two are not particularly associated with touch. Each receptor converts energy from the stimulus into an electrical signal, which is carried to the brain or spinal cord. Sensation is disturbed in many neurological diseases.

SENSORY ASSESSMENT TECHNIQUES

If a patient demonstrates sensory impairment, there are a number of assessment techniques that can be utilized. The patient always closes their eyes during these tests.

- The **tactile sense** can be evaluated by touching the patient with a cotton swab at various points and asking when the patient feels the prodding; this can separate normal from abnormal tactile sensation.
- The sense of **temperature** is assessed by placing warm or cold glasses against the patient's skin.
- **Vibratory sense** can be evaluated by placing a vibrating tuning fork against a limb.
- **Proprioception** can be tested by moving one of the patient's toes or fingers and asking the patient to identify the digit.
- **Pain discrimination** is assessed by pricking with an open safety pin and having the person describe the location and feeling (sharp or dull) of the prick. There is also a test called **two-point discrimination** in which two skin pricks (in this case usually with toothpicks) are done, and the individual must determine the distance between them.

PERCEPTION

Perception is a complex process involving observation, integration, and understanding of stimuli. Different types of stimuli are processed in either the right or left parietal lobe of the cerebral cortex. For example, spatial and textural information is processed in the **right lobe**, whereas reading and writing are understood through processing in the **left lobe**. Many perception defects are associated with brain injuries. Problems related to **body image or arrangement** are common, including asomatognosia (ignorance of one's own body parts and structure), inability to discriminate between left and right, visual spatial neglect (lack of response on affected side), anosognosia (denial of one's paralysis), and finger agnosia (inability to distinguish specific fingers). Various types of **spatial relation disorders** are also prevalent, such as problems distinguishing distances, distinguishing an object from its background, or distinguishing similar forms. Agnosia (the partial or total loss of recognition of familiar objects) and apraxia (the incapacity to perform complex movements) are also perception problems.

MANAGEMENT OF PERCEPTION DEFICITS

There are some broad approaches that can be used to **manage perception deficits**. These include a **sensorimotor approach**, which attempts to organize the thought pattern by controlling sensory stimulation and the desired motor response, and the **functional approach**, which uses repetition of tasks to foster their relearning. Another general method utilized is to make the connection between similar applications in slightly different tasks, known as **transfer of training**. Specific defects call for special types of management as well. For example, patients with visual spatial neglect most often are unaware of the left side of their body; this means the nurse's job is to modify the milieu and increase the patients' awareness of the environment on that side through techniques that stimulate their senses there. Objects may need to be tagged for people with spatial relation disorders. Other senses may need to be incorporated into identification of objects for patients with agnosia.

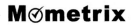

Safety Concerns

BURN INJURIES
TYPES AND CLASSIFICATIONS
Burn injuries may be chemical, electrical, or thermal, and are assessed by the area, percentage of the body burned, and depth:

- **First-degree burns** are superficial and affect the epidermis, causing erythema and pain.
- **Second-degree burns** extend through the dermis (partial thickness), resulting in blistering and sloughing of epidermis.
- **Third-degree burns** affect underlying tissue, including vasculature, muscles, and nerves (full thickness).

Burns are classified according to the **American Burn Association's criteria**:

- **Minor**: Less than 10% body surface area (BSA). 2% BSA with third degree without serious risk to face, hands, feet, or perineum.
- **Moderate**: 10-20% combined second- and third-degree burns (children younger than 10 years or adults older than 40 years). 10% or less full thickness without serious risk to face, hands, feet, or perineum.
- **Major**: 20% BSA; at least 10% third-degree burns. All burns to face, hands, feet, or perineum that will result in functional/cosmetic defect. Burns with inhalation or other major trauma.

SYSTEMIC COMPLICATIONS
Burn injuries begin with the skin but can affect all organs and body systems, especially with a major burn:

- **Cardiovascular**: Cardiac output may fall by 50% as capillary permeability increases with vasodilation and fluid leaks from the tissues.
- **Urinary**: Decreased blood flow causes kidneys to increase ADH, which increases oliguria. BUN and creatinine levels increase. Cell destruction may block tubules, and hematuria may result from hemolysis.
- **Pulmonary**: Injury may result from smoke inhalation or (rarely) aspiration of hot liquid. Pulmonary injury is a leading cause of death from burns and is classified according to the degree of damage:
  - *First*: Singed eyebrows and nasal hairs with possible soot in airways and slight edema
  - *Second*: (At 24 hours) Stridor, dyspnea, and tachypnea with edema and erythema of upper airway, including area of vocal cords and epiglottis
  - *Third*: (At 72 hours) Worsening symptoms if not intubated and if intubated, bronchorrhea and tachypnea with edematous, secreting tissue
- **Neurological**: Encephalopathy may develop from lack of oxygen, decreased blood volume and sepsis. Hallucinations, alterations in consciousness, seizures, and coma may result.
- **Gastrointestinal**: Ileus and ulcerations of mucosa often result from poor circulation. Ileus usually clears within 48-72 hours, but if it returns it is often indicative of sepsis.
- **Endocrine/metabolic:** The sympathetic nervous system stimulates the adrenals to release epinephrine and norepinephrine to increase cardiac output and cortisol for wound healing. The metabolic rate increases markedly. Electrolyte loss occurs with fluid loss from exposed tissue, especially phosphorus, calcium, and sodium, with an increase in potassium levels. Electrolyte imbalance can be life-threatening if burns cover >20% of BSA. Glycogen depletion occurs within 12-24 hours and protein breakdown and muscle wasting occurs without sufficient intake of protein.

MANAGEMENT

Management of burn injuries must include both wound care and systemic care to avoid complications that can be life threatening. **Treatment** includes:

- Establishment of airway and treatment for inhalation injury as indicated:
  - Supplemental oxygen, incentive spirometry, nasotracheal suctioning
  - Humidification
  - Bronchoscopy as needed to evaluate bronchospasm and edema
  - β-Agonists for bronchospasm, followed by aminophylline if ineffective
  - Intubation and ventilation if there are indications of respiratory failure (This should be done prior to failure. Tracheostomy may be done if ventilation >14 days.)
- Intravenous fluids and electrolytes, based on weight and extent of burn. Parkland formula: Fluid replacement (mL) in first 24 hours = (mass in kg) × (body % burned) × 400
- Enteral feedings, usually with small lumen feeding tube into the duodenum
- NG tube for gastric decompression to prevent aspiration
- Indwelling catheter to monitor urinary output. Urinary output should be 0.5-2 mL/kg/hr
- Analgesia for reduction of pain and anxiety
- Topical and systemic antibiotics
- Wound care with removal of eschar and dressings as indicated

PHASES OF BURN CARE AND THE WOUND HEALING PROCESS

The first phase of burn care is the **emergent or resuscitative stage**, generally performed at the injury site or in the emergency room, in which critical issues are addressed. This can involve airway clearance, fluid replacement, infection control procedures, and general support. The **acute phase** is considered to be the time from burn injury to stabilization and coverage of full-thickness lesions with skin. The goals during this phase are stabilization of all relevant systems, wound care, control of infections, nutritional support, and maintenance of functionality and mobility. Wound healing depends on the thickness of the burn. Partial-thickness burns heal through marginal cell migration to form fresh epithelium in about 2–3 weeks. Full-thickness burns heal through the release of phagocytes by white blood cells to clear the wound area, collagen secretion, and epithelial cell migration to restore capillary networks and circulation. Then the patient enters the **rehabilitative phase**, in which issues such as life and workplace reentry, body image, minimizing muscle tightening from scarring, and maintaining range of motion and strength are addressed.

INTERVENTIONS FOR IMPAIRED SKIN INTEGRITY AFTER BURNS

During the **acute phase** of a burn injury, any necessary debridement, scab removal, and grafting are performed. During the **rehabilitative phase**, the nurse is primarily responsible for wound care and maintaining skin integrity. This usually involves use of topical agents such as 1% silver sulfadiazine or mafenide acetate to avoid infection of the fragile skin area. Skin dryness can be addressed with topical emollients made up of both water and lipids because these will both absorb and slow down evaporation. Agents to control pruritus (itchiness) are usually necessary. Both systemic drugs such as antihistamines and topical antipruritic lotions incorporating menthol, camphor, or anesthetics are helpful. The patient should be instructed to stay out of the sun or cover up when outside for at least a half-year to avoid sunburn and permanent hyperpigmentation of the burned area. A related issue is the possible imbalance of nutritional requirements due to loss of bodily fluids.

INTERVENTIONS FOR IMPAIRED PHYSICAL MOBILITY RESULTING FROM BURN INJURIES

Depending on the severity and site of burns, appropriate **positioning** of the patient can be important to preserve elements of mobility. The goals of proper position during the acute phase are minimization of edema and maintenance of joint alignment and tendon balance to avoid contracture. The main emphasis during the rehabilitative stage is **contracture prevention**. When the patient is lying flat, contracture formation can be hindered by using various pillows, a neck roll or brace, braces to keep the knee extended, and/or a footboard

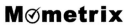

with a pad. Since joints often become stiff and muscles can subsequently tighten, a daily **exercise routine** incorporating a full set of range-of-motion exercises should be instituted. A **splint** may be used temporarily to maintain joint structures. A customized **compression garment** usually needs to be ordered and worn constantly by the patient for up to 2 years to prevent and/or reduce hypertrophy scarring.

NURSING DIAGNOSES AND INTERVENTIONS RELATED TO THE REHABILITATIVE PHASE OF BURN RECOVERY

The other nursing diagnoses and interventions related to the rehabilitative phase of burn recovery are either related to pain management, ineffective health maintenance, or psychosocial adjustment. **Chronic pain** is managed through prescribed medications, making the patient comfortable, and implementing alternative techniques. The rehabilitation nurse can help the patient with **ineffective health maintenance** by educating them about lifestyle changes and self-care techniques. **Psychosocial issues** can include a disturbed body image, social isolation, and changes in family dynamics. The patient may experience post-trauma syndrome prompted by injury flashbacks. Depending on the severity and location of the burn, a return to sexuality may be difficult, or going back to work in a previous capacity may be affected. The nurse can serve as a support and educational resource.

DRUGS FOR BURN TREATMENT

There are several commonly used drugs for the deterrence and treatment of infections that can result from second- or third-degree burns. All are topically applied. The first is **silver sulfadiazine** (SSD) in a 1% concentration. After wounds have been cleaned and debrided, SSD is spread over the area under sterile conditions once or twice daily. **Nanocrystalline silver** has also proven effective in deterring infection and promoting healing. Another drug is **mafenide acetate**, which is available as either an 8.5% cream, or a powder that must be diluted to a 5% solution in either sterile water or saline. This is an alternative to SSD. Mafenide acetate is applied one to two times a day to the area. It is contraindicated for patients with sulfite allergies or kidney failure. **Bismuth-impregnated gauze** is a petroleum-impregnated dressing that is especially effective in treating grafts and partial-thickness burns, and is applied once in a single layer over the burn site.

FALLS

Falls are the most commonly occurring adverse event in the hospital setting. Confusion and agitation are factors that contribute to an increased risk for falling. In addition, impaired balance or gait, orthostatic hypotension, altered mobility, a history of falling, advanced age, and the use of certain medications are risk factors. Approximately 30% of patient falls result in injury, some of which can significantly contribute to an increase in morbidity and mortality, including fractures and subdural hematomas. Both physical and environmental factors contribute to patient falls, some of which are preventable. Fall prevention strategies include utilization of a standardized fall risk assessment to determine the patient's level of risk and subsequent care planning and interventions individualized to the patient. Fall prevention should also be balanced with progressive mobility.

NURSING INTERVENTIONS TO DECREASE RISK OF FALLS FOR ELDERLY PATIENTS

If the patient is a new admission or has been recently moved, the nurse's main job is to **orient** the patient to the new environment and make it patient-friendly. If it is known that the individual has a history of falls or physical weakness, additional **environmental adaptations**—such as a bedside commode, bed alarm devices, and anti-slip mats—are needed. The nurse needs to closely watch the patient during **ambulation**. If the patient has **postural hypotension**, then elastic stockings and at least 1.5 liters of hydration per day are required. If the patient is or could be **incontinent**, regular voiding and easy access to the bathroom are indicated. The nurse needs to assess and monitor the patient's **drug use**, including regular use of pain medications if necessary. If the individual has **visual impairments**, lighting must be adequate, the environment must be unobstructed, and the patient's glasses must be usable. Patients with **altered mental status** need relaxing environments and close supervision. Those with **emotional or other psychosocial problems** should be assessed by a professional and given appropriate treatments.

CONDITIONS THAT MAKE OLDER ADULTS SUSCEPTIBLE TO FALLS

About 7 out of 10 inadvertent deaths in older adults at least 75 years of age are associated with **falls**. Many chronic illnesses increase susceptibility to falls. Only a small proportion of those sustaining falls resulting in **hip fractures** regain functionality with ADLs. Conditions associated with falls include **neurological diseases** and **attacks** such as a stroke, musculoskeletal disorders and muscle weakness, sensory problems (particularly of balance or sight), and cardiovascular abnormalities. Certain **genitourinary issues** such as incontinence can contribute to falls because of unsafe practices dealing with them. Older adults often have **respiratory issues**, such as low blood oxygenation or pneumonia, increasing their risk for falls. Much of the increased risk for falls in the aging population is related to **medication usage** (narcotics, diuretics, antidepressants, and the like) or **psychological factors** such as confusion or anxiety. Restrictive clothing and improper use of assistive equipment such as wheelchairs or walkers also increase the risk for falls.

INFECTION CONTROL

NOSOCOMIAL INFECTIONS

Nosocomial infections are those that are healthcare-associated or hospital-acquired. The following is a list of common nosocomial infections.

- *Enterococci* infections include urinary infections, bacteremia, endocarditis as well as infections in wounds and the abdominal and pelvic areas.
- *Enterobacteriaceae* cause about half of the urinary tract infections and a quarter of the postoperative infections.
- *Escherichia coli* primarily causes urinary tract infections (especially related to catheters), diarrhea, and neonatal meningitis but it can also lead to pneumonia, and bacteremia (usually secondary to urinary infection).
- Group B β-hemolytic *Streptococci* (GBS) has increasingly been a cause of infections in neonatal units, causing pneumonia, meningitis, and sepsis. GBS infections may occur as wound infections after Cesarean sections, especially in those immunocompromised.
- *Staphylococcus aureus* is a major cause of nosocomial post-operative infections, both localized and systemic, and from indwelling tubes and devices.
- Methicillin-resistant *Staphylococcus aureus (MRSA)* is a common cause of surgical infections.
- *Clostridioides difficile* causes more nosocomial diarrhea cases than any other microorganism.
- *Candida*, a yeast fungal pathogen, can overgrow and lead to mucocutaneous or cutaneous lesions and sepsis.
- *Aspergillus* spp., filamentous fungi, produce spores that become airborne and can invade the respiratory tract, causing pneumonia.

CATHETER-RELATED INFECTIONS

Intravenous catheter-related infections are a significant cause of morbidity and mortality in the hospital setting. Usually, these infections are due to *Staphylococcus aureus, enterococcus*, or fungal infection such as *Candida*. These infections are important because they may progress and eventually lead to bacteremia, infective endocarditis, septic pulmonary emboli, septic shock, osteomyelitis, or superficial thrombophlebitis. Therefore, vigilance should be maintained to prevent these infections. The patient may exhibit fevers, chills, and discomfort around the catheter site. The site itself may show purulence or erythema. The subclavian vein is the preferred intravenous site and the femoral is the least-preferred site due to high infection rates. Infections are diagnosed with blood cultures and catheter tip cultures. Initial treatment includes removal of the catheter and antibiotic treatment. Antibiotics should be empiric at first, then directed toward culture results. Treatment duration should be 2 weeks at first, but 4-6 weeks if there is a complicated infection.

INFECTION CONTROL MEASURES

Standard infection control measures are designed to prevent transmission of microbial substances between patients and/or medical providers. These measures are indicated for everyone and include frequent handwashing, gloves whenever bodily fluids are involved, and face shields and gowns when splashes are anticipated. For more advanced control with tuberculosis, SARS, vesicular rash disorders (such as VZV), and most recently COVID-19, **airborne precautions** should be instituted to prevent the spread of tiny droplets that can remain suspended in the air for days and travel throughout a hospital environment. Therefore, negative pressure rooms are essential, and providers and patients should wear high-efficiency N95 masks and be fitted in advance. For disorders such as influenza or other infections spread by droplets (spread by cough or sneeze) basic surgical masks should be worn (**droplet precautions**). For **contact precautions** in the setting of fecally-transmitted infection or vesicular rash diseases, gowns/gloves should be used and contact limited. White coats are not a substitute for proper gowning. In the case of a *Clostridioides difficile* infection, contact precautions should be used in addition to washing hands with soap and water (rather than alcohol-based hand sanitizer) after patient contact.

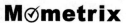

Ability to Communicate Effectively

MICROANATOMY AND NEUROPHYSIOLOGY OF LINGUISTICS

Linguistics, or **language functions**, are directed by the left hemisphere of the brain in the vast majority of individuals. On the simplest level, there are three major neuroanatomical areas involved with language function: the angular gyrus, Wernicke's area, and Broca's area. It is believed that the **angular gyrus**, located at the temporoparietal-occipital intersection, relates visual impressions to the spoken word. This information is then transferred to **Wernicke's area** in the back of the superior temporal gyrus, where sound pattern recognition occurs. Adults learning a second language utilize another brain region called **Broca's area**. There is also evidence that other parts of the brain are summoned in the processing of language. For example, the secondary region of the auditory cortex appears to be utilized by hearing-impaired individuals for sign language usage.

COMPONENTS OF SPEECH AND LEVELS OF LANGUAGE PRODUCTION

Speech is both expressive and receptive. In other words, it is either produced or comprehended. Both aspects are necessary for effective communication. There are also levels of **language construction**. The most basic level is **automatic language**, which is a routine response such as prayers or curse words. **Imitation** is a more advanced form of language because it entails processing of what is heard before a trite or imitative response is given. The highest plane of language formation is called **symbolic language**, which involves independent creative intention, correct syntactic organization, and application of the rules of tense and plurality.

PRAGMATICS

The term "pragmatics" refers to the study of language in actual use beyond just words and grammar. While most language is controlled by the left cerebral hemisphere, the **right hemisphere** contributes to the components of pragmatics, and these can be impaired if there is damage to that side. These components include prosody, kinesics, and facial recognition and expression. **Prosody** (or prosodia) is the rhythm of speech that conveys nuances of meaning, attitudes, and emotions. It includes things such as intonation, pauses, accents, emphases, and melody. **Kinesics** is the study of communication using body language, in particular gestures or movements that accentuate or enhance verbal communication. **Pantomime** is a variation using only gestures. Both brain hemispheres seem to be involved in the understanding and use of gestures and pantomime, but the specifics are unclear at present. **Facial recognition and expression** also contribute to pragmatics by communicating emotions and mood.

STAGES OF NORMAL LANGUAGE DEVELOPMENT

Up to about 1 year of age, most children are in a language-less stage. Newborns can only express **reflex sounds** such as crying, screaming, or whimpering. By about 4 months old, an infant can generally laugh, voice vowel and some consonant sounds, and produce repetitive babble or alternating consonant and vowel sounds like "dada." In the next few months, other consonants appear, and the pitch of the infant's voice begins to resemble adult speech. Most infants reach **semantic stage 2** by age 8 months to 1 year. At this stage, the infant can understand a few words, and in the next few months progresses to partially intelligible speech, particularly single words about actions, objects, or location. **Stage 3**, the semantic language or substantive word stage, is usually reached in phases between about 18 and 36 months. During this time, the percentage of intelligible speech increases to about 75%; the child's vocabulary increases to several hundred words, and they begin to understand syntax and spatial relationships. Most children are able to understand syntax (**stage 4**) by about age 3, and certain remaining distorted sounds are mastered over the next few years.

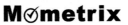

ATTENTION NETWORKS INVOLVED WITH ADVANCED LANGUAGE SKILLS

Advanced language skills involve the integration of several cognitive networks. **Attention networks** control patterns of communication. Attention has two components:

- A **selective orientation** physically or mentally, which is mediated by the thalamus.
- A **detachment from tasks**, which is controlled by the right side of the parietal region.

There is another network related to **declarative memory or personal history**. This also has two sets of connections:

- **Domain-independent** or short-term memory is centered in the left hippocampus and associated temporal regions.
- **Domain-specific** or long-term memory is stored in various areas of parietal, temporal, and occipital lobes.

Both hemispheres participate in long-term memory, with the left primarily involved with language and mathematics and the right with more experiential features. There are also **executive attention networks** involved with vigilance, detection, and working memory. Vigilance is mainly controlled by right frontal areas and the brain stem's locus coeruleus; detection is mainly controlled by the anterior cingulate cortex and basal ganglia; and working memory is mainly controlled by the anterior cingulate and lateral regions of frontal lobes.

CONCEPT FORMULATION

Concept formulation and storage is mediated by **memory networks**. Concept formation requires categorization and analysis of relationships, logical reasoning, and the ability to abstract from information gleaned. The **executive attention networks** of detection and working memory are accessed for concept formulation rather than new stimuli. The **prefrontal cortex regions** are important for advanced language skills such as concept formulation, with the left one related to learning and the right prefrontal cortex involved with recall. Young children have not developed enough networks to analyze relationships and form concepts, but concept formation and problem solving usually begin prior to school age and continue throughout life unless impaired.

APHASIA

BROCA'S APHASIA

The term *aphasia* refers to any type of linguistic deficit precipitated by brain damage. People with **Broca's aphasia** generally comprehend the spoken word, but many other functions associated with verbalization are impaired. This aphasia results from brain damage at or near **Broca's area**, and it is primarily characterized by **agrammatism** (syntactic loss) as well as partial or total **inability to move the right side**. These individuals do not have fluent speech, and their abilities to read, write, repeat, and sometimes name objects are impaired. They may have trouble responding to verbal commands with the left side of the face or the left arm as well. **Transcortical motor aphasia** often mimics Broca's aphasia, but in this case, repetition capabilities are preserved, and the site of damage is generally near Broca's area or the supplementary motor area (SMA), causing a disconnect between the two.

Functional Health Patterns

WERNICKE'S APHASIA

Wernicke's aphasia can result from brain damage to **Wernicke's area**. Here the major defect is **verbal comprehension**. Reading, writing, repetition, and naming functions are impaired as well. Interestingly, people with Wernicke's aphasia are able to speak with ease, inflect properly, and use proper syntax. However, they use incorrect words and nonsensical words or phrases, and make phonetic substitutions. They may also have other **sensory deficits** such as loss of visual fields. These deficits make communication with the individual difficult, and the people in contact with the affected individual (including the nurse) must rely on techniques such as gesturing and using facial changes to get their point across. **Transcortical sensory aphasia** can imitate Wernicke's aphasia, except that repetition is functional and the area of damage is the border zone of the parietotemporal intersection.

GLOBAL APHASIA AND MIXED TRANSCORTICAL APHASIA

Global or **total aphasia** is a marked incapacity to comprehend verbal or written language or to write. **All language abilities**, including speech, are impaired (except possibly **naming**), and the person also has loss of use of the **right side** as well as **visual field and sensory deficits**. Global aphasia is caused by injury to massive regions in the frontal and parietotemporal language parts of the brain.

Mixed transcortical aphasia can resemble global aphasia except that the person has intact repetition abilities. This type of aphasia is usually caused by oxygen deprivation or head injury to the cortical areas around—but not directly within—the language centers. These individuals only repeat what they have heard and do not speak otherwise.

With global aphasia, the best method to improve communication is to use **alternative forms of communication**, such as gestures and pictures. People with only **expressive aphasia** may benefit from repetition of sounds or words, whereas those with only **receptive aphasia** may have some understanding if the speech is slow and clear, but they may also need alternative forms of communication.

OTHER TYPES OF APHASIAS

Another type of deficit is **conduction aphasia**, primarily characterized by intact verbal comprehension and fluent but highly **paraphrasic or repetitive language production**. It is caused by damage in the **supramarginal gyrus** of the brain. Writing ability is generally impaired, and there may be other sensory losses. The most prevalent type of deficit is **anomic aphasia**, which is primarily characterized by the inability to spontaneously **locate the correct word** to use while most other language facilities are intact. Anomic aphasia is generally caused by injury to the **left temporoparietal junction region** if severe, but mild cases can result from many types of damage. The inability to comprehend speech while retaining most other language functions is known as **pure word deafness**, also considered a type of aphasia. Here, repetition is also affected generally, and the injured area of the brain is usually the **superior temporal region** or the **superior temporal gyri**. Imaging studies show that some degree of spontaneous recovery from aphasias after injuries is possible.

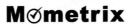

APROSODIAS

Aprosodias are deficits in expression or comprehension of the **nuances of meaning** in verbal communication.

- **Motor aprosodia** is characterized by intact comprehension of both prosody and gesturing, but poor expression thereof, resulting in flat, monotone speaking patterns accompanied by left-sided hemiplegia and sensory deficits. It is usually caused by right frontal or anteroinferior parietal brain damage.
- **Sensory aprosodia** is characterized by poor understanding of prosody and gestures but intact ability to use these features in expression. The main defect is right-sided posterotemporal or posteroinferior parietal damage. Other senses such as position and vibration may be affected.
- Prosodic and kinesic expression and comprehension are all diminished in **global aprosodia**, which is generally caused by a large lesion affecting several right lobes and possibly hemorrhaging. These people can also have left-side hemiplegia, visual defects, and other sensory loss.

There are three types of possible transcortical aprosodias: motor, sensory, and mixed. In the **motor version**, the spontaneous affective prosody and gesturing are both compromised, as well as some prosodic comprehension. Comprehension of nuances and gestures is affected in **transcortical sensory aprosodia**, whereas both expression and comprehension of these features are absent in the mixed condition. Interestingly, the ability to express prosodic repetition is retained in all of these. Areas of damage in transcortical aprosodias have been postulated but not proven. Other possible aprosodias are **conduction type**, where the only defect is poor affective prosodic repetition, and **anomic aprosodia**, mainly characterized by inability to understand gestures.

DYSPHONIA AND DYSARTHRIA

Dysphonia is diminished or total loss of capacity to vocalize as a result of dysfunction of the vocal cords or associated nerves. Reduced voice sounds can be due to nerve damage, laryngeal carcinoma or polyps, or muscle paralysis or spasms.

Dysarthria is difficulty articulating speech due to a lack of muscle control. Both central and peripheral system motor problems can result in dysarthria. There are several types, with the most prevalent type being **flaccid dysarthria**, characterized by breathy and nasal sounds and caused by damage to motor centers in the brain stem and/or cranial nerves VII, IX, X, and XII. **Hypokinetic** and **hyperkinetic** forms of dysarthria are characterized respectively by slow and muffled or rapid and irregular speech patterns. **Spastic dysarthria** or bulbar palsy is due to corticobulbar injury; the person has weak or no speech movement and unclear articulation. Cerebellar damage can result in **ataxic dysarthria**, in which the person has episodes of explosive speech followed by barely audible words. Patients may have **mixed dysarthrias** as well.

OTHER TYPES OF SPEECH DISORDERS

Stuttering—repetitive sounds interspersed with halting in an attempt at pronunciation—is a common speech-related disorder, especially in boys. Several motor areas of the right hemisphere of the brain have been implicated during stuttering, as well as the cerebellum, while certain parts of the cortex are unfazed. It has therefore been postulated that stuttering may be due to high levels of **dopamine and serotonin** in language processing and vocal areas accompanied by left cerebral dominance. Other disorders include vocal tics, repetitive speech, echoing, extremely high or low pitch or loudness, abnormal nasal quality, broken words, inability to express thoughts in a direct manner, and more.

ADDITIONAL LANGUAGE PROBLEMS

Dyslexia is a common problem characterized by the impaired ability to **understand written language**; many areas of the brain have been found to contribute to dyslexia. Several types of language delay or general communication problems can be identified in childhood. Many of these problems can be connected to **chromosomal abnormalities**. Delayed language development in association with global intellectual disability can be found in children with **Down syndrome**. Another disorder, called **Angelman syndrome**, is

153

characterized by no speech plus intellectual disability. Language postponement can be associated with **developmental aphasias**. In children with **infantile autism**, communication is absent or highly abnormal.

ASSESSMENTS FOR LANGUAGE DISORDERS

ASSESSMENT FOR APPREHENSION AND EXPRESSION OF PRAGMATICS

The examiner should observe the patient's speech in terms of use of **affective prosody** and **expression of suitable emotion and attitudes**. The examiner should test the person's ability to recognize **nuances** by delivering a seemingly neutral declarative sentence in a particular tone and seeing if the patient can repeat it using the same tone. Another good assessment tool is to stand outside the patient's visual field while delivering the same type of sentence to see if they can **identify** the voice affect utilized. The patient's ability to understand **visual gestures** can be evaluated by making a statement in a neutral tone of voice while conveying emotion through use of facial gestures, and then asking the patient to categorize or describe the suggested emotion.

ASSESSMENT FOR APHASIA

The nurse should observe the patient's **speech** in terms of fluency, speed, grammar, and responses. The nurse should check the person's ability to **comprehend** verbal language (by asking the patient to follow increasingly complex commands) and written language (by asking the patient to follow written instructions). The clinician should ask the patient to **name objects** in the room. The clinician should test the ability to **repeat** a simple sentence. Lastly, the person's **writing ability** should be evaluated by having them complete two exercises: to write a spontaneous idea, and to write down a statement that has been spoken.

ASSESSMENT FOR DYSARTHRIA AND OTHER LANGUAGE DISORDERS IN CHILDREN

There are a number of questions the nurse should ask the parent of a child with **dysarthria**. Most of the queries should be about the presence of stammering, omission of certain sounds, substitution of wrong consonants, recent voice changes, and difficulties understanding the child. In addition, the clinician needs to observe the patient's **speech pattern** during dialogue or reading aloud for types of articulation errors. The clinician might also have the patient reiterate sounds that are **lingual** ("la-la-la"), **labial** ("me-me-me"), and **guttural** ("k-k-k"). **Muscle tone** and **movement of the face, palate, and tongue** should be clinically observed, and motor function tests for the facial, vagus, and hypoglossal nerves should also be performed. There are a number of general questions to ask the parent of a child with any language disorder, centered on the timeline of speech, omissions, grammatical errors, ability to multitask, and facility in responding to questions.

ASSESSMENT FOR COGNITIVE NETWORKS

The examiner should observe the patient's degree of **arousal** and the patient's ability to **focus** their attention. Short-term and long-term language and non-language memory need to be assessed. **Short-term memory** can be evaluated by studying whether the patient is oriented or confused in some way, and also by asking questions to see whether the patient is able to learn new information. Similarly, questions related to **long-term memory** should be asked. The clinician should look at aspects of the patient's ability to form **concepts**, such as the facility to categorize, think clearly, and formulate abstract concepts. The executive functions of vigilance, detection, and working memory should also be evaluated. A person exhibiting **vigilance** will actively search their environment. Cognitive assessment of the **detection function** encompasses things such as looking to see if the patient is motivated, expresses emotion, and is aware of their current pattern of communication. **Working memory** is concerned with the ability to sustain attention or concentrate over time.

THERAPEUTIC ENVIRONMENT FOR REHABILITATION OF COMMUNICATION DISORDERS

A therapeutic rehabilitation environment for patients with communication disorders is one that is quiet, tranquil, unhurried, and uncluttered, but not completely isolated. The main goal is to provide a setting that makes the patients' attempts at communication **less stressful**. Inherent in this concept is the **identification of stressors** and their **elimination**. For people whose comprehension is relatively intact but who have trouble with expression, the clinician's role is to provide a pleasant environment and many opportunities for social

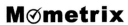

interaction such as group activities. The nurse should praise the individual for any communication attempts and utilize **all means of communication**, such as gestures and sign language, in addition to speech. For patients who have comprehension problems, the room should be as quiet as possible. For these patients, boundaries need to be set for the amount and duration of communication and group activities, to avoid fatigue. Any interaction that creates anxiety or stress should be stopped.

FACILITATING COMMUNICATION IN AFFECTED PATIENTS

Efforts to facilitate communication in affected patients are generally tailored to the individual and the type of deficit involved. However, there are some general guidelines.

- **Communications** with the patient should be spontaneous, topical, frequent, and relatively brief.
- **Gestures** and other aids should be incorporated if needed, and the person should be given sufficient time to respond.
- There are many tactics for patients whose ability to comprehend is intact, such as **cueing**, having the patient **describe** what the nurse is doing, **expanding** on statements the patient has made, and encouraging the patient to **verbalize** in any manner they wish.
- The patient should be allowed to make mistakes and should only be interrupted if they become very perturbed.
- People with **aphasia** or **aprosodia** have difficulty understanding as well, which means further measures are necessary. Their environment must be quiet to allow for communication, and one must secure their attention first. Other people need to speak to them slowly, clearly, and directly, incorporating gestures and reinforcing their responses when correct. Generally, comprehension is addressed before language production.

DYSARTHRIA THERAPY

Dysarthria therapy can be approached medically and may include treatment of the fundamental neurological disorder, laryngeal surgery (particularly for phonation), use of various pharmacological agents or injections (such as Teflon or Botox), respiratory support, or use of artificial devices. The **speech pathologist** is usually instrumental in diagnosis of articulation problems and the design of **exercises** to improve various speech errors. These include exercises to strengthen palatal, laryngeal valve, or respiratory muscles to improve resonance, phonation, and respiration, respectively. **Behavioral management** is another approach, which can range from compensation techniques such as breathing exercises and biofeedback to general procedures to improve the patient's speaking, listening, and interacting. Modalities that circumvent or support actual speech and/or writing are known as **augmentative and alternative communication (AAC) devices** and include things such as printed signs, pictorial illustrations, symbols, sign language, speech synthesizers, and picture books and charts.

PASSY MUIR VALVE

The Passy Muir valve (PMV) is a small tracheostomy and ventilator swallowing and speaking valve that attaches to the hub of a tracheostomy or the tubing of a ventilator circuit. Before the PMV is inserted, the tracheostomy tube should be secured and the cuff deflated. The PMV is attached by twisting into place in a clockwise direction—one-quarter turn—and removed by twisting counterclockwise. The PMV allows air to flow in during inspiration, but closes during expiration so that air can flow out around the tracheostomy or endotracheal tube and over the vocal cords, allowing the production of speech and restoring physiological PEEP (positive end-expiratory pressure). Because the PMV creates a closed system, the positive pressure can help individuals cough up secretions more effectively. Most individuals find they have increased sense of smell and of taste and can swallow more effectively with a PMV. Individuals may have some anxiety about initial use but usually adapt quickly. Some may require the assistance of a speech language pathologist and/or respiratory therapist to improve breath support for speaking and swallowing, especially if they have not used their voice for a long period of time. Contraindications to the PMV include foam-filled or inflated tracheotomy cuffs, paralysis of vocal cords, and severe obstruction of the airway or risk of aspiration.

Functional Health Patterns

HELPING A CHILD LEARN LANGUAGE

Initially **limiting and reinforcing vocabulary taught** is helpful for teaching a child language. For example, relating a limited number of words to a specific activity that the child performs is useful. Making the child **verbally express a word** rather than gesture before action is helpful. The clinician or other adult should always speak at a level a bit higher than that of the child and show the child ways to **extend** what they have already said. The emphasis should be on **meaning**, not linguistics. Children (or adults) who cannot read or write are said to have **alexia** or **agraphia** respectively. These individuals are generally taught in a traditional classroom setting supplemented with homework projects.

DIAGNOSES, INTERVENTIONS, AND DESIRED OUTCOME FOR COMMUNICATION PROBLEMS

The general nursing diagnosis for a patient with communication problems is **impaired verbal communication**, according to the North American Nursing Diagnosis Association (NANDA). The desired nursing outcome is achievement of **effective communication**, both receptive and expressive. The achievement of this goal can be furthered by interventions such as providing a therapeutic and supportive environment to overcome the speech deficit and managing the patient's environment and energy levels. The NANDA also recognizes four other possible **nursing diagnoses**:

- Impaired written, emotional, and/or gestural communication, with many of the same interventions and goals as impaired verbal communication.
- Impaired social interaction, where the nurse's role is socialization enhancement.
- Anxiety, where the main goal is to reduce the patient's anxiety in order to allow the patient to cope and relax.
- Deficient knowledge, where the nurse serves primarily to educate the patient and the patient's family about procedures and the disease process.

GOALS FOR TREATMENT OF COMMUNICATION DEFICITS

The caregiving process for individuals with communication deficits can be objectively **documented**. There are goals for both the patient with communication deficits and the patient's family members.

- The patient should **participate** in some type of activity designed to enhance communication skills.
- The patient should eventually be able to control and express their frustrations.
- The patient should be able to **function** relatively independently and **communicate** to others the things they cannot do alone.
- The patient needs to see himself or herself in a positive light, be receptive to social interaction, and develop the best possible pattern of communication.
- The effectiveness of **family support** can be verified by how well the family can explain aspects of the patient's problem, such as cause, prognosis, facilitation modalities, safety requirements, methods for recovery, and the necessity for independence of the patient.

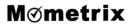

Optimal Nutrition and Hydration

ASSESSMENT OF NUTRITIONAL STATUS

Assessment of nutritional status begins with an assessment of the patient's intake. The patient is asked to report intake for the previous 24 hours. This may indicate the need for a **food diary** over a period of time:

- Compare the patient's nutritional intake with the requirements of the USDA's MyPlate.
- Measure height and weight and check against a BMI table to help determine nutritional status.
- Measure waist circumference.
- Assess the patient for physical signs of poor nutrition, such as muscle wasting, obesity, hair breakage and loss, poor skin turgor, ulcers, bruising, and loss of subcutaneous tissue.
- Assess mucous membranes and condition of teeth, abdomen, extremities, and thyroid gland.

Nutritional status is connected to endocrine disease, infections, other acute and chronic diseases, digestion, absorption, excretion, and storage of nutrients, so these areas must also be assessed. Blood testing should include proteins, transferrin, electrolytes, vitamins A and C, carotene, and CBC. Test urine for creatinine, thiamine, riboflavin, niacin, albumin, and iodine.

SIGNS OF NUTRITIONAL DEFICIENCIES

The physical assessment is an important part of nutritional assessment to determine **malnutrition** or problems with **self-feeding**.

- **Hair** may be dry and brittle or thinning.
- **Skin** may show poor turgor, ecchymosis, tears, pressure areas, ulcerations, abrasions, or other compromises.
- The **mouth** may show dry mucous membranes. Lips may be scaly (riboflavin deficiency), have cheilosis, and be cracking at the corners. Gums may be swollen or bleeding, teeth loose or needing care, or dentures poorly fitting. The tongue may be inflamed, dry, cracked, or have sores.
- **Nails** may become brittle. Spoon-shaped or pale nail bed indicates low iron.
- **Hands** may be impaired or arthritic, making eating difficult.
- **Vision** may be compromised so that people can't see to prepare food or have difficulty feeding themselves.
- **Mental status** may be impaired to the point that people can't understand diet instructions or prepare or eat meals.
- **Motor skills** may decrease, including hand-mouth coordination or the ability to hold utensils.

ASSESSING NUTRITIONAL STATUS OF HOSPITALIZED PATIENTS

Assessing the nutritional status of the hospital inpatient is an important part of forming a care plan. The two screening tools that are most commonly used are the **Subjective Global Assessment (SGA)** and the **Prognostic Nutritional Index (PNI)**. The SGA provides a nutritional assessment based on both the patient history and current symptoms. The patient is asked about any changes in weight and is also asked questions about his or her diet. The presence of symptoms that may lead to weight loss and poor nutritional status, such as diarrhea, nausea, and vomiting, as well as water retention (edema) and muscle wasting (cachexia), is also included in the SGA. The PNI is also used as an indicator of malnutrition and is especially helpful in determining how well a patient will recover from surgery. The PNI assesses nutritional status through the measurement of serum proteins such as albumin and transferrin combined with a skinfold measurement and a cutaneous hypersensitivity test as an indicator of immune function.

ISSUES WITH PEDIATRIC NUTRITION

MALNUTRITION

Protein malnutrition (kwashiorkor or **hypoalbuminemia)** is characterized by inadequate protein but adequate fats and carbohydrates. It can result from chronic diarrhea, renal disease, infection, hemorrhage, burns, traumatic injuries, or other illnesses. Onset is usually rapid with loss of visceral protein while skeletal muscle mass is retained, so it may be difficult to detect on a physical exam. **Symptoms** include:

- Hypoalbuminemia and anemia
- Edema
- Delayed healing of wound, immunoincompetence.

Protein-calorie malnutrition (marasmus), inadequate protein and calories, is usually more obvious. Visceral protein is usually intact, as is immune function, because weight loss is gradual. However, children are often very thin or emaciated from loss of skeletal muscle mass. **Symptoms** include:

- Decreased basal metabolism, hypothermia
- Lack of subcutaneous fat, decreased tissue turgor
- Bradycardia

Mixed protein-calorie malnutrition (combination) is common in hospitalized patients and has an acute onset with low visceral protein as well as rapid loss of weight, skeletal muscle mass, and fat.

FEEDING AND SWALLOWING DISORDERS

Feeding and swallowing disorders in pediatric patients can include problems with sucking, chewing, and swallowing. Those especially at risk are children with brain injuries, neuromuscular disorders, congenital defects (heart, cleft lip, cleft palate), preterm birth, developmental disorders (autism, intellectually disabled), reflux, muscle weakness, head and neck cancers, stroke, and respiratory distress. **Interventions** include:

- Dysphagia assessment to determine what phase of swallowing is impaired: oral phase, pharyngeal phase, or esophageal phase
- Swallowing exercises and feeding therapy to strengthen muscles or improve awareness of food and fluid in the mouth
- Modification of diet to accommodate problems, such as by thickening liquids and changing textures of food
- Medications, such as proton pump inhibitors (PPIs) or H2 antagonists, to treat reflux
- Surgical repair, such as for cleft lip and cleft palate
- Use of different feeding equipment, such as modified utensils
- Feeding tube, which may be placed until the child is able to take oral foods and fluids

ALTERATIONS IN HUNGER/THIRST AND INABILITY TO SELF-FEED

Alterations in hunger and/or thirst can result from physical or psychological conditions. Brain injuries can result in some patients not feeling hunger and eating inadequately, and others not feeling satiation and overeating. The hypothalamus governs feelings of hunger and thirst, so hypothalamic lesions may be characterized by changes in appetite. Some medications (antibiotics, antipsychotics, chemotherapeutic agents) may impair the sense of taste. Chemotherapeutic agents often cause xerostomia, ulcerations, and mucositis, all of which make eating difficult. Infections of the mouth, such as oral candidiasis, may make oral tissue swollen and painful. Some patients, such as those with anorexia and bulimia, have distortions of body image that affect their attitude about and intake of food.

Inability to self-feed most often relates to injuries (fractures, pain, amputations), disabilities (stroke, paralysis, cerebral palsy), or neuromuscular disease (muscular dystrophy). The condition may be temporary or permanent. In some cases, the child can self-feed with assistive devices or better pain control.

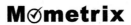

Factors Contributing to Malnutrition and Dehydration

Many neurological diseases can cause **dysphagia** and, therefore, a lack of nourishment and dehydration. Dysphagia is the inability to swallow in a normal manner. It can cause aspiration or inhalation of fluids or food into the lungs, predisposing the person to aspiration pneumonia, choking, dehydration, and nutritional deficits. Many other factors can contribute to malnutrition. These include polypharmacy (the use of multiple conflicting medications, common in the elderly population), alcohol use, poor dentition, depression, functional disability or frailty, and failure to eat enough. As people age, they lose some sense of thirst and also retain less water in their kidneys, creating a propensity toward **dehydration**. Certain diseases change the person's appetite and nutritional intake. **Stressful situations**, such as burns or other traumas, increase the individual's metabolic rate and promote loss of nutrients, and therefore these people need more calories, vitamins, and minerals. Elderly patients generally have a **low basal metabolic rate**, decreased glucose tolerance, and often excess weight. Anyone who is **obese** (BMI≥30) is at increased risk for many disease states.

Metabolic Patterns

Metabolic Syndrome

Metabolic syndrome is defined by a cluster of abnormalities in an individual, including hyperglycemia or insulin resistance, hypertension, dyslipidemia, and obesity. The diagnostic criteria generally used to identify metabolic syndrome were developed by the National Cholesterol Education Program Adult Treatment Panel III (ATP III). The guidelines for diagnosis require the presence of at least three of the following:

- Excessive abdominal circumference, defined as a waistline of >40 inches for men or >35 inches for women
- Elevated triglyceride level of ≥150 mg/dL
- Decreased HDL cholesterol levels of <40 mg/dL for men and <50 mg/dL for women
- Elevated blood pressure reading of ≥130/85 mmHg
- Elevated fasting glucose level of ≥100 mg/dL

Nursing Diagnoses, Interventions, and Goals

Since metabolic syndrome encompasses several abnormalities, possible **nursing diagnoses** are quite diverse. Some of the more common diagnoses directly related to health with metabolic syndrome are decreased cardiac output, risk of infection, ineffective renal tissue perfusion, and risk of peripheral neurovascular dysfunction. Electrolyte and fluid management can both increase cardiac output and improve renal function. Infection risk can be diminished through immunization, vaccination, infection control, and nutritional support. Exercise, already discussed previously in relation to the obesity component of metabolic syndrome, can also reduce risk of peripheral neurovascular dysfunction. People with metabolic syndrome may be at risk for activity intolerance, falls, unsafe health behavior, or ineffective coping. Often, their caregivers are at risk for role strain. It is the nurse's role to educate the patient about the disease and its management.

Obesity

Obesity and other classifications of weight are defined by the **body mass index (BMI)**. BMI is calculated as an individual's weight (w) in kilograms divided by the square of their height (h) in meters:

$$BMI = \frac{w}{h^2}$$

The following BMI ranges classify individuals:

- **Underweight**—BMI <18.5
- **Normal**—BMI of 18.5–24.9
- **Overweight**—BMI of 25.0–29.9
- **Obese class I**—BMI of 30.0–34.9

Functional Health Patterns

- **Obese class II**—BMI of 35.0–39.9
- **Obese class III**—BMI ≥40

Anyone overweight or in an obesity class is at increased risk for many health problems; overweight individuals with waist circumferences of greater than 40 inches for men, or 35 inches for women, are more at risk than BMI would indicate. Weight reduction, increased physical activity (such as walking), and reduction in caloric intake are suggested for people in any of these latter categories.

DIABETES MELLITUS TYPES 1 AND 2

Diabetes mellitus is the most common metabolic disorder. Over 6% of adults have diabetes, but only 4% of adults are diagnosed. Insulin resistance tends to increase in older adults, so there is less ability to handle glucose. Type II is more common in older adults, with incidence increasing with age.

- **Type I:** Immune-mediated form with insufficient insulin production because of the destruction of pancreatic beta cells
  - **Symptoms** include pronounced polyuria and polydipsia, short onset, obesity or recent weight loss, and ketoacidosis present on diagnosis.
  - **Treatment** includes insulin as needed to control blood sugar, glucose monitoring 1–4 times daily, diet with carbohydrate control, and exercise.
- **Type II:** Insulin resistant form with defect in insulin secretion
  - **Symptoms** include long onset, obesity with no weight loss or significant weight loss, mild or absent polyuria and polydipsia, ketoacidosis or glycosuria without ketonuria, androgen-mediated problems such as hirsutism and acne (adolescents), and hypertension.
  - **Treatment** includes diet and exercise, glucose monitoring, and oral medications.

> **Review Video: Diabetes Mellitus**
> Visit mometrix.com/academy and enter code: 501396
>
> **Review Video: Diet, Exercise, and Medications for Diabetes**
> Visit mometrix.com/academy and enter code: 774388
>
> **Review Video: Diabetes: Complications**
> Visit mometrix.com/academy and enter code: 996788

INSULIN USED TO TREAT GLYCEMIC DISORDERS

There are a number of different types of **insulin** with varying action times. Insulin is used to metabolize **glucose** for those whose pancreas does not produce insulin. People may need to take a combination of insulins (short- and long-acting) to maintain glucose control. Duration of action may vary according to the individual's metabolism, intake, and level of activity:

- **Humalog** (Lispro H) is a fast-acting, short-acting insulin with onset in 5–15 minutes, peaking between 45 and 90 minutes and lasting 3–4 hours.
- **Regular** (R) is a relatively fast-acting insulin with onset in 30 minutes, peaks in 2–5 hours, and lasts 5–8 hours.
- **NPH** (N) insulin is intermediate-acting with onset in 1–3 hours, peaking at 6–12 hours, and lasting for 16–24 hours.
- **Insulin Glargine** (Lantus) is a long-acting insulin with onset in 3–6 hours, no peak, and lasting for 24 hours.
- **Combined NPH/Regular** (70/30 or 50/50) has an onset of 30 minutes, peaks at 7–12 hours, and lasts 16–24 hours.

ORAL HYPOGLYCEMIC AGENTS TO TREAT TYPE II DIABETES

Oral hypoglycemic agents are **anti-diabetic treatments** generally used in the treatment of Type II Diabetes. There are five classic categories of oral hypoglycemic agents: sulfonylureas, biguanides, meglitinides, competitive inhibitors of alpha-glucosidases (located in the intestinal brush border), and thiazolidinediones. More recently, two additional novel classes of oral hypoglycemics, DPP-4 inhibitors and SGLT2 inhibitors, were introduced with proven effectiveness when used in conjunction with changes in diet and exercise. Some examples of sulfonylurea oral hypoglycemic agents include the first-generation agents tolbutamide, tolazamide, chlorpropamide, and acetohexamide; and second-generation agents glyburide, glimepiride, and glipizide. The biguanide oral hypoglycemic agent is metformin. Metformin has the distinct advantage of not causing weight gain or hypoglycemic reactions. The meglitinide agent is repaglinide. Examples of alpha-glucosidase inhibitors are acarbose and miglitol. Alpha-glucosidase inhibitors bind tightly to intestinal alpha-glucosidases and decrease the postprandial rise in glucose levels. The only available thiazolidinedione oral hypoglycemic agent is currently pioglitazone; troglitazone was removed from US market in 2000, and rosiglitazone was removed from US market in 2011. Examples of DPP-4 inhibitors include linagliptin, vildagliptin, sitagliptin, and saxagliptin. Examples of SGLT2 inhibitors include canagliflozin, dapagliflozin, and empagliflozin.

FLUID AND ELECTROLYTE BALANCE

SODIUM

Sodium (**Na**) regulates fluid volume, osmolality, acid-base balance, and activity in the muscles, nerves, and myocardium. It is the primary **cation** (positive ion) in extracellular fluid (ECF), necessary to maintain ECF levels that are needed for tissue perfusion:

- Normal range: 135-145 mEq/L
- Hyponatremia: <135 mEq/L
- Hypernatremia: >145 mEq/L

Hyponatremia may result from inadequate sodium intake, excess sodium loss through diarrhea, vomiting, or NG suctioning, or illness, such as severe burns, fever, SIADH, and ketoacidosis.

- **Symptoms**: Irritability to lethargy and alterations in consciousness, cerebral edema with seizures and coma, dyspnea to respiratory failure.
- **Treatment**: Identify and treat the underlying cause and provide Na replacement.

Hypernatremia may result from renal disease, diabetes insipidus, and fluid depletion.

- **Symptoms**: Irritability to lethargy to confusion to coma; seizures; flushing; muscle weakness and spasms; thirst.
- **Treatment**: Identify and treat the underlying cause, monitor Na levels carefully, and give IV fluid replacement.

POTASSIUM

Potassium (**K**) is the primary **electrolyte** in intracellular fluid (ICF), with about 98% inside cells and only 2% in ECF, although this small amount is important for neuromuscular activity. Potassium influences activity of the skeletal and cardiac muscles. Its level is dependent upon adequate renal functioning because 80% is excreted through the kidneys and 20% through the bowels and sweat:

- Normal range: 3.5-5.5 mEq/L
- Hypokalemia: <3.5 mEq/L. Critical value: <2.5 mEq/L
- Hyperkalemia: >5.5 mEq/L. Critical value: >6.5 mEq/L

A healthy NPO patient will need about 40 mEq of K per day to maintain serum K levels. Expect alterations in renal disease and other disease processes.

Hypokalemia is caused by alkalosis, decreased intake associated with starvation, nephritis, and loss of potassium through diarrhea, vomiting, gastric suction, and diuresis.

- **Symptoms**: Lethargy and weakness; nausea and vomiting; paresthesia and tetany; muscle cramps with hyporeflexia; hypotension; dysrhythmias with EKG changes: PVCs or flattened T-waves.
- **Treatment**: Treatment involves identifying and treating the underlying cause and replacing K. When possible, oral replacement is preferable to IV, as it allows slower adjustment of K levels. When given IV, K should be given no faster than 20 mEq/hour via central line if possible. If given peripherally, 10 mEq/hour is preferable for patient comfort.

Hyperkalemia is caused by renal disease, adrenal insufficiency, metabolic acidosis, severe dehydration, burns, hemolysis, and trauma. It rarely occurs without renal disease but may be induced by treatment (such as NSAIDs and potassium-sparing diuretics). Untreated renal failure results in reduced excretion. Those with Addison's disease and deficient adrenal hormones suffer sodium loss that results in potassium retention.

- **Symptoms**: The primary symptoms relate to the effect on the cardiac muscle: ventricular arrhythmias with increasing changes in EKG lead to cardiac and respiratory arrest, weakness with ascending paralysis and hyperreflexia, diarrhea, and increasing confusion.
- **Treatment**: Treatment includes identifying the underlying cause and discontinuing sources of increased K. Calcium gluconate to decrease cardiac effects. Sodium bicarbonate, insulin, and hypertonic dextrose shift K into the cells temporarily. Cation exchange resin (Kayexalate) to decrease K. Peritoneal dialysis or hemodialysis to remove excess K.

Note: When a tourniquet is on, a patient opening and closing their hand can lead to falsely elevated K levels.

CALCIUM

More than 99% of calcium (**Ca**) is in the skeletal system with 1% in serum, but it is important for transmitting nerve impulses and regulating muscle contraction and relaxation, including the myocardium. Calcium activates enzymes that stimulate chemical reactions and has a role in the coagulation of blood:

- Normal range: 8.2-10.2 mg/dL
- Hypocalcemia: <8.2. Critical value: <7 mg/dL
- Hypercalcemia: >10.2 mg/dL. Critical value: >12 mg/dL

Hypercalcemia may be caused by acidosis, kidney disease, hyperparathyroidism, prolonged immobilization, and malignancies. Crisis carries a 50% mortality rate.

- **Symptoms**: Increasing muscle weakness with hypotonicity; anorexia; nausea and vomiting; constipation; bradycardia and cardiac arrest.
- **Treatment**: Identify and treat underlying cause, loop diuretics, IV fluids, phosphate.

Hypocalcemia may be caused by damage to the parathyroid resulting in hypoparathyroidism (directly decreasing calcium production), vitamin D resistance or inadequacy, or liver/kidney disease.

- **Symptoms**: Muscle cramping or spasms; seizures; numbness or tingling of the feet, hands, or lips; tetany if severe.
- **Treatment**: Identify and treat underlying cause, replace calcium by administering IV calcium gluconate in acute circumstances or increasing oral Vitamin D and calcium in chronic cases.

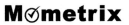

PHOSPHORUS

Phosphorus, or phosphate, (**PO$_4$**) is necessary for neuromuscular and red blood cell function, the maintenance of acid-base balance, and provides structure for teeth and bones. About 85% is in the bones, 14% in soft tissue, and <1% in ECF.

- Normal range: 2.4-4.5 mEq/L
- Hypophosphatemia: <2.4mEq/L
- Hyperphosphatemia: >4.5 mEq/L

Hypophosphatemia occurs with severe protein-calorie malnutrition, hyperventilation, severe burns, diabetic ketoacidosis, and excess antacids with magnesium, calcium, or aluminum.

- **Symptoms**: Irritability, tremors, seizures to coma; hemolytic anemia; decreased myocardial function; respiratory failure.
- **Treatment**: Identify and treat underlying cause and replace phosphorus.

Hyperphosphatemia occurs with renal failure, hypoparathyroidism, excessive intake, neoplastic disease, diabetic ketoacidosis, muscle necrosis, and chemotherapy.

- **Symptoms**: Tachycardia; muscle cramping; hyperreflexia and tetany; nausea and diarrhea.
- **Treatment**: Identify and treat underlying cause, correct hypocalcemia, and provide antacids and dialysis.

MAGNESIUM

Magnesium (**Mg**) is the second most common intracellular electrolyte (after potassium) and activates many intracellular enzyme systems. Mg is important for carbohydrate and protein metabolism, neuromuscular function, and cardiovascular function, producing vasodilation and directly affecting the peripheral arterial system:

- Normal range: 1.7-2.2 mg/dL
- Hypomagnesemia critical value: <1.2 mg/dL
- Hypermagnesemia critical value: >4.9 mg/dL

Hypomagnesemia occurs with chronic diarrhea, chronic renal disease, chronic pancreatitis, excess diuretic or laxative use, hyperthyroidism, hypoparathyroidism, severe burns, and diaphoresis.

- **Symptoms**: Neuromuscular excitability or tetany; confusion, headaches, dizziness; seizure and coma; tachycardia with ventricular arrhythmias; respiratory depression.
- **Treatment**: Identify and treat underlying cause, provide magnesium replacement. IV magnesium is a vasodilator, 2 g over 60 mins.

Hypermagnesemia occurs with renal failure or inadequate renal function, diabetic ketoacidosis, hypothyroidism, and Addison's disease.

- **Symptoms**: Muscle weakness, seizures, and dysphagia with decreased gag reflex; tachycardia with hypotension.
- **Treatment**: Identify and treat underlying cause, IV hydration with calcium, and dialysis.

> **Review Video: Fluid and Electrolytes**
> Visit mometrix.com/academy and enter code: 384389

Functional Health Patterns

163

SWALLOWING

PHYSIOLOGICAL PROCESSES

Food is ingested through the **oral cavity**, comprising the lips, the hard and soft palates of the maxilla (upper jaw), the mandible (lower jaw), tonsils, salivary glands, tongue, teeth, and gums. There are also various types of **sensory cells** (mechanoreceptive, thermoreceptive, and chemoreceptive) that innervate the oral cavity and promote swallowing or deglutition. The **larynx**, also known as the voice box, is a cartilaginous structure beginning with the epiglottis at the base of the tongue. The **epiglottis** moves during swallowing to protect the trachea. The muscular tube between the soft palate and the esophagus is the **pharynx**. It is composed of three parts: the nasopharynx above the soft palate, the oropharynx at the back of the mouth, and the hypopharynx at the lower end of the pharynx, leading into the esophagus. Its muscle fibers aid the propulsion of food in the correct direction. The **esophagus** itself is a bare muscular tube with sphincters at either end. The **upper esophageal sphincter (UES),** consisting of the **cricopharyngeus muscle**, prevents air from entering the stomach and decreases gastric reflux.

Initially, food undergoes an **oral preparatory phase** in which it is taken into the mouth, mixed with saliva, and processed according to consistency. The tongue then compresses against the hard palate and moves the food toward the back, near the oropharynx. This is known as the **oral phase**. Both the oral preparatory and oral phases are voluntary, with open airways and nasal breathing. In the **pharyngeal stage**, the mass of chewed food is propelled down toward the esophagus along the pharynx through a series of reflex actions. The airway or larynx is cut off for less than a second by the downward angulation of the epiglottis, and entry to the esophagus is controlled by the cricopharyngeal sphincter. After entry into the esophagus, food is forced down by involuntary peristaltic waves into the stomach. The complete **swallowing process** takes an average of about 5–10 seconds. If the respiratory passages are not isolated properly, other motor responses usually initiate the gag reflex, which propels food up and out. This gag reflex is often weak or absent in individuals with dysphagia.

CRANIAL NERVES STIMULATED DURING DEGLUTITION

During swallowing (deglutition), six cranial nerves carry information from the involved structures to the brain for assimilation and coordination. The first three cervical nerves are also implicated in eating and deglutition. The **trigeminal (V) cranial nerve** is associated with both motor control of the mandibular muscles and sensory functions in both jaws. The **facial (VII) cranial nerve** controls motor functions in salivary glands and those involving facial expression; it is also associated with frontal taste buds. The **glossopharyngeal (IX) nerve** regulates the stylopharyngeus muscle (which moves the pharynx and larynx), posterior taste buds, and feeling in the soft palate. The **vagus (X) nerve** controls sensory responses in the membrane of the larynx, pharynx, and trachea. The last two nerves, the **spinal accessory (XI) nerve** and the **hypoglossal (XII) nerve**, regulate motor functions of the sternocleidomastoid muscle and intrinsic tongue muscles, respectively.

DIFFERENCES IN THE ACT OF SWALLOWING BETWEEN AGE GROUPS

In infants, the swallowing process is a constantly evolving neuromuscular process. In actuality, most fetuses can swallow by as early as 11 weeks gestation. At birth, infants have usually developed a sucking reflex, which initiates swallowing for about the first 7 months of life. They have a relatively small oral cavity and a highly positioned larynx, leading to a pattern of inhalation, swallowing, and then exhalation. Their tongue often raises and lowers or protrudes. As the oral cavity enlarges, these actions usually subside by about 9 months of age. In children, the ability to feed themselves independently must be learned and employs many motor skills. Children with neurological impairments often find self-feeding difficult, especially if they have been tube-fed for a long period or have issues related to posture or lip or mouth control. While healthy adults usually have no trouble swallowing, there are alterations that can be found in older individuals. The tongue loses motor function and strength, making swallowing slower and weaker, particularly in people over age 60.

NEUROLOGICAL DISEASES LINKED TO POOR DEGLUTITION

Poor deglutition or dysphagia is highly associated with having a **stroke**, particularly a brain stem stroke. The deglutition phase affected can be related to the side where the stroke occurred, though there have been studies

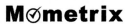

showing that both the oral and pharyngeal phases of swallowing can be impacted by strokes in both the left and right hemispheres. People with **amyotrophic lateral sclerosis (ALS)** typically have oral preparatory or pharyngeal issues such as poor tongue control, poor tongue mobility, and incomplete chewing (impacting peristalsis) or pharyngeal weakness (causing aspiration). Patients with **Parkinson's disease** have problems with all stages of swallowing, starting with the oral phase. Multiple stage deficits are common with most neuromuscular diseases, including head traumas, multiple sclerosis, and myasthenia gravis. **Cerebral palsy** is primarily linked to a poor suck and other unsuitable reflexes during the oral preparatory phase. There are also anatomical variations that can cause poor deglutition, such as cleft palates or lips and muscular pouches near the cricopharyngeal muscle. Surgery or tubes in the area can also affect the ability to swallow.

POSTURAL CHANGES TO IMPROVE DEGLUTITION

The **head down/chin tuck position** is suggested most often, as it allows the epiglottis to cover more of the airway to prevent aspiration and also lowers the pressure at the cricopharyngeal muscle. **Holding the head back** (with or without turning) allows food to travel more quickly through the oral cavity; these are good positions for people with tongue use problems. For patients with impairments on one side, the head is often **turned toward the affected side** in order to close the pharynx on that side and permit the food to move down the opposite portion; this also relaxes the cricopharyngeal muscle. If the head is **tilted toward the more functional side** instead, food proceeds down that side, mainly due to gravity. **Turning the head and keeping the chin down** protects the larynx by directing the food path. Gravity can also be eliminated as a factor by having the patient lie on their **side with the head propped up**, which is a position often used for people with deficient peristaltic movement or laryngeal elevation. Tumblers with cutouts, scoop dishes, and other special utensils can be utilized to maintain postures.

SWALLOWING TECHNIQUES TO IMPROVE DEGLUTITION

For patients with a late pharyngeal swallow or impaired closure of the vocal cords, a **supraglottic swallow** is suggested because it enhances airway protection and closure of the epiglottis. With or without food in the mouth, the patient inhales, holds their breath, and swallows. Then the patient either coughs or clears the throat before the next inhalation. Another technique called the **Mendelsohn maneuver** is recommended for individuals who have insufficient laryngeal elevation or opening of the cricopharyngeal sphincter. In this maneuver, the patient places their hand on their larynx and swallows to get a sense of the larynx position afterward. The patient then usually puts food in their mouth and swallows while holding the larynx in the predetermined highest position during the swallow. Both of these exercises are generally repeated several times at each session, with 3–4 sessions a day. Patients who cannot move the back of their tongue well are taught **effortful swallows** to enhance the tongue base.

CHARACTERISTICS OF FOOD THAT AFFECT CAPACITY TO SWALLOW

Thicker liquids pass through the oral cavity and pharynx more slowly than thinner liquids. The **region of swallowing deficit** dictates the preferred liquid consistency. Thicker liquids are recommended for people with **inadequate laryngeal elevation**, to protect the larynx, while thinner liquids are suggested for those who have **difficulty clearing the pharynx** or those with **cricopharyngeal sphincter problems**. The **bolus size** of food or liquid is also important. Patients susceptible to aspiration should be given smaller volumes, while others may need larger boluses in order to initiate transit in the oral phase, or augment elevation and closure of the larynx and opening of the junction into the esophagus. Some patients have increased sensory stimulation with cold, hot, or sour foods.

DYSPHAGIA

NURSING DIAGNOSES, INTERVENTIONS, AND OUTCOMES

Recommendations for nursing diagnoses, interventions, and outcomes for patients with dysphagia cover three main areas: airway issues, nutritional deficits, and impaired swallowing. If the patient is determined to be at risk for **aspiration** or has **failed airway clearance**, the nurse's interventional role is to initiate safety measures against possible aspiration and swallowing therapy. If the patient is not receiving adequate **nutrition** to meet body requirements, the nurse should institute nutritional therapy to improve nutritional

Functional Health Patterns

status and intake of foods, fluids, and nutrients. If the individual cannot **swallow** properly, again, the nurse should take aspiration precautions and initiate swallowing therapy to improve the swallowing status of the oral, pharyngeal, and esophageal stages. People with eating or deglutition problems may also have other issues that should be documented and attended to, such as impaired ability to speak or inability to perform self-care and ADLs. Specific goals should be developed and carried out by the nurse along with the patient and family.

DIAGNOSTIC TESTS

The universal diagnostic test for identification of dysphagia is the **bedside swallow examination (BSE)**. In the BSE, the medical professional (such as a speech therapist) places their four fingers (not the thumb) on the submandibular area, the hyoid bone, the thyroid notch, and the cricoid cartilage while the patient swallows to see whether the tongue and larynx move up and forward. More detailed analysis can be obtained by doing either a **videofluoroscopic swallowing study (VFSS)** or a **video endoscopic swallowing study (VESS)**. In the VFSS, the person ingests a barium-containing mixture, and the eating and swallowing process is videotaped. In the VESS, a fiber optic nasopharyngoscope is used to observe deglutition (usually enhanced with dye) of normal secretions, fluids, and foods of various consistencies. This latter test is also known as the **fiberoptic endoscopic evaluation of swallowing (FEES)**, and often sensory differences are also evaluated by injecting air-pulsed stimuli through the endoscope. Another technique, called **manometry**, may be used to diagnose abnormal peristaltic patterns in the pharynx and esophagus through insertion of pressure measurement transducers.

SPECIFIC NURSING INTERVENTIONS FOR FEEDING PATIENTS

When feeding a patient with dysphagia, the nurse should sit down with the patient in a quiet, well-lit room during feeding and constantly be attuned to signs of aspiration or respiration/voice changes. There are specific recommendations for **body position** of the patient with dysphagia while eating and swallowing. The person should be seated upright during and for about a half hour after the meal to prevent reflux. The patient should place their arms on the table for support. Usually, the patient's head is flexed downward and chin tucked in to protect the airway and avoid aspiration. The nurse may need to put their palm on the patient's forehead to help support the patient's head. The patient should consume the meal **slowly**, taking up to 45 minutes and allowing the sensory awareness of the food. At first, only small bites of soft foods are suggested. Generally, the food should be placed firmly with a teaspoon toward the **back of the tongue**. If the person has paralysis or other issues on one side, the food should be put on the unaffected side. It may be necessary to take the spoon out and have the person move the food back, or possibly physically seal the lips to initiate the swallowing reflex.

DIETARY MODIFICATIONS AND ADMINISTRATION OF MEDICATIONS

Liquid and food **consistencies** are important considerations for the feeding of patients with dysphagia and should be selected according to the nature of the swallowing disorder. The Academy of Nutrition and Dietetics (AND) has developed standardized classifications to define both. Liquid consistencies are classified as **thin** (water, broth, milk, most juices, supplements, coffee, and tea), **nectar-like** (nectars and prune juice), **honey-like**, and **spoon thick**. The latter two refer to consistencies created by the addition of a thickening agent. Food consistency is divided into four levels through which patients proceed. **Level 1 foods**, such as those that have been pureed, do not necessitate much chewing. **Level 2 foods** have been mechanically changed to be consistent and semi-solid and therefore require limited chewing capacity. **Level 3 foods** are soft but require more chewing, and foods classified as **level 4** are normal foods that have solid consistency. Constipation can be averted through the addition of bran or prune juice. Medications are usually given in custard or a gelatin product.

FEEDING TUBES

Feeding tubes are indicated when a patient with dysphagia cannot obtain adequate nutrition **orally,** and the tube should be removed once the patient can re-establish normal nutrition. The tubes are often used initially during treatment but should not be used long-term. **Fine bore nasogastric tubes** are recommended. If feeding tubes are needed for a month or longer, they are usually surgically positioned. Problems with feeding tubes

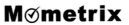

can include irritation, swelling, bleeding, aspiration, peritonitis, diarrhea, and displacement of the tube. Some medications may be administered through the tube. Patients receiving **enteral nutrition** need to be checked every day for evidence of edema or dehydration. Intake and output, including characteristics of fluid and stool output, need to be evaluated daily as well. Less frequent measurements should include chemistries, serum electrolyte levels, blood urea nitrogen (BUN), blood counts, and weight.

REHABILITATION TEAM

A patient with dysphagia has a team of health care providers involved in their treatment. A **doctor** is ultimately accountable for the patient's management, refers the patient to rehabilitation team members, and prescribes dietary changes. The **nurse** generally conducts a patient history, physical examination, self-feeding, and swallowing studies, and monitors essential parameters such as caloric intake, weight, hydration, and nourishment. The nurse is also the primary link between all team members and the patient and family. Other important team members are as follows: the **physical therapist**, who is responsible for devising exercises to promote the tone of any muscles used for eating; the **occupational therapist**, who educates the patient about use of adaptive devices or exercises to improve hand movement; the **speech pathologist**, who usually does the bedside swallow test, suggests the compensatory postures and swallowing techniques to use, and addresses speech problems; and the **dietitian**, responsible for the diet plan and monitoring of nutritional status.

GENERAL SKIN ASSESSMENT

Skin color varies according to ethnicity. Color changes should be assessed to determine if they are local or extend over the entire body, and if they are permanent or transient. Pallor may indicate stress, impaired oxygenation, and vasoconstriction. Erythema may indicate vasodilation, local inflammation, and blushing. Cyanosis indicates impaired oxygenation, and jaundice indicates increased bilirubin.

Temperature is typically assessed by touching the skin with the back of the hand. Skin should be warm and equal bilaterally. Hypothermia may indicate impaired circulation, intravenous infusion, and immobilized limb (such as in a cast). Hyperthermia may indicate fever, infection, and excessive exercise.

> **Review Video: Skin Assessment**
> Visit mometrix.com/academy and enter code: 794925

EFFECTS OF AGE ON SKIN

Age is an important consideration when evaluating the skin because the characteristics of the skin change as people age.

- An **infant's** skin is thinner than an adult's because, while the epidermis is developed, the dermis layer is only about 60% of that of an adult and continues to develop after birth. The skin of premature infants is especially friable, allowing for transepidermal water loss and evaporative heat loss.
- During **adolescence**, the hair follicles activate, the thickness of the dermis decreases about 20%, and epidermal turnover time increases, so healing slows.
- As people **continue to age**, Langerhans' cells decrease in number, making the skin more prone to cancer, and the inflammatory reactions decrease. The sweat glands, vascularity, and subcutaneous fat all decrease, interfering with thermoregulation and contributing to dryness and irritation of the skin. The epidermal-dermal junction flattens, resulting in skin that is prone to tearing. The elastin in the skin degrades with age and solar exposure. The thinning of the hypodermis can lead to pressure ulcers.

> **Review Video: Integumentary System**
> Visit mometrix.com/academy and enter code: 655980

Functional Health Patterns

ASSESSMENT CHARACTERISTICS OF ARTERIAL, NEUROPATHIC, AND VENOUS ULCERS

The assessment process is important in delineating between the arterial, neuropathic, or venous origin of the ulcer. Characteristics of each must be known and closely examined:

Location

- **Arterial**: Ends of toes, pressure points, traumatic nonhealing wounds
- **Neuropathic**: Plantar surface, metatarsal heads, toes, and sides of feet
- **Venous**: Between knees and ankles, medial malleolus

Wound Bed

- **Arterial**: Pale, necrotic
- **Neuropathic**: Red (or ischemic)
- **Venous**: Dark red, fibrinous slough

Exudate

- **Arterial**: Slight amount, infection common
- **Neuropathic**: Moderate to large amounts, infection common
- **Venous**: Moderate to large amounts

Wound Perimeter

- **Arterial**: Circular, well-defined
- **Neuropathic**: Circular, well-defined, often with callous formation
- **Venous**: Irregular, poorly-defined

Pain

- **Arterial**: Very painful
- **Neuropathic**: Pain often absent because of reduced sensation
- **Venous**: Pain varies

Skin

- **Arterial**: Pale, friable, shiny, and hairless, with dependent rubor and elevational pallor
- **Neuropathic**: Ischemic signs (as in arterial) may be evident with comorbidity
- **Venous**: Brownish discoloration of ankles and shin, edema common

Pulses

- **Arterial**: Weak or absent
- **Neuropathic**: Present and palpable, diminished in neuroischemic ulcers
- **Venous**: Present and palpable

PRESSURE ULCERS

Pressure ulcers occur when pressure from the weight of the body causes a decrease in perfusion, affecting arterial and capillary blood flow and resulting in ischemia. Ulcers may then develop from pressure, shearing, and friction. Common pressure points include the occiput, scapula, sacrum, buttocks, ischium, and heels. Patients with a decreased level of consciousness, brain/spinal cord injuries, peripheral neuropathies, malnutrition, dehydration, PVD, or impaired mobility are at a higher risk for pressure ulcers. Critically ill patients are at an increased risk due to prolonged immobility, sedation, and often incontinence of urine and

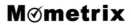

stool. In addition, patients on vasopressors are at a higher risk due to the constriction of the peripheral circulation.

Signs and symptoms: Early stages include redness, tenderness, and firmness at the site of the ulcer. Once the ulcer progresses to severe tissue injury, bone, muscle, or tendons may be exposed, and there may be a yellow or black wound base in addition to pain and drainage at the site.

Diagnostics: Skin and wound assessment, including staging of the ulcer.

Treatment: Wet-to-Dry dressings, Wound VAC therapy, and hyperbaric oxygen may be used; a wound care consult is often advised.

Prevention: Begins with a risk assessment; the Braden scale is a commonly used scale. A score of 16 or below indicates that the patient is at risk. At-risk patients or patients with active ulcers should be placed on a turning and positioning schedule or on a specialty bed to relieve pressure. Moisture barriers and skin protectants may also be utilized.

NATIONAL PRESSURE INJURY ADVISORY PANEL STAGING

Pressure ulcers result from pressure or pressure with shear and/or friction over bony prominences. The **National Pressure Injury Advisory Panel (NPIAP) stages** include:

- **Suspected deep tissue injury**: Skin discolored, intact or blood blister
- **Stage I**: Intact skin with non-blanching reddened area
- **Stage II**: Abrasion or blistered area without slough but with partial-thickness skin loss
- **Stage III**: Deep ulcer with exposed subcutaneous tissue; tunneling or undermining may be evident with or without slough
- **Stage IV**: Deep ulcer, full thickness, with necrosis into muscle, bone, tendons, and/or joints
- **Unstageable**: Eschar and/or slough prevents staging prior to debridement

Patients should be placed on pressure-reducing support surfaces and turned at least every two hours, avoiding the area(s) with a pressure ulcer. Wound care depends on the stage of the wound and the amount of drainage but includes irrigation, debridement when necessary, antibiotics for infection, and appropriate dressing.

Functional Health Patterns

Patients should be encouraged to have adequate protein and iron in their diets to promote healing and to maintain adequate hydration.

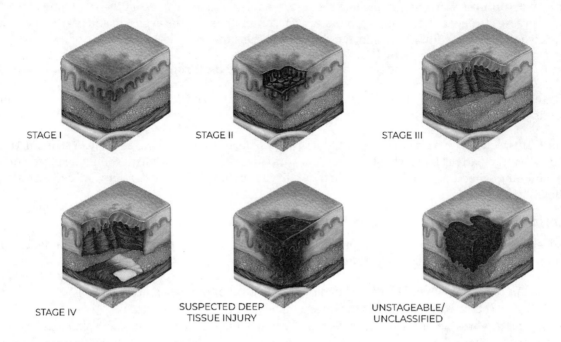

STAGE I   STAGE II   STAGE III

STAGE IV   SUSPECTED DEEP TISSUE INJURY   UNSTAGEABLE/ UNCLASSIFIED

ASSESSMENT OF PRESSURE ULCERS

When assessing an ulcer, it is necessary to determine if it is a non-pressure or pressure ulcer because the treatment protocol may vary depending upon whether the ulcer is caused by pressure, venous or arterial insufficiency, or neuropathic disorders. The clinical basis for this determination should be clearly outlined.

- The ulcer should be classified according to the stage and the characteristics, including size (length, width, and depth).
- Pain associated with the ulcer should be described.
- Photographs should be taken if a protocol is in place.
- Ulcers should be monitored daily and any changes carefully documented.
- The ulcer should be evaluated for signs of infection.

It is important to differentiate between colonization, which is very common, and infection, which usually presents with symptoms such as periwound erythema, induration, and increased pain as well as delayed healing of the wound. Wound culture and blood tests should be done if there are indications of infection. Treatment should be determined according to the characteristics of the wound.

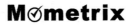

BRADEN SCALE

The Braden scale is a risk assessment tool that has been validated clinically as predictive of the risk of patients developing pressure sores. It was developed in 1988 by Barbara Braden and Nancy Bergstrom and is in wide use. The scale scores six different areas, with five areas scored 1-4 points and one area 1-3 points. The lower the score, the greater the risk.

Area	Score of 1	Score of 2	Score of 3	Score of 4
Sensory perception	Completely limited	Very limited	Slightly limited	No impairment
Moisture	Constantly moist	Very moist	Occasionally moist	Rarely moist
Activity	Bed	Chair	Occasional walk	Frequent walk
Mobility	Immobile	Limited	Slightly limited	No limitations
Nutritional pattern	Very poor	Inadequate	Adequate	Excellent
Friction and shear	Problem	Potential problem	No apparent problem	

CAUSES OF PRESSURE ULCERS

PRESSURE INTENSITY, PRESSURE DURATION, AND TISSUE TOLERANCE

Pressure ulcers, also known as decubitus ulcers, are caused primarily by pressure, but there are numerous additional considerations:

- **Pressure intensity**: Capillary closing pressure (10-32 mmHg) is the minimal pressure needed to collapse capillaries, reducing tissue perfusion. This pressure can be easily exceeded in the sitting or supine position if weight is not shifted.
- **Duration of pressure**: Low pressure for long periods and high pressure for short periods can both result in pressure ulcers.
- **Tissue tolerance**: The tissue tolerance is the ability of the skin to tolerate and redistribute pressure, preventing anoxia. Both extrinsic and intrinsic factors can affect tissue tolerance. Extrinsic factors include shear (the skin stays in place but the underlying tissue slides), friction (moving the skin against bedding or other objects), and moisture. Intrinsic factors include poor nutrition, advanced age, low blood pressure, stress, smoking, and low body temperature.

SHEAR AND FRICTION

Shear occurs when the skin stays in place and the underlying tissue in the deep fascia over the bony prominences stretches and slides, damaging vessels and tissue and often resulting in undermining. Shear is one of the most common causes of ulcers, which are often described as pressure ulcers but are technically somewhat different, although the effects of shearing are often combined with pressure. The most common cause of shear is elevation of the head of the bed over 30°. Friction against the sheets holds the skin in place while the body slides down the bed, resulting in pressure and damage in the sacrococcygeal area. The underlying vessels are damaged and thrombosed, leading to undermining and deep ulceration.

Friction is a significant cause of pressure ulcers because it acts with gravity to cause shear. Friction by itself results only in damage to the epidermis and dermis, such as abrasions or denudement referred to as "sheet burn." Friction and pressure can combine, however, to form ulcers.

MEASURES TO CONTROL SHEAR AND FRICTION

Because **shear** and **friction** are primary factors in the development of pressure ulcers, measures to reduce them are essential:

- The head of the bed should never be elevated more than 30°; however, bed-bound patients may not be able to feed themselves at this angle. If the bed is elevated higher, the patient should be carefully positioned, using a pull sheet or overhead trapeze to make sure the patient is at the right position. The bed should be lowered as soon as possible.

Note: Elevating the foot of the bed to prevent sliding and shear simply increases pressure to the sacrococcygeal area, solving one problem by creating another.

- Making sure that the skin is dry; using fine cornstarch-based powders may help prevent the skin from "sticking" to the sheets.
- Pull sheets or mechanical lifting devices should be used to lift, move, or transfer the patient.
- Medical treatments may reduce restlessness.
- Heel and elbow protectors provide protection.

MANAGEMENT OF PRESSURE ULCERS

MEASURES TO PROMOTE MOBILITY

Mobility is a problem for many patients with pressure ulcers because their restricted mobility is often the cause of the ulcers in the first place. However, promoting mobility to the extent possible improves circulation, aids healing, and decreases risk of developing further pressure ulcers:

- Bed-bound patients must be repositioned on a scheduled basis and should receive passive ROM exercises and active bed exercises if tolerated daily. The patient's head should be elevated only to 30° for short periods of time.
- Patients with limited mobility should be evaluated by physical and occupational therapists in order to develop an individualized plan for activities. Patients may need assistive devices, such as walkers, canes, or wheelchairs. Because the wound must be protected without compromise to circulation, the amount and type of mobility or exercises must be designed with respect to the area and stage of the ulcer as well as underlying pathology or co-morbid conditions.

MEASURES TO CONTROL FECAL INCONTINENCE

Control of fecal incontinence is necessary to prevent deterioration of tissue that can increase the risk of pressure ulcers and to prevent contamination of existing pressure ulcers:

- Assess incontinence to determine cause and whether it is temporary, related to health problems, or chronic.
- Determine the type of incontinence:
  - Passive, in which the person is unaware.
  - Urge, which is the inability to retain stool.
  - Seepage, after a bowel movement or around a blockage.
- Use medications as indicated to control diarrhea or constipation.
- Place on a bowel-training regimen with scheduled bowel movements, using suppositories, stool softeners, and bulk formers as indicated, according to cause of incontinence. Use skin moisture barriers and absorbent pads or briefs as needed
- Modify diet as needed with foods to control diarrhea or constipation.
- Ensure adequate fluid intake.
- Consider fecal pouches or fecal containment devices if incontinence cannot be otherwise controlled.

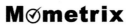

MEASURES TO CONTROL URINARY INCONTINENCE

Control of urinary incontinence is necessary to prevent deterioration of the tissue that can increase the risk of pressure ulcers:

- Assess incontinence to determine cause and whether it is temporary, related to health problems, or chronic.
- A temporary Foley catheter may be used in some cases while tissue heals, but long-term use is contraindicated because of the danger of infections.
- Medications may be indicated to treat urinary infections or frequency. Scheduled toileting with reinforcement may help to decrease incidence.
- Use absorbent pads or adult diapers that wick liquid away from the body, and establish a regular schedule for changing.
- Cleanse soiled skin with no-rinse wipes, as they are less drying to skin than soap and water.
- Use skin moisture barrier ointments to protect skin from urine.
- Use protective and support devices as needed.
- Avoid positioning on ulcers.

PRESSURE REDUCTION SURFACES

Pressure reduction surfaces redistribute pressure to prevent pressure ulcers and reduce shear and friction. There are various types of support surfaces for beds, examining tables, operating tables, and chairs. Functions of pressure reduction surfaces include temperature control, moisture control, and friction/shear control. **General use guidelines** include:

- Pressure redistribution support surfaces should be used for patients with stage II, III, and IV ulcers, as well as for those that are at risk for developing pressure ulcers.
- Chairs should have gel or air support surfaces to redistribute pressure for chair-bound patients, critically ill patients, or those who cannot move independently.
- Support surface material should provide at least an inch of support under areas to be protected when in use to prevent bottoming out. (Check by placing hand palm-up under the overlay below the pressure point.)
- Static support surfaces are appropriate for patients who can change position without increasing pressure to an ulcer.
- Dynamic support surfaces are needed for those who need assistance to move or when static pressure devices provide less than an inch of support.

ELEMENTS OF WOUND ASSESSMENT

LOCATION AND SIZE

Wound location should be described in terms of anatomic position using landmarks (such as sternal notch, umbilicus, lateral malleolus), correct medical terminology, and directional terms:

- Anterior (in front)
- Posterior (behind)
- Superior (above)
- Inferior (below)

Wound size should be carefully described through actual measurement rather than association (the size of a dime). Measurements should be done with a disposable ruler in millimeters or centimeters. The current standard for measurement:

$$length \times width \times depth = dimension$$

Functional Health Patterns

However, a clear description requires more detail. The measurement should be done at the greatest width and greatest length. More than two measurements may be needed if the wound is very irregularly shaped. The depth of the wound should be measured by inserting a sterile applicator and grasping or marking the applicator at skin level and then measuring the length below. Ideally, the wound should be photographed as well, following protocols for photography.

WOUND BED TISSUE

Wound bed tissue should be described as completely as possible, including color and general appearance:

- **Granulation tissue** is slightly granular in appearance and deep pink to bright red and moist, bleeding easily if disturbed.
- **Clean non-granular tissue** is smooth and deep pink or red and is not healing.
- **Hypergranulation** is excessive, soft, flaccid granulating tissue that is raised above the level of the periwound tissue, preventing proper epithelization, and may reflect excess moisture in the wound.
- **Epithelization** should appear at wound edges first and then eventually cover the wound. It is dry and light pink or violet in color.
- **Slough** is necrotic tissue that is viscous, soft, and yellow-gray in appearance and adheres to the wound.
- **Eschar** is hard dark brown or black leathery necrotic tissue that accumulates with death of the tissue.

WOUND MARGINS

Wound margins and the tissue surrounding the wound should be described carefully and with correct terminology:

- **Color** should be described using color descriptions and such terms as blanched, erythematous (red), or ecchymosed (purple, green, yellow).
- **Skin texture** may be normal, indurated (hardened), or edematous (swollen). Note if there is cellulitis or maceration evident.
- **Wound edges** may be diffuse (without clear margins), well defined, or rolled. A healing ridge may be evident if granulation has begun. Note if the wound is closed (as with a surgical incision) or open (as with dehiscence or ulcerations). Note if wound edges are attached or unattached (indicating undermining or tunneling).
- **Tunneling or undermining** should be assessed by probing the wound margins with a moist sterile cotton applicator, using clock face locators (toward the head is 12 o'clock, for example). Tunneling may be described as extending from 3 o'clock to 4 o'clock. A large area is usually described as undermining. The size should be measured or estimated as closely as possible.

DISTRIBUTION, DRAINAGE, AND ODOR

Distribution of lesions should be clearly delineated if there is more than one lesion over an area. The arrangement of the lesions can be helpful for diagnosis and treatments.

- Linear (in a line)
- Satellites (small lesions around a larger one)
- Diffuse (scattered freely over an area)

Drainage may vary considerably from nothing at all to copious outpourings of discharge.

- Serous drainage is usually clear to slightly yellow.
- Serosanguineous drainage is a combination of serous drainage and blood.
- Sanguineous drainage is bloody.
- Purulent discharge may be thick and milky, yellow, brownish, or green, depending upon the infective agent.

Odor requires more subjective assessment, but the odor and type of discharge together can provide useful information. Some infective agents, such as *Pseudomonas*, produce distinctive odors, which may be described in various ways: musty, foul, sweet.

WOUND HEALING, TREATMENT, AND DRESSINGS
PRIMARY, SECONDARY, AND TERTIARY HEALING

Primary healing (healing by first intention) involves a wound that is surgically closed by suturing, flaps, or split or full-thickness grafts to completely cover the wound. Primary healing is the most common approach used for surgeries or repair of wounds or lacerations, especially when the wound is essentially "clean."

Secondary healing (healing by second intention) involves leaving the wound open and allowing it to close through granulation and epithelialization. Debridement of the wound is done to prepare the wound bed for healing. This approach may be used with contaminated "dirty" or infected wounds to prevent abscess formation and allow the wound to drain.

Tertiary healing (healing by third intention) is also sometimes called delayed primary closure because it involves first debriding the wound and allowing it to begin healing while open and then later closing the wound through suturing or grafts. This approach is common with wounds that are contaminated, such as severe animal bites, or wounds related to mixed trauma.

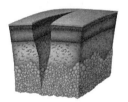 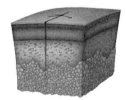 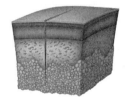

PHASES OF WOUND HEALING

There are **four phases of wound healing**:

1. **Hemostasis** is the first phase of wound healing, occurring within minutes of injury. After the wound occurs, the blood vessels constrict to decrease bleeding. Platelets gather to form a clot and then secrete factors, which cause the production of thrombin. This stimulates fibrin formation from fibrinogen. The resultant clot is a strong one, which becomes the serosanguinous crust (scab) for the wound. Platelets secrete cytokines, including platelet-derived growth factor that begins the healing process.
2. The **inflammation phase** occurs next and lasts about four days normally. Blood vessels in the area leak plasma and neutrophils into the wound, causing erythema, edema, and increased warmth. Any debris or microorganisms are destroyed by the neutrophils and localized mast cells through phagocytosis. When fibrin is broken down, it attracts macrophages to the area. They also destroy microorganisms and secrete growth factors to stimulate the next phase of healing.
3. The **proliferative phase** occurs over about days 5-20 in normal healing. During the proliferative phase, fibroblasts secrete collagen to manufacture a framework within the wound. New capillaries sprout from damaged vessel ends in a process called angiogenesis. Keratinocytes cause epithelialization in which new skin cells form at the edges of the wound, migrating inward to meet in the center of the defect. Approximately five days after a wound occurs, the fibroblasts and myofibroblasts contract to bring the wound edges closer, resulting in a smaller defect.

175

4. **Remodeling or maturation** of a wound begins about 21 days after the wound occurs and continues over the next year. Collagen is deposited, eventually resulting in a stiff, strong scar that has 70-80% of the tensile strength of normal skin. Blood vessels in the newly formed tissues gradually disappear from the scar during this phase.

WOUND CLEANSING WITH EACH DRESSING CHANGE

Microorganisms, contaminants, and cellular debris in a wound can significantly delay healing and increase inflammation. Antiseptics such as hydrogen peroxide, acetic acid, povidone-iodine, or sodium hypochlorite (Dakin solution) are toxic to developing fibroblasts and interfere with healing over time. They are sometimes used and rinsed with saline for a short period of time to control heavily infected wounds. The current standard is to use irrigation to deliver normal saline in a manner forceful enough to break the adhesion of debris to the wound bed yet gentle enough to prevent injury to developing cells. Pressures of at least 5-15 psi delivered by mechanical irrigators are needed for effective cleansing. Higher pressures can cause penetration of the fluid into tissues. Irrigation using a 12 mL syringe and a 22 G needle will deliver a force of 13 psi. The use of a 35 mL syringe and a 19 G needle will deliver 8 psi and is more effective than using a bulb syringe when mechanical irrigation is not available.

CLEANSING A WOUND BY SOAKING

Soaking is a beneficial way to cleanse a wound that has a large amount of necrotic debris or contamination. Contamination must be removed from new wounds to avoid excess inflammation that will delay wound healing. Soaking softens any necrotic tissue and helps to ease it away from the healthy tissue at the bottom of the wound bed. It also helps to loosen contaminants that are embedded in the wound. Antiseptic agents should not be used in the soaking solution. Soaking may be accomplished using any container that will hold the wound area, or by whirlpool. The container must be disinfected well prior to and after the soaking. It may take several soaks to remove tough, dry eschar, and once the necrotic material has been removed, soaking should be discontinued, as it will then delay healing.

IRRIGATING A WOUND FOR CLEANSING PURPOSES

When **irrigating a wound** for cleansing purposes, the area beneath the wound should be covered to prevent contamination of the bed linens:

1. Place a basin beneath the wound to catch the returned solution.
2. Wash hands and wear gloves.
3. Use pulsatile lavage or a syringe to deliver water or saline with a force of 5-15 psi to the wound bed. Using pressure >15 psi forcefully injects irrigating fluid into newly formed tissues and risks inoculating microorganisms into deeper tissues. Highly contaminated or infected wounds may require pressure at the higher range of 15 psi to cleanse. Use low pressure (5-8 psi) to cleanse healthy wounds so new capillaries are not damaged.
4. Flush undermined, tunneled areas well, and then massage over the area of tunneling or undermining to dislodge debris and encourage the fluid to return.
5. Repeat as needed until the return fluid is free of debris.
6. Finish by packing these areas as ordered.

CLEANSING A SHALLOW WOUND BY SCRUBBING

Scrubbing is sometimes combined with a cleansing solution to initially cleanse a wound to remove debris. It is best performed using a very porous, soft sponge and a nonionic surfactant cleansing solution to avoid damaging the wound bed as much as possible. Even so, damage to the wound bed is often unavoidable, so scrubbing may be done initially to a traumatic wound, but the practice should not be continued after the wound is clean and beginning to heal because it can disrupt the development of granulation tissue and damage areas of epithelialization. When scrubbing, one should begin cleansing in the center of the wound and work in a circle toward the edges of the wound, avoiding recleansing an area to prevent recontamination of the center of the wound.

PERIWOUND CLEANSING

The stratum corneum of the **periwound skin** is not as stable as normal skin. Periwound skin has more skin debris, such as water-insoluble proteins, amino acids, urea, ammonia, microorganisms, and cholesterol, than other tissue. Microorganisms up to 10 cm away from the wound edge can be more numerous and differ from those found in the wound bed, so cleansing prevents wound contamination. The microorganism level increases when the amount of protein on the periwound surface is increased. This area must be cleansed along with the wound when dressing changes are done. Cleansing reduces bacterial counts within and around the wound for about 24 hours. Normal saline may not remove these substances adequately. A skin cleanser that is mild and will not harm skin or strip away intercellular lipids may be used on the periwound area.

BASIC DRESSING REQUIREMENTS

The **basic dressing requirements**, regardless of the type, are the following:

- Maintain a moist environment in order to promote healing.
- Absorb wound drainage and prevent leakage.
- Increase wound temperature to promote healing.
- Provide a protective barrier to prevent mechanical injury to the wound.
- Provide a protective barrier to prevent colonization and infection with microorganisms.
- Allow exchange of gases and fluids.
- Retain and absorb odor of the wound or drainage.
- Remove easily without causing additional trauma to the wound or disrupting the healing process.
- Debride wound of dead tissue and exudate.
- Provide protection without toxicity or causing sensitivity reactions.
- Provide a sterile protective covering for the wound.

The dressing that directly covers the wound may be inadequate to absorb large amounts of drainage, so sometimes additional secondary dressings are needed.

WOUND DRESSING SELECTION

The proper **dressing** for a wound may change over time depending on wound characteristics:

- The wound environment's moisture content may call for a dressing that either wicks away too much moisture or provides moisture to a dry wound to enhance epithelialization.
- Slough and dry eschar calls for a dressing that will enhance debriding.
- The presence of tunneling or undermining will require a packing material.
- Some wounds need dressings that are absorbent and deodorizing to control exudate.
- Control and prevention of infection is important in some wounds.
- Dressings must allow oxygen, water, and carbon dioxide to be exchanged between the environment and the wound.
- Dressings need to provide warmth as well.
- Dressings must not adhere to or harm the wound tissues but must be kept in place reliably without harming the skin around the wound.

Functional Health Patterns

CATEGORIES OF DRESSINGS AND METHODS OF SECURING DRESSINGS

Dressings are considered primary if they are next to the wound surface and secondary if they are used to cover the primary or to secure the dressing. There are **three main types of dressings** to consider when determining which will be the most effective for a particular type of wound:

- **Traditional topical dressings** are used primarily to cover the wound, such as gauze and tulle.
- **Interactive dressings**, such as polymeric films, are generally transparent so that the wound can be observed and are permeable to water vapor and oxygen but provide an effective barrier for microorganisms, such as hyaluronic acid, hydrogel, and foam dressings.
- **Bioactive dressings** provide substances that directly promote wound healing, such as hydrocolloids, alginates, collagens, and chitosan.

Securing a dressing depends on the health of the surrounding skin and the type of dressing. Skin protection and tape may be appropriate. Some are self-adherent. Tubular dressings or wraps can help to secure dressings with fragile skin.

IMPACT OF ANTICHOLINERGICS ON SWALLOWING

Anticholinergic medications inhibit the neurotransmitter acetylcholine by blocking its action and thereby stopping or decreasing nerve impulse transmission of the parasympathetic nervous system. The result is the relaxing of smooth muscle tissue, like that found in the bladder and GI tract, decreasing spasms. These drugs are often administered in the treatment of incontinence, Parkinson's disease, cardiovascular disease, psychiatric conditions, and allergies. One of the most common side effects of anticholinergic medications is dysphagia, and because these medications are commonly prescribed to the elderly population, they enhance a risk that is already present in this demographic.

Anticholinergic effects are cumulative and include urinary retention, dry mouth, dry eyes, and constipation. CNS effects include sedation, confusion, hallucinations (auditory and visual), and increased risks of falls. Effects that more directly lead to dysphagia include relaxation of the lower esophageal sphincter, dry mouth leading to difficulty with appropriately moistening food in preparation for swallowing, interference with peristalsis due to the drug's impact on smooth muscle tissue, and oral muscle weakness. Patients on anticholinergics should be closely monitored for difficulties in any phase of the swallowing process, and for signs of aspiration.

> **Review Video: Cholinergic and Anticholinergic Drugs**
> Visit mometrix.com/academy and enter code: 245811

POTENTIALLY HARMFUL INTERACTIONS BETWEEN MEDICATIONS AND SPECIFIC FOODS OR NUTRITIONAL STATUS

Certain medications and herbal preparations can affect nutritional status. Some medications cause **accelerated depletion of essential nutrients**, such as furosemide (a diuretic that increases excretion of fluids, including sodium, potassium, and calcium) and cholestyramine (which prompts excretion of folic acid, vitamin B12, the fat-soluble vitamins, iron, and calcium). Others impede **absorption of essential nutrients** in the gastrointestinal tract, such as phenobarbital and similar compounds that affect calcium absorption, or the habitual use of antacids or potassium, which depletes a number of vitamins and minerals. Likewise, some foods hinder or occasionally enhance **absorption of certain medications**. Examples include amino acids or carbohydrates, which respectively decrease or increase assimilation of levodopa, phenytoin, and theophylline. Enteric coatings on pills can be worn off through ingestion of hot beverages, alcohol, or milk. It is also important to establish the patient's use of herbals because many have potentially harmful side effects.

Elimination Patterns

ASSESSMENT OF KIDNEYS AND URINARY TRACT

Assessment of kidneys and urinary tract includes:

- Assess the health history for family urinary system disease and risk factors, such as previous urinary disease, increased age, immobility, hypertension, diabetes, chemical exposure, chronic disease, radiation to the pelvis, STDs, alcohol or drug use, and complications of pregnancy and delivery.
- Determine daily fluid intake.
- Question symptoms such as flank or abdominal pain, hesitancy, urgency, difficulty or straining with voiding, difficulty emptying the bladder, urinary incontinence, fatigue, SOB, exercise intolerance from anemia, fever, chills, blood in the urine, and GI symptoms.

Physical assessment includes vital signs, kidney and bladder palpation, and percussion over the bladder after urination:

- Palpate for ascites and edema.
- Measure the DTRs and check gait and ability to walk heel-to-toe.
- Examine the genitalia and check the urethra and vagina for herniation, irritation, or tears.

Urine specimen is obtained via clean catch midstream technique for analysis and culture if indicated. Blood is taken for a CBC, and in males, prostate-specific antigen (PSA) levels will also be measured via blood specimen.

Functional Health Patterns

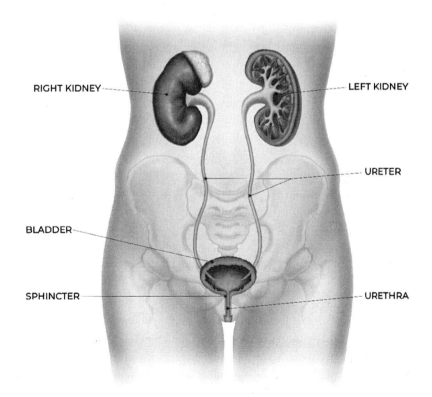

RIGHT KIDNEY — LEFT KIDNEY — URETER — BLADDER — SPHINCTER — URETHRA

Review Video: <u>Urinary System</u>
Visit mometrix.com/academy and enter code: 601053

KIDNEY REGULATORY FUNCTIONS REGARDING FLUID BALANCE

Kidney regulatory functions include maintaining **fluid balance**. Fluid excretion balances intake with output, so increased intake results in a large output and vice versa:

- **Osmolality** (the number of electrolytes and other molecules per kg/urine) measures the concentration or dilution. With dehydration, osmolality increases; with fluid retention, osmolality decreases. With kidney disease, urine is dilute and the osmolality is fixed.
- **Specific gravity** compares the weight of urine (weight of particles) to distilled water (1.000). Normal urine is 1.010-1.025 with normal intake. High intake lowers the specific gravity, and low intake raises it. In kidney disease, it often does not vary.
- **Antidiuretic hormone** (ADH/vasopressin) regulates the excretion of water and urine concentration in the renal tubule by varying water reabsorption. When fluid intake decreases, blood osmolality rises, and this stimulates the release of ADH, which increases reabsorption of fluid to return osmolality to normal levels. ADH is suppressed with increased fluid intake, so less fluid is reabsorbed.

CHRONIC KIDNEY DISEASE

Chronic kidney disease (CKD) occurs when the kidneys are unable to filter and excrete wastes, concentrate urine, and maintain electrolyte balance because of hypoxic conditions, kidney disease, or obstruction in the urinary tract. It results first in azotemia (increase in nitrogenous waste in the blood) and then in uremia (nitrogenous wastes cause toxic symptoms). When >50% of the functional renal capacity is destroyed, the kidneys can no longer carry out necessary functions, and progressive deterioration begins over months or years. Symptoms are often non-specific in the beginning, with loss of appetite and energy.

Symptoms and complications are as follows:

- Weight loss
- Headaches, muscle cramping, general malaise
- Increased bruising and dry or itchy skin
- Increased BUN and creatinine
- Sodium and fluid retention with edema
- Hyperkalemia
- Metabolic acidosis
- Calcium and phosphorus depletion, resulting in altered bone metabolism, pain, and retarded growth
- Anemia with decreased production on RBCs. Increased risk of infection
- Uremic syndrome

Treatment includes:

- Supportive/symptomatic therapy
- Dialysis and transplantation
- Diet control: low protein, salt, potassium, and phosphorus
- Fluid limitations
- Calcium and vitamin supplementation
- Phosphate binders

ESRD

Patients with **end-stage renal disease** (ESRD) must monitor their diet and fluid intake carefully as instructed by a renal dietitian. Guidelines recommend a daily intake of 1.0–1.5 g/kg protein, 2–3 g sodium, 60–90 milliequivalents of potassium, 600–800 mg phosphorus, and fluid intake of 1.0–1.2 liters. Urine output is also monitored (if the individual is still producing urine). **Dialysis regimens** affect blood glucose levels in patients with diabetes because glucose is incorporated into dialysate fluid, and blood pressure is often decreased after dialysis. Therefore, patients on medications for hypertension should be careful about taking those medications

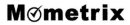

immediately prior to dialysis. ESRD patients may require a myriad of medications, including antihypertensive agents, iron supplements, insulin, phosphate binders (for stool elimination), antidepressants, or human growth hormone (generally children). **Epoetin alfa** (and iron) is usually injected intravenously or subcutaneously during the dialysis process to bolster erythropoietin levels and red blood cells, in order to minimize risks for anemia. Currently, mild to moderate **exercise** is suggested (if possible) for ESRD patients. These individuals are prone to psychosocial and emotional problems due to the impact of the disease on their quality of life and time/travel constraints required for maintaining their dialysis regimen.

> **Review Video: End-Stage Renal Disease**
> Visit mometrix.com/academy and enter code: 869617

RENAL DIALYSIS
PERITONEAL DIALYSIS

Renal dialysis is used primarily for those who have progressed from renal insufficiency to uremia with end-stage renal disease (ESRD). It may also be temporarily for acute conditions. People can be maintained on dialysis, but there are many complications associated with dialysis, so many people are considered for renal transplantation. There are a number of different approaches to **peritoneal dialysis:**

- **Peritoneal dialysis:** An indwelling catheter is inserted surgically into the peritoneal cavity with a subcutaneous tunnel and a Dacron cuff to prevent infection. Sterile dialysate solution is slowly instilled through gravity, remains for a prescribed length of time, and is then drained and discarded.
- **Continuous ambulatory peritoneal dialysis:** a series of exchange cycles is repeated 24 hours a day.
- **Continuous cyclic peritoneal dialysis:** a prolonged period of retaining fluid occurs during the day with drainage at night.

Peritoneal dialysis may be used for those who want to be more independent, don't live near a dialysis center, or want fewer dietary restrictions.

> **Review Video: End-Stage Renal Disease**
> Visit mometrix.com/academy and enter code: 869617

HEMODIALYSIS

Hemodialysis, the most common type of dialysis, is used for both short-term dialysis and long-term for those with ESRD. Treatments are usually done three times weekly for 3-4 hours or daily dialysis with treatment either during the night or in short daily periods. **Hemodialysis** is often done for those who can't manage peritoneal dialysis or who live near a dialysis center, but it does interfere with work or school attendance and requires strict dietary and fluid restrictions between treatments. Short daily dialysis allows more independence, and increased costs may be offset by lower morbidity. A vascular access device, such as a catheter, fistula, or graft, must be established for hemodialysis, and heparin is used to prevent clotting. With hemodialysis, blood is circulated outside of the body through a dialyzer (a synthetic semipermeable membrane), which filters the blood. There are many different types of dialyzers. High flux dialyzers use a highly permeable membrane that shortens the duration of treatment and decreases the need for heparin.

MICTURITION

Micturition (urination) begins when the bladder is filled with urine, after the urine is filtered through the kidneys and then passes to the bladder through the ureters. The urine is stored in the bladder until a threshold volume, typically 200–300 mL, is reached. In this filling stage, pressure builds up, and continence is maintained by sympathetic control mechanisms such as the release of the α-adrenergic neurotransmitter **norepinephrine**, which contracts the internal sphincter, and **β-receptors** that depress contraction of the detrusor muscle. Micturition proceeds when pressure increases and a feeling of fullness is achieved through parasympathetic release of the cholinergic neurotransmitter **acetylcholine** at the bladder base. The bladder

Functional Health Patterns

181

neck opens and the bladder contracts. Acetylcholine is also released through somatic innervation at the external sphincter. **Emptying** or voiding then occurs through the urethra.

NERVOUS SYSTEM CONTROL

The processes of micturition and maintenance of continence are primarily controlled by messages to the **cerebral cortex region** as well as other central nervous system centers in the **thalamus** and in the **basal ganglia**. Patients who have had a stroke or who have a brain tumor or trauma, multiple sclerosis, or dementia, have damage to their cerebral cortex. The brain stem is specifically impacted in individuals with Parkinson's disease, and some strokes can occur there as well. Spinal cord damage can cause paraplegia and multiple sclerosis. Lower spinal injuries or tumors in the S2 to S4 sacral region can cause a condition called sacral bladder, and even some peripheral neuropathies (such as those caused by diabetes) can affect the efferent control of micturition. Continence is also controlled by the **complex reflex arc**, in which the brain stem centers, notably the **pons**, synchronize urethral sphincter relaxation and detrusor muscle contraction.

NERVE FIBERS IN THE LOWER URINARY TRACT

There are three types of peripheral nervous system nerve fibers that supply the lower urinary tract and other areas: parasympathetic, sympathetic, and somatic fibers. **Parasympathetic nerve fibers** control unconscious and involuntary bodily functions. The main parasympathetic fibers innervating the lower urinary tract comprise the pelvic nerve, which initiates bladder contraction; other parasympathetic nerve fibers facilitate voiding by augmenting urine transport in the ureters, contracting the detrusor muscle, and opening the internal sphincter. **Sympathetic nerve fibers** control other autonomic functions such as stress responses and changes in muscle tone. They aid bladder storage by slowing down urine transport in the ureters, easing the detrusor muscle, and constricting the internal sphincter, all in opposition to parasympathetic functions. **Somatic nerve fibers** are under voluntary control and are either efferent, stimulating motor responses in the external sphincter and pelvic floor via the pudendal nerve, or they are afferent, transmitting sensory responses from the bladder to the spinal cord.

CHANGES OVER A LIFESPAN THAT CAN AFFECT THE PROCESS OF VOIDING

Infants do not have a fully developed **central nervous system**. Their voiding cycle cannot be voluntarily controlled and occurs entirely through activation of the **complex reflex arc**. Between ages 2 and 3, the CNS matures, and the child can eventually voluntarily control the reflex arc and when they void. **Pubertal maturational changes** strengthen pelvic muscles for further control; in boys, the prostate gland grows, and in girls, estrogen is released. The **pelvic floor** can be briefly or permanently weakened in adult women during childbirth. The **prostate gland** in men continues to grow in adulthood, especially when they reach middle age, which augments their urethral resistance and can enlarge or stress the bladder, causing urine retention. In women, estrogen is depressed after menopause, which suppresses the urethral resistance and can lead to withering of pelvic floor structures, propensity to infection, and incontinence. Some older adults are prone to overactive bladder. **Overactive bladder** may result when the detrusor contracts too often involuntarily or when an increased urgency to void occurs due to late realization of the need to void.

URINARY INCONTINENCE

Urinary incontinence occurs more commonly in women than men and can range from an intermittent leaking of urine to a full loss of bladder control. Causes of urinary incontinence may include neurologic injury (including cerebral vascular accidents), infections, weakness of the muscles of the bladder, and certain medications, including diuretics, antihistamines, and antidepressants. **Stress incontinence** is defined as an involuntary leakage of urine with sneezing, coughing, laughing, lifting, or exercising. **Urge incontinence** is defined as an uncontrollable need to urinate on a frequent basis. **Total incontinence** is the full loss of bladder control.

Signs and symptoms: Urinary frequency and urgency may accompany the inability to control urine. If urinary incontinence is severe, incontinence-associated dermatitis may occur, predisposing the patient to skin breakdown and the development of pressure ulcers.

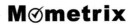

Diagnosis: Physical assessment and presence of symptoms. Ultrasound, urinalysis, urodynamic testing, and cystoscopy may be used to determine the underlying cause.

TOILETING AND ASSISTIVE DEVICES

There are many types of **absorbent pads** and **underwear** that patients with micturition issues can wear. Easily opened clothing closers (such as Velcro) or aids such as reachers or zipper pulls are available. There are options for **hygiene management**, such as bidets, special types of gender-specific urinals and bedpans, and external collection (often occlusive) devices. There are also **urinary drainage bags** and **unique commode configurations**, such as over-the-toilet, bedside, or riser. For women with incontinence issues, there are a number of devices that either support the bladder neck or inhibit bladder prolapse, such as rings and donuts. For men, penile clamps are available. In addition, numerous **catheterization devices** are sold as adjuncts to perform associated functions, such as holding the catheter, assisting with clothing management, or spreading the labia in women.

POST-VOID RESIDUAL

A post-void residual (**PVR**) is a measurement of the difference between the amount of urine voided and the residual volume in the bladder. It is viewed as a good diagnostic test for the **adequacy of bladder voiding**. PVR is usually taken using a bladder scanner. The patient voids into a collecting device while breathing deeply and contracting the pelvic muscles. The urine volume is documented. The individual then lies down, and within 10 minutes, either a bladder scan or a sterile catheterization is performed to verify the residual volume, which is also recorded. The total volume is the sum of the voided volume plus the residual volume after voiding (PVR). **Adequate bladder voiding** is defined as a PVR of <50 mL, versus **incomplete bladder voiding**, which is a PVR >200 mL.

BLADDER TRAINING

Bladder training usually requires the person to keep a toileting diary for at least three days so patterns can be assessed. There are a number of different approaches:

- **Scheduled toileting** is toileting on a regular schedule, usually every 2-4 hours during the daytime.
- **Habit training** involves an attempt to match the scheduled toileting to a person's individual voiding habits, based on the toileting diary. This is useful for people who have a natural and fairly consistent voiding pattern. Toileting is done every 2-4 hours.
- **Prompted voiding** is often used in nursing homes and attempts to teach people to assess their own incontinence status and prompts them to ask for toileting.
- **Bladder retraining** is a behavioral modification program that teaches people to inhibit the urge to urinate and to urinate according to an established schedule, restoring normal bladder function as much as possible. Bladder training can improve incontinence in 80% of cases.

PROMPTED VOIDING

Prompted voiding is a communication protocol for people with mild to moderate **cognitive impairment**. It uses positive reinforcement for recognizing being wet or dry, staying dry, urinating, and drinking liquids.

- Ask patient **every two hours** (8 a.m. to 4-8 p.m.) whether they are wet or dry.
- Verify if they are correct and give **feedback**, "You are right, Mrs. Brown, you are dry."
- **Prompt** patient, whether wet or dry, to use the toilet or urinal. If yes, assist them, record results, and give positive reinforcement by praising and visiting for a short time. If no, repeat the request again once or twice. If they are wet, and decline toileting, change and tell them you will return in two hours and ask them to try to wait to urinate until then.
- Offer **liquids** and record amount.
- **Record** results of each attempt to urinate or wet check.

Functional Health Patterns

183

BLADDER RETRAINING

Bladder retraining teaches people to control the urge to urinate. It usually takes about three months to rehabilitate a bladder muscle weakened from frequent urination, causing a decreased urinary capacity. A short urination interval is gradually lengthened to every 2-4 hours during the daytime as the person suppresses bladder urges and stays dry.

- The patient keeps a **urination diary** for a week.
- An individual program is established with **scheduled voiding times and goals**. For example, if a patient is urinating every hour, the goal might be every 80 minutes with increased output.
- The patient is taught **techniques** to withhold urination, such as sitting on a hard seat or on a tightly rolled towel to put pressure on pelvic floor muscles, doing five squeezes of pelvic floor muscles, deep breathing, and counting backward from 50.
- When the patient consistently meets the goal, a **new goal** is established.

THE KNACK TO CONTROL URINARY INCONTINENCE

The **knack** is the use of precisely timed muscle contractions to prevent **stress incontinence**. It is "the knack" of squeezing up before bearing down. The knack is a preventive use of **Kegel exercises**. Women are taught to contract the pelvic floor muscles right before and during events that usually cause stress incontinence. For example, if a woman feels a cough or sneeze coming, she immediately contracts the pelvic floor muscles and holds until the stress event is over. This contraction augments support of the proximal urethra, reducing the amount of displacement that usually takes place with compromised muscle support, thereby preventing incontinence. It is particularly useful if used before and during stress events, such as coughing, sneezing, lifting, standing, swinging a golf club, or laughing. Studies have shown that women who are taught this technique for mild to moderate urinary incontinence and use it consistently are able to decrease incontinence by 73-98%.

SURGERY FOR URINARY INCONTINENCE

Stress incontinence is sometimes treated surgically, depending upon the underlying cause (hypermobility or sphincter issues). Either some type of **suspension** is inserted or a **sling or artificial sphincter** is used. Urge incontinence due to instability of the detrusor can be managed by using **plastic surgery** to enlarge the bladder. Overflow issues can be treated by **surgical removal of an obstruction** or **intermittent catheterization**. **Transurethral sphincterotomy** can be used to manage neurogenic bladder dysfunction, detrusor-sphincter dyssynergia, and other issues. Other surgical techniques include **augmentation enterocystoplasty**, which uses part of the small intestine, bowel, or other tissue to create continent diversions. **Sacral nerve stimulators** can be implanted at the S2-S3 level to help communicate the need to urinate from the spinal cord to the brain.

CLASSES OF DRUGS USED TO CONTROL BLADDER ELIMINATION

Bladder incontinence is generally treated with **anticholinergic agents** such as oxybutynin (Ditropan and others) or tolterodine (Detrol). The **conjugated estrogen**, Premarin, applied vaginally or as a patch, can also be used in women to control bladder incontinence. The **α-adrenergic agonist pseudoephedrine** (Sudafed) can act to alleviate stress incontinence as well. Overflow often occurs in men with enlarged benign prostates. This can be controlled with a number of **α-adrenergic antagonists** such as tamsulosin (Flomax), **antiandrogens** such as finasteride (Proscar), or the plant extract *Serenoa repens* (saw palmetto), a **phytotherapeutic agent**. Atonic bladder, in which there is a lack of bladder muscle tone, can be treated with the **cholinergic bethanechol** (Urecholine).

CLEAN INTERMITTENT CATHETERIZATION

Intermittent catheterization can generally be performed safely using clean techniques with new sterile catheters at intervals of 6 hours or greater. If the patient has not voided between catheterizations, the volume limit is **500 mL**. If more than 500 mL is voided during a catheterization, then catheterization may have to be more frequent. The patient's privacy must be protected during the procedure. The nurse, caregiver, or family member performing the catheterization washes their hands, lowers the patient's clothing to expose the urinary

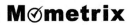

opening, and dons clean gloves. The individual performing the catheterization then applies lubricant on the catheter tip and creates access to the opening by either pulling back the man's foreskin or spreading the woman's labia with fingers or a spreader. The urinary collection device, if utilized, is positioned. The catheter is inserted, and urine is drained into the collection device or toilet. Diminishing flow can be aided by **manual pressure**. The catheter is removed, the lubricant is wiped off, and the region is washed. If the patient is male, his foreskin should be returned to normal position. The nurse/caretaker stores or discards supplies and washes their hands.

PATIENT EDUCATION FOR CLEAN INTERMITTENT CATHETERIZATION

FEMALES

When teaching **clean intermittent catheterization (CIC) for females**, the following steps should be included:

1. Gather supplies; wash hands.
2. Sit on toilet or stand with one foot on toilet.
3. Clean vulva and urethral opening with soap and water or individually packaged wipes containing benzalkonium chloride, wiping top to bottom.
4. Lubricate catheter with water-soluble lubricant (or water).
5. Spread labia with second and fourth fingers of one hand; feel for meatus with middle finger.
6. Gently insert catheter into meatus, guiding it upward. Insert 2–3 inches until urine flows; then slowly insert another inch.
7. When drainage ceases, withdraw catheter incrementally, making sure bladder is empty.
8. Wash reusable catheter with soap and hot water. Rinse completely and dry. Store in a clean, dry place or carrying case/Ziploc bag. Reusable catheters last about 2–4 weeks but should be soaked in a white vinegar solution once weekly.
9. If there are signs of infection or incomplete emptying, observe urine flow or drain urine into a container and measure.

MALES

When teaching the procedure for **CIC for males**, the following should be included:

1. Gather supplies; wash hands.
2. Sit on toilet or chair with container near.
3. Clean end of penis and urethral opening with soap and water or individually packaged wipes containing benzalkonium chloride.
4. Lubricate catheter with water-soluble lubricant (or water).
5. Hold penis by the sides, perpendicular to the body or pointing slightly upward.
6. Gently insert catheter into meatus, guiding it through the penis. There may be resistance when the catheter passes the prostate. Deep breathing and relaxing may help to advance the catheter. Do not force past a blockage.
7. When urine flow begins, insert the catheter 1 inch more.
8. When drainage ceases, withdraw catheter incrementally, making sure bladder is empty.
9. Wash reusable catheter with soap and hot water. Rinse completely and dry. Store in a clean, dry place or carrying case/Ziploc bag. Reusable catheters last about 2–4 weeks but should be soaked in a white vinegar solution once weekly.

Functional Health Patterns

NEUROGENIC BLADDER DYSFUNCTION

There are five types of neurogenic bladder dysfunction. Three of these result from central nervous system damage: uninhibited, reflex, and autonomous.

- **Uninhibited neurogenic bladder** is characterized by numerous uninhibited contractions and complete voiding without residual volume. It is caused primarily by lesions in the brain or subcortical areas.
- People with **reflex neurogenic bladder** have little or no awareness of their voiding pattern, which occurs as a reflex instead of voluntarily. The etiology is upper spinal cord injury involving both motor and sensory tracts of regions down to about T11.
- **Autonomous neurogenic bladder** is the unawareness of fullness, dribbling, and involuntary emptying due to bladder overflow as a result of lower neural damage to the sacral reflex arc.

MOTOR AND SENSORY PARALYTIC BLADDERS

These are two other types of neurogenic bladder. Motor and sensory paralytic bladders result from damage to the efferent or afferent portions, respectively, of the micturition reflex arc, usually at the S2-S4 level.

- Individuals with **motor paralytic bladder** have the feelings of fullness and emptiness, but their motor functions and tone are diminished. Thus, they generally have difficult or incomplete urination. Common etiologies are a herniated disc, trauma to the pelvis, or poliomyelitis.
- People with **sensory paralytic bladder** cannot sense voiding needs, but they can generally initiate voiding. They tend to have high-volume but infrequent voiding patterns. This type of bladder can result from damage during childbirth in mothers with diabetes, peripheral vascular disease, and pelvic trauma.

EFFECTS OF SPINAL SHOCK ON BLADDER FUNCTION

When an individual suffers spinal injury, they temporarily develop **spinal shock** or loss of all reflex capabilities below the level of the spinal lesion. The patient initially has no control over urinary voiding and cannot tell when the bladder is full. As a result, the bladder becomes over-distended. These are symptoms that resemble **autonomous neurogenic bladder**, which is generally associated with injury to the sacral reflex arc. The nurse's main role during this period is handling of **urinary retention**. Once the patient recovers from spinal shock, the true area of CNS injury and consequent type of neurogenic bladder can be pinpointed more accurately.

INTERVENTIONAL PROCEDURES FOR URINARY RETENTION

Patients can suffer from urinary retention due to spinal cord damage, an enlarged prostate, or neurogenic bladder dysfunction. The immediate goal is to safely void the bladder. The primary intervention is **urinary catheterization**, either as an indwelling device inserted within the urethra or an artificial surgically created opening in the pubic area, both of which provide constant draining. This urinary catheterization can also be **intermittent**, in which a catheter is inserted and removed at regular intervals, usually in order to maintain manageable volumes. In a hospital setting, sterile technique is strongly recommended during insertion and removal in order to thwart **catheter-associated urinary tract infections (UTIs)**. If this is not possible, as when insertion takes place at home, techniques that maintain as clean an environment as possible may suffice; examples include use of small-bore catheters, irrigation methods, topical ointments, and avoidance of unnecessary catheter changes.

AUTONOMIC DYSREFLEXIA

Autonomic dysreflexia is characterized by an acute onset of high blood pressure that occurs with central cord lesions at/above T6. This is often preceded by a painful stimulus that occurs below the spinal cord injury. The hypertension is accompanied by an intense headache, sweating above the level of the spinal injury with cool, clammy skin below the injury, and a decreased heart rate. Normally, the autonomic nervous system maintains homeostasis through negative feedback between the opposing sympathetic (dilated pupils, increased HR,

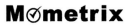

vasoconstriction) and parasympathetic (constricted pupils, decreased HR, vasodilation) nervous systems. When one is active, the other is not. The parasympathetic nerves leave the central nervous system at the midbrain, the base of the brain (cranial nerves), and at the lumbar area. The sympathetic nerves leave between T5 and L2 with major output at the splanchnic outflow (T5-T6). Spinal cord injury causes the two systems to work independently and disrupts feedback, so when a painful stimulus ascends to the splanchnic outflow, a sympathetic response causes vasoconstriction below the injury, resulting in hypertension with severe headache. The parasympathetic system can't counteract this through the feedback loop. Instead, the brainstem stimulates the vagus nerve to slow the heart and dilate vessels above the injury, but this response cannot travel below the injury.

SYMPTOMS AND MANAGEMENT

Autonomic dysreflexia can result in encephalopathy and shock if undiagnosed and untreated. Autonomic dysreflexia occurs only after initial spinal shock has resolved. Onset is often very sudden and constitutes a medical emergency. Common causes include distended bladder, fecal impaction, pressure sores, tight clothing, hyperthermia, and other painful stimuli.

Symptoms	Treatment
Hypertension, severe pounding headache, increased ICP, and/or rupture of cerebral vessel	Elevate head immediately to reduce blood pressure
Bradycardia, other cardiac arrhythmias	Identify and rectify cause (check bladder, bowels, skin, clothing, temperature)
Diaphoresis, piloerection, flushing of skin below level of injury and pallor above	If related to bladder distention, catheterize and drain the bladder slowly
Nasal congestion	If initial treatment is not successful in reversing symptoms, then give medications (IV antihypertensives)
Blurred vision, spots in visual field	
Seizures	

PATIENT AND CAREGIVER EDUCATION

For patients with spinal cord injuries occurring above T6, **education** regarding symptoms, prevention, and management of autonomic dysreflexia is needed. This education should be done frequently and again at transition of care. Autonomic dysreflexia usually doesn't occur in the first few weeks following a spinal cord injury but often occurs within the **first year following injury**, often placing the patient at home or in a long-term care facility the first time they experience the complication. Patients should be taught that headache accompanied by diaphoresis and hypertension are common **symptoms** of autonomic dysreflexia, and blurred vision, flushing, and nausea may present as well. Blood pressure should be monitored, and the body should be checked for any items causing irritation. If possible, the patient should be assisted to rapidly but safely sit up to try to induce orthostatic hypotension. Nifedipine sublingually can be used for severe episodes or episodes that don't respond to other interventions.

GASTROINTESTINAL SYSTEM
INNERVATION OF THE GASTROINTESTINAL TRACT

The gastrointestinal (**GI**) tract is made up of bundles of smooth muscles that form layers. Individual muscle fibers are innervated and function as a unit. The electrical activity between muscle fibers produces either slow and rhythmic **waves** or **contractions** to aid mixing and transport, or spikes to preserve pressure and tone. In the wall of the gut, there is a contained **enteric** or **intrinsic nervous system**. This intrinsic system consists of two networks, an outer motor or myenteric plexus and an inner sensory or submucosal plexus. The former influences movement within the GI tract, while the latter regulates GI secretions and area blood flow. **Parasympathetic nerve signals** from the brain via the vagus nerve are also transmitted to certain parts of the GI tract, most notably the esophagus, stomach, and pancreas (a digestive and endocrine gland), to increase activity. Sympathetic nerve fibers from the spinal cord innervate the entire tract to decrease activity within the canal.

Functional Health Patterns

ORGANIZATION OF THE GASTROINTESTINAL TRACT

The GI tract is the passage between the mouth and anus involved with **digestion** and **waste elimination**. Food is taken in through the mouth and descends through the esophagus into the stomach. Food is digested as it goes through the stomach, duodenum, jejunum, and then the ileum of the small intestine. Nutrients and water are later absorbed as the food goes through the small intestine and colon. The colon consists of the cecum and ascending, transverse, descending, and sigmoid colons. The alimentary tract is completed by passage through the rectum and elimination at the anus. There are **secretory glands** throughout the GI tract that lubricate the walls of the canal for easy food passage, and others up to the ileum that aid digestion. The tract itself is made up of **smooth muscle fiber layers** under electrical and neural control.

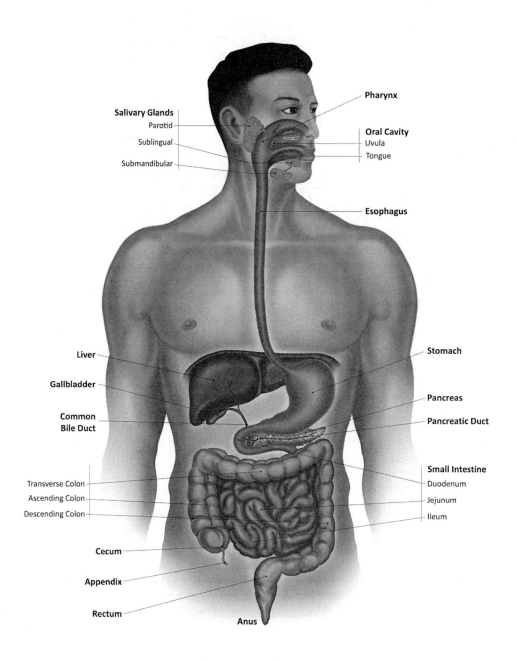

ASSESSMENT OF THE GASTROINTESTINAL SYSTEM

Assessment of the gastrointestinal system includes the following:

- Ask about personal and family history of gastrointestinal problems and risk factors, such as alcoholism, smoking, drug and medicine use, and poor dietary habits.
- Ask about symptoms, such as GI discomfort, flatus, nausea, vomiting, diarrhea, and abdominal pain.
- Determine the defecation pattern and ask about weight fluctuations.

When performing a **physical assessment**, one must assess oral mucosa, tongue, teeth, pharynx, thyroid and parathyroid glands, skin color, moisture, turgor, nodules or lesions, bruises, scars, abdominal shape, and bowel sounds, assessing the abdomen in all 4 quadrants using the stethoscope diaphragm. The number of sounds heard determine if the intestines are functioning:

- **Absent**: no sounds in 3-5 minutes
- **Hypoactive**: only one sound in 2 minutes
- **Normal**: sounds heard every 5-20 seconds
- **Hyperactive**: 5-6 sounds in <30 seconds

One should examine the anal region for fissures, inflammation, tears, and dimples. Blood may be drawn for liver function studies, lipid profile, iron studies, CBC.

> **Review Video: Gastrointestinal System**
> Visit mometrix.com/academy and enter code: 378740

DIAGNOSES AND SUITABLE INTERVENTIONS FOR PROBLEMS RELATED TO BOWEL ELIMINATION

A patient with bowel incontinence can have one of the five types of **neurogenic impairments**. The incontinence could also be due to other factors such as loss of muscle tone in the GI tract, pressure in the GI tract from gas, habitual laxative use, and poor bowel habits. The nurse's role in managing incontinent patients is to provide **bowel incontinence care**, **management**, and **training** in order to eventually achieve control, proper elimination, and skin integrity. If the patient has **true constipation**, the nurse is responsible for management of the problem as well as fluids and nutrition. Some people merely have perceived constipation; a big part of the nurse's role in this case is education. Others can be at risk for development of constipation as previously discussed, and here the clinician should incorporate all of the concepts discussed as well as medication management. For patients with diarrhea, nursing interventions include management of the problem as well as medications taken, general bowel habits, fluids and electrolytes, perianal care, and skin inspections.

> **Review Video: Diagnostic Procedures of the GI System**
> Visit mometrix.com/academy and enter code: 645436

BOWEL DYSFUNCTIONS

HISTORY AND PHYSICAL EXAMINATION FOR BOWEL DYSFUNCTIONS

The **history portion of the examination** of a patient with bowel dysfunction needs to incorporate questions about the patient's present and past bowel routines, such as frequency, volume, texture of stool, degree of continence, perception of filling, ability to control movements, and use of laxatives. **Dietary and drinking habits**, particularly the amount of fiber ingested, should be noted. **Medications** the patient is taking should be documented, especially those that might have side effects or actually elicit constipation. The presence of **bowel syndromes** or other diseases that can affect bowel motility or secretions should be included in a medical history. The clinician should test to determine **neural function** in the bowel area. The clinician should check the patient's **abdomen** by inspection, auscultation, and palpation for distention and movement, bowel sounds, muscle function, and presence of impacted stool. A **rectal examination** is also performed to appraise the tone and strength of the anal sphincter and to look for lesions or stool.

Functional Health Patterns

NEUROGENIC BOWEL DYSFUNCTION

Neurogenic bowel dysfunction falls into five categories similar to those for urinary dysfunction: uninhibited, reflex, and autonomous neurogenic bowels, plus motor and sensory paralytic bowels. Incontinence rarely occurs with the latter two with damage in the S2 to S4 region. A person with **motor paralytic bowel** has saddle sensation but absent bulbocavernosus and anal reflexes, while the opposite is generally true in the sensory version. **Uninhibited neurogenic bowel** results from neural lesions in the cortical and subcortical regions above C1. All sensations and reflexes normally associated with defecation are intact, but the brain cannot decipher these signals; voluntary control of the anal sphincter is diminished, and involuntary elimination can occur. Spinal cord lesions can result in either **reflex** or **autonomous neurogenic bowel** depending on the level affected—above or at T12 to L1, or below T12 to L1, respectively. In both versions, patients cannot control defecation or their anal sphincter, but the sacral involvement in autonomous neurogenic bowel means they also have no spinal reflex arc and are incontinent between mass bouts of elimination.

DESIRED NURSING OUTCOMES

There are some general nursing outcomes expected when managing a patient with bowel dysfunctions. The individual should eventually establish a **regular bowel movement pattern** every day to every three days under control, at established times, and without use of measures to promote it. Eventually the texture of the patient's stool should be normalized, and episodes of incontinence should be diminished or eliminated. The nurse is responsible for establishing an **exercise schedule** and a **diet plan** with enough fluid and fiber for the patient such that these goals are achieved without introducing other complications. There are also outcomes specific to the various types of neurogenic bowel. For the person with **uninhibited neurogenic bowel**, the main goal is the establishment of a regular pattern. For someone with **reflex neurogenic bowel**, measures that encourage reflex movement into the rectal area are indicated. For patients with **autonomous neurogenic bowel**, the main objectives are, predictably, firm stools and a relatively empty colon.

TESTS TO CLASSIFY BOWEL DYSFUNCTION

Neurogenic bowel dysfunction can cause altered bowel elimination or bladder incontinence. There are three common tests that might be done to classify the type of impairment. The first tests the person's **perception** of the defecation urge by use of a pinprick or soft touch to the perianal region. The **bulbocavernosus reflex** is evaluated by grabbing either the penis or clitoris and observing whether the external anal sphincter contracts. Contraction of the bulbocavernosus and ischiocavernosus muscles can be felt as well. An individual with an upper motor neuron injury should have a positive reflex, while someone with lower motor neuron or areflexic damage should be unresponsive. This reflex is generally absent during spinal shock. The skin near the external anal sphincter can also be pricked to see if it contracts, known as the **anal "wink" reflex**.

CONSTIPATION AND IMPACTION

Constipation is a condition with bowel movements less frequent than normal for a person, or hard, small stool that is evacuated fewer than 3 times weekly. Food moves through the GI from the small intestine to the colon in semi-liquid form. Constipation results from the colon, where fluid is absorbed. If too much fluid is absorbed, the stool can become too dry. People may have abdominal distension and cramps and need to strain for defecation.

Fecal impaction occurs when the hard stool moves into the rectum and becomes a large, dense, immovable mass that cannot be evacuated even with straining, usually as a result of chronic constipation. In addition to abdominal cramps and distention, the person may feel intense rectal pressure and pain accompanied by a sense of urgency to defecate. Nausea and vomiting may also occur. Hemorrhoids will often become engorged. Fecal incontinence, with liquid stool leaking about the impaction, is common.

MEDICAL PROCEDURES TO EVALUATE CAUSES OF CONSTIPATION

Medical procedures to evaluate causes of constipation should be preceded by a careful history as this may help to define the type and guide the choice of diagnostic procedures. Most tests are necessary only for severe constipation that does not respond to treatment. Medical **diagnostic procedures** may include the following:

- **Physical exam** should include rectal exam and abdominal palpation to assess for obvious hard stool or impaction.
- **Blood tests** can identify hypothyroidism and excess parathyroid hormone.
- **Abdominal x-ray** may show large amounts of stool in the colon.
- **Barium enema** can indicate tumors or strictures causing obstruction.
- **Colonic transit studies** can show defects of the neuromuscular system.
- **Defecography** shows the defecation process and abnormalities of anatomy.
- **Anorectal manometry studies** show malfunction of anorectal muscles.
- **Colonic motility studies** measure the pattern of colonic pressure.
- **Colonoscope** allows direct visualization of the lumen of the rectum and colon.

DIARRHEA

Diarrhea is rapid passage of waste through the large intestine resulting in frequent, excessive, and watery bowel movements. Excessive amounts of water and electrolytes are lost, which can lead to cardiac issues, renal failure, and even death. The most common cause of diarrhea is some type of **infection in the gastrointestinal tract**. The infection irritates the bowel and intensifies secretions and motility there. Diarrhea can also be triggered by situations that directly **suppress absorption** and **augment stool volume and fluid level**, such as lactose intolerance or taking hyperosmolar drugs. Other times the main disruption is primarily **increased motility**, which can be found in people with diabetes, irritable bowel syndrome, or ulcerative colitis. Generally, diarrhea is considered acute if it persists for less than a month, and chronic otherwise.

DIARRHEA IN INFANTS AND CHILDREN

Diarrhea is common in infants and children and can be caused by a variety of different infections and conditions. Diarrhea accounts for about 20% of hospitalizations of children <2 and causes about 500 deaths in children <4 in the United States each year. Because of the potential for loss of fluids, electrolytes, and nutrition, and the danger of ulceration and bleeding, diarrhea should be monitored carefully to determine the **cause**:

- **Osmotic**: Increased fluid in the stool and may be related to lactose intolerance and overfeeding.
- **Secretory**: Inhibited electrolyte (ion) absorption or increased electrolyte secretion related to bacterial endotoxins.
- **Motility disorders**: Interfere with absorption of fluids, including bile salt or pancreatic enzyme deficiencies.
- **Inflammatory**: Related to Crohn's disease or ulcerative colitis.
- **Viral/bacterial**: The most common cause of diarrhea in children. A wide range of viral and bacterial pathogens can cause mild to severe life-threatening diarrhea.

Functional Health Patterns

ULCERATIVE COLITIS

Ulcerative colitis is superficial inflammation of the mucosa of the colon and rectum, causing ulcerations in the areas where inflammation has destroyed cells. These ulcerations, ranging from pinpoint to extensive, may bleed and produce purulent material. The mucosa of the bowel becomes swollen, erythematous, and granular. Patients may present emergently with **severe ulcerative colitis** (having >6 blood stools a day, fever, tachycardia, anemia) or with **fulminant colitis** (>10 blood stools per day, severe bleeding, and toxic symptoms) These patients are at high risk for megacolon and perforation.

Symptoms:

- Abdominal pain
- Anemia
- F&E depletion
- Bloody diarrhea/rectal bleeding
- Diarrhea
- Fecal urgency
- Tenesmus
- Anorexia
- Weight loss
- Fatigue
- Systemic disorders: Eye inflammation, arthritis, liver disease, and osteoporosis as immune system triggers generalized inflammation

Treatment:

- Glucocorticoids
- Aminosalicylates
- Antibiotics if signs/symptoms of toxicity
- D/C anticholinergics, NSAIDS, and antidiarrheals
- If fulminant: Admitted & monitored for deterioration. Kept NPO, and given IV F&E replacement. NGT for decompression if intestinal dilation is present. Knee-elbow position to reposition gas in bowel. Colectomy for those with megacolon or who are unresponsive to therapy.

Review Video: <u>Ulcerative Colitis</u>
Visit mometrix.com/academy and enter code: 584881

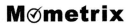

CROHN'S DISEASE

Crohn's disease manifests with inflammation of the GI system. Inflammation is transmural (often leading to intestinal stenosis and fistulas), focal, and discontinuous with aphthous ulcerations progressing to linear and irregular-shaped ulcerations. Granulomas may be present. Common sites of inflammation are the terminal ileum and cecum. The condition is chronic, but patients with severe or fulminant disease (fevers, persistent vomiting, abscess, obstruction) often present emergently for treatment.

Symptoms:

- Perirectal abscess/fistula in advanced disease
- Diarrhea
- Watery stools
- Rectal hemorrhage
- Anemia
- Abdominal pain (commonly RLQ)
- Cramping
- Weight loss
- Nausea and vomiting
- Fever
- Night sweats

Treatment:

- Triamcinolone for oral lesions, aminosalicylates, glucocorticoids, antidiarrheals, probiotics, avoid lactose, and identify and eliminate food triggers.
- For patients who present with toxic symptoms: hospitalization for careful monitoring, IV glucocorticoids, aminosalicylates, antibiotics, and bowel rest. Parenteral nutrition for the malnourished.
- For repeated relapses (refractory):
  - Immunomodulatory agents (azathioprine, mercaptopurine, methotrexate) or Biologic therapies (infliximab).
  - Bowel resection if unresponsive to all treatment or with ischemic bowel.

Functional Health Patterns

193

BOWEL TRAINING

Bowel training for defecation includes keeping a bowel diary to chart progress:

- **Scheduled defecation** is usually daily, but for some people 3-4 times weekly, depending on individual bowel habits. Defecation should be at the same time, so work hours and activities must be considered. Defecation is scheduled for 20-30 minutes after a meal when there is increased motility.
- **Stimulation** is necessary. Drinking a cup of hot liquid may work, but initially many require rectal stimulation, inserting a gloved, lubricated finger into the anus and running it around the rim of the sphincters. Some people require rectal suppositories, such as glycerine. Stimulus suppositories, such as Dulcolax (bisacodyl), or even Fleet enemas are sometimes used, but the goal is to reduce use of medical or chemical stimulants.
- **Position** should be sitting upright with knees elevated slightly if possible and leaning forward during defecation.
- **Straining** includes attempting to tighten abdominal muscles and relax sphincters while defecating.
- **Exercise** increases the motility of the bowel by stimulating muscle contractions. **Walking** is one of the best exercises for this purpose, and the person should try to walk 1 or 2 miles a day. If the person is unable to walk, then other activities, such as chair exercises that involve the arms and legs and bending can be very effective. Those who are bed bound need to turn from side to side frequently and change position.
- **Kegel exercises** increase strength of the pelvic floor muscles. Kegel exercises for urinary incontinence and fecal incontinence are essentially the same, but the person tries to pull in the muscles around the anus, as though trying to prevent the release of stool or flatus. The person should feel the muscles tightening while holding for 2 seconds and then relaxing for 2 seconds, gradually building the holding time to 10 seconds or more. Exercises should be done 4 times a day.

MANAGEMENT STRATEGIES FOR CONSTIPATION AND FECAL IMPACTION

Management strategies for constipation and impaction include:

- **Enemas** and **manual removal of impaction** may be necessary initially.
- Add **fiber** with bran, fresh/dried fruits, and whole grains, to 20-35 grams per day.
- Increase **fluids** to 64 ounces each day.
- **Exercise** program should include walking if possible, and exercises on a daily basis.
- Change in **medications** causing constipation can relieve constipation. Additionally, the use of stool softeners, such as Colace (docusate), or bulk formers, such as Metamucil (psyllium), may decrease fluid absorption and move stool through the colon more quickly. Overuse of laxatives can cause constipation.
- Careful **monitoring** of diet, fluids, and medical treatment, especially for irritable bowel syndrome.
- **Pregnancy-related constipation** may be controlled through dietary and fluid modifications and regular exercise.
- **Delayed toileting** should be avoided and bowel training regimen done to promote evacuation at the same time each day. During travel, stool softeners, increased fluid, and exercise may alleviate constipation.

PURPOSE OF FIBER IN THE DIET

Most constipation is caused by insufficient **fiber** in the diet, especially if people eat a lot of processed foods. An adequate amount of fiber is 20-30 grams daily. There are both soluble and insoluble forms of fiber, and both add bulk to the stool and are not absorbed into the body. Some foods have both types:

- **Soluble fiber** dissolves in liquids to form a gel-like substance, which is why liquids are so important in conjunction with fiber in the diet. Soluble fiber slows the movement of stool through the gastrointestinal system. Food sources include bananas, potatoes, dried beans, nuts, apples, oranges, and oatmeal.

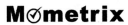

- **Insoluble fiber** changes little with the digestive process and increases the speed of stool through the colon, so too much can result in diarrhea. Food sources of insoluble fiber include wheat bran, whole grains, seeds, skins of fruits, vegetables, and nuts.

BOWEL TRAINING PROGRAM FOR REFLEX NEUROGENIC BOWEL

Patients with reflex neurogenic bowels have upper motor neuron injuries and lack of cortical control of bowel functions. Initially, these spinal cord injury patients usually experience **spinal shock**, and **manual stool removal** is generally indicated. Once shock abates, a **bowel program** can be instituted. Since constipation between occasional bouts of incontinence is the primary concern, the time for evacuation is generally lengthy. Once bowel sounds are heard and the person has been put on a suitable high-fiber diet, sufficient fluids, and some physical activity, they are given a daily **suppository** (preferably glycol-based) to stimulate reflexive elimination. This suppository is inserted 15–30 minutes before scheduled elimination, but longer times may be required. Eventually suppository use can be cut back to every 2 or 3 days. The patient should use the toilet if feasible. The patient may have weak abdominal muscles, indicating additional use of softeners, bulking agents, or stimulant laxatives. People with higher levels of injury may experience potentially fatal **hyperreflexia**, which can be abated with rectal ointments.

BOWEL TRAINING PROGRAM FOR UNINHIBITED NEUROGENIC BOWEL

Patients with uninhibited neurogenic bowel, such as those who have experienced a stroke or other cerebrovascular event, can usually return to continence with a good **bowel training program**. The timing of the program should be consistent and set based on habits and expediency. The patient should be consuming a healthy, fiber-rich diet and plenty of fluids. The patient's colon should be empty upon initiation of the regimen. The patient is given **stool softeners** such as docusate sodium, docusate calcium, or some form of dioctyl sodium sulfosuccinate daily if needed, plus **suppositories** on an as-needed basis. If these do not work alone, a **laxative** (such as senna or bisacodyl) may be added to facilitate peristalsis. Since laxatives typically take 12 hours to be effective, that should be taken into account. **Bulking agents** such as psyllium products, alfalfa tablets, or calcium polycarbophil should only be added if the person has inadequate bowel tone, not in the case of impaction. The nurse should keep a bowel record and initiate program changes slowly.

BOWEL TRAINING PROGRAM FOR AUTONOMOUS NEUROGENIC BOWEL

People with autonomous neurogenic bowel as a result of lower spinal cord injuries do not have spinal reflex responses. They have decreased bowel tone and propulsive ability. Thus, they are incontinent between expulsions due to their inability to control their external sphincter. Evacuation can be aided through use of **suppositories** placed relatively high against the rectal wall and/or manual manipulation. The main goal of the bowel program is to establish a relatively **firm stool texture** by use of dietary fiber and/or bulking agents. During evacuation, the person should sit on the toilet, bend forward, and perform the **Valsalva maneuver** (straining) and possibly abdominal massage to increase intra-abdominal pressure.

CORRECT POSITIONING DURING DEFECATION

A patient should be seated during defecation to facilitate the process. In addition, it is recommended to have the patient sit in a **squat position** in which the knees are a little above the hips and the feet are completely on the floor. This position puts pressure on the **abdomen** and also lines up the **rectum and anus**. If the patient has weak abdominal muscles, then binders, massage to the area, or breathing exercise can be used as adjuncts to increase pressure in the area. Use of bedpans during the process is not advocated unless absolutely necessary, and then the patient should eventually be weaned from using them. An incontinence pad may be used for patients with skin issues or those who have lost sensation in the buttocks region.

ACHIEVING A CLEAN BOWEL

The term "clean bowel" refers to one that does not contain **impacted feces**. Achieving a clean bowel is one of the parts of an **interventional bowel program**. It is generally achieved by some sort of manual procedure or use of laxatives or rectally administered enemas. **Laxatives** are substances that escalate small bowel and colon motility. They are usually administered orally, are effective within 8–12 hours, and include mixtures of milk of

Functional Health Patterns

magnesia, magnesium citrate, oil suspensions, or bisacodyl. **Enemas** are used less often to establish a clean bowel because they can eventually compromise the elasticity of colon walls. **Suppositories** are sometimes inserted rectally to instigate reflex emptying of the bowel as adjuncts. Most act within an hour of insertion, and the group includes glycerin, sodium bicarbonate, potassium bitartrate, and bisacodyl-based products. **Small-volume enemas** consisting of stool softeners and/or bulk formers are sometimes used to help achieve a clean bowel by initiating evacuation. The main manual procedure is **digital stimulation** using a gloved, lubricated hand against the inside of the anal sphincter wall to relax it.

CLASSES OF DRUGS USED TO CONTROL BOWEL ELIMINATION

Constipation is treated with various types of **laxatives** to promote elimination. Some of these, such as psyllium (Metamucil) or calcium polycarbophil (FiberCon and others), act by bulking the stool (bulk forming). Most other laxatives act by irritating the lower colon, which stimulates elimination. **Irritant laxatives** can be emollients, stimulants, hyperosmolar, or saline-derived. **Emollients** are basically softeners with docusate compounds formed with sodium (Colace), potassium, or calcium. **Stimulants** include senna (Senokot) and bisacodyl (Dulcolax). Glycerin, given in either suppository form or as a rectal liquid, is a **hyperosmolar** or highly concentrated solution; lactulose (Chronulac and others) falls into this category as well. Oral magnesium citrate is a **saline-derived product** used to evaluate the bowel.

> **Review Video: Gastrointestinal Medications**
> Visit mometrix.com/academy and enter code: 455152

PATIENT EDUCATION REGARDING OSTOMY CARE

Patient education regarding ostomy care involves a variety of focuses. First, assess the patient's readiness and ability to learn and manage their own care. Provide emotional support and allow the individual to express their feelings. Consider individuals with special needs, such as those with limited cognitive or physical ability, as they may need modifications or assistance. People who are hard of hearing, vision-impaired, or illiterate may need video or audiotapes or illustrated instructions. Do **step-by-step instruction** of main tasks; begin with **simple steps** such as draining and clamping the pouch, and continue until the person has mastered the main tasks: emptying the pouch, removing the pouch, cleansing and caring for the skin, measuring the stoma, applying a new pouch, and disposing of the old pouch.

Conduct **ongoing assessments** over time and **evaluate** the individual's ability to manage pouching while in the rehab facility and again before discharge. If in community rehab nursing, assess these abilities on initial intake of patient to services, after returning home from any hospital stays, and periodically to ensure that all questions are answered and problems have been resolved.

Sleep and Rest Patterns

STAGES OF SLEEP

During sleep, an individual undergoes 5–6 cycles of the **pattern of sleep**. Each pattern is divided into four stages. The first three stages are associated with **slow or non-rapid eye movement (non-REM) sleep**, while the last stage is characterized by **rapid eye movement (REM) sleep**.

- In the relatively short **stage 1**, muscles relax, eye movements shift slowly from side to side, and blinking diminishes. The individual transitions from awake to asleep in this stage.
- The majority of sleep is spent in **stage 2**, which is a somewhat deeper sleep during which the heart and respiratory rates slow and muscles continue to relax. There are short bursts of brain activity during this stage, amid otherwise slower brain activity.
- **Stage 3** is a deep sleep with slow eye movement during which the heart rate, respiratory rate, and body temperature are at their lowest.

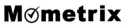

- The last stage, **stage 4**, is rapid eye movement or REM sleep, which is the period where people experience dreams, brain activity is high, and respiratory/heart rates increase to close to awake levels.

Each stage has characteristic wave patterns on polysomnography, which is a procedure combining electroencephalogram, electrooculogram, and electromyogram techniques.

PHYSIOLOGY OF SLEEP

The brain's sleep center is situated in the portion of the midbrain called the **midline raphe system**, which controls noradrenergic and cholinergic responses. In the course of non-REM stage sleep, secretion of various **hormones** is either enhanced (growth and luteinizing hormones) or suppressed (adrenocorticotropic and thyroid-stimulating hormones). By deep sleep in stage 3, **vital functions** such as blood pressure and respiration are minimized, while **cardiovascular tone** is augmented. The **homeostatic mechanisms** initiated during sleep are designed to gradually take the person through the following stages in sequence: wakefulness, deep sleep, REM sleep, and wakefulness again. Sleep restores vigor. If normal patterns are disrupted through unhealthy habits or use of some medications, this restoration cannot occur properly. Sleep-wake cycles are also affected by an individual's **circadian or daily rhythm**.

ASSESSMENT OF PATIENT'S SLEEP PATTERN

Sleep assessment should be included when evaluating patients. This means asking them appropriate **questions** (possibly through use of a questionnaire) as well actually **observing** their hourly sleep pattern. The nurse should question patients about difficulties experienced when falling asleep and during sleep, and whether they feel refreshed upon awaking. They should be asked whether they have a regular time schedule for going to sleep and waking up, whether they use medications to induce sleep, and if and when they consume alcohol or stimulants. It is also important to question the patient about snoring, in particular snoring that can be heard through a closed door, or periods of apnea (where a partner has witnessed the patient stop breathing in their sleep), as these may indicate the presence of obstructive sleep apnea. Questions addressing daytime drowsiness or napping, the frequency and reasons for getting up at night, and whether the patient can go back to sleep, should be included. The **hourly objective sleep evaluation** is important because the nurse can document how long the patient sleeps and whether they get up during that period in order to adjust factors that might facilitate sleep, such as room temperature or noise levels.

FACTORS THAT CAN DEPRIVE PEOPLE OF SLEEP

The leading causes of **sleep deprivation** are **psychological** in nature and include illness, stressors, or marital issues. Sleep problems are also often experienced by shift workers because their work requires them to sleep at times not attuned to the population at large or their natural **circadian rhythm**. Thus, in order to establish a regular sleep pattern during the daytime, they need to take additional measures, such as using blackout shades, sleep masks, and a cool and quiet room to sleep in. The room temperature and noise level, type of bed, and sleep partner practices can affect anyone's ability to sleep. People can also be deprived of sleep if they are in pain, have certain health issues such as pregnancy, or have consumed certain foods or medications prior to bedtime, as well as during periods of jetlag.

HEALTH CARE ISSUES THAT CAN AFFECT THE QUALITY OR AMOUNT OF SLEEP

Pain and the medications used to relieve pain can affect the quality of sleep. In particular, **narcotic analgesics** do not appear to affect the time spent sleeping, but they do disrupt both deep and REM sleep. This causes sleepiness during the day and agitation during sleep. **Cardiopulmonary problems** manifest as general or prone shortness of breath and associated issues such as sleep apnea and hypertension. In **sleep apnea**, muscles in the upper airway relax and collapse, causing oxygen levels to be depressed. Eventually, the individual wakes up periodically gasping for breath. People with **urinary frequency or urgency issues**, whether due to infection, use of diuretics, or an innate physical problem, awaken during the night and the sleep cycle is disrupted. Position changes during sleep and spasticity in patients with **musculoskeletal problems** can cause arousal and changes in the sleep cycle. Patients with **Alzheimer's disease** and patients with alterations in cognition have an impaired circadian rhythm, which causes nocturnal sleeplessness and

Functional Health Patterns

197

other problems. Older people often have difficulty getting enough deep sleep and REM sleep because later sleep stages become shorter as individuals **age**.

HEALTHY ROUTINES TO ENCOURAGE NORMAL SLEEP PATTERNS

The duration of a good night's sleep ranges from well **over half a day** in infants and toddlers to **between 7 and 9 hours** for an adult. In order to achieve this on a regular basis, an individual should try to go to bed and wake at the same times daily. Institution of **bedtime routines** such as a warm bath, relaxation exercises, playing music, or reading is helpful. **Exercise** done earlier in the day, but not right before bed, promotes better sleep. A number of **dietary** or other practices should be avoided close to bedtime, including excessive fluid intake, the nervous system depressant alcohol, stimulants such as caffeine or nicotine, spicy foods, and heavy meals in general. If the individual cannot fall asleep quickly, they should get up and do something else.

EFFECTS OF ALCOHOL AND DIET ON SLEEP

Patients may use alcohol as a "sleep aid," believing that it helps them to fall asleep and stay asleep. While alcohol may aid the patient in falling asleep, resulting in longer duration of sleep, it also results in **lower sleep quality**. Drinking alcohol reduces the amount of time spent in REM sleep (considered the restorative part of sleep), and the more a person drinks before sleeping, the more interruptions in REM are noted. This leads to daytime drowsiness and fatigue.

Eating meals close to bed can also result in difficulty falling and staying asleep. Patients should be taught that eating initiates metabolism, causing blood glucose levels to rise, which is followed by the pancreas releasing insulin. This can lead to a blood glucose drop below baseline, which leads to the adrenals secreting cortisol, a stress hormone. Another dietary consideration is that gastroesophageal reflux disease (GERD) is aggravated by heavy meals before lying down. Patients with GERD should avoid citrus fruits, caffeinated beverages, and dairy products close to bedtime. Most patients should try to eat at least 2–3 hours before bedtime.

MEDICATIONS THAT INDUCE SEDATION

There are a number of **tricyclic antidepressants** that induce sedation in addition to managing depression or mood disturbances. Some of these produce **heavy sedation**, such as amitriptyline, amoxapine, doxepin, and nortriptyline. People taking the selective serotonin reuptake inhibitors fluvoxamine or paroxetine also become quite drowsy, as do those taking the α2-adrenergic blocker antidepressant mirtazapine or the serotonin inhibitor and antagonist nefazodone. **REM sleep** is depressed by use of monoamine oxidase inhibitors such as phenelzine. Other tricyclic antidepressants, selective serotonin reuptake inhibitors, and the dopamine uptake inhibitor bupropion, have less powerful sedative effects.

NATURALLY OCCURRING SUBSTANCES AND DIETARY SUPPLEMENTS THAT CAN IMPACT SLEEP

The amino acid **tryptophan** can induce sleep if ingested on an empty stomach prior to bed. Milk and potatoes are good sources of tryptophan, but the synthetic version is not recommended due to possible safety issues. **Melatonin**, a hormone derived from serotonin, is secreted from the pineal gland in the brain. It is involved in both pigmentation and regulation of biorhythms with maximum amounts available at bedtime. Melatonin in herbal supplement form is being evaluated as a sleep enhancer. Other **herbal supplements** being touted as sleep inducers are under investigation. The calming agents valerian root, lavender, and chamomile, and the antidepressant St. John's wort, are among the most promising, but they have not been definitively proven to have value as sleep aids or been investigated for their sleep pattern effects.

DYSSOMNIAS

Dyssomnias are abnormal sleep patterns categorized as either **insomnia**, the inability to fall asleep or remain asleep long enough to be rested, or **hypersomnia**, extreme sleepiness and extended periods of sleep. Insomnia can have a myriad of underlying causes, as previously discussed. Nursing interventions include environmental control, relaxation measures, management of neurological symptoms, medication administration, and toileting assistance. Hypersomnia is generally caused by some sort of brain disturbance, such as lesions in the hypothalamus, intracranial pressure, encephalitis, depression, or metabolic abnormalities such as

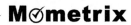

hypoglycemia. **Narcolepsy** is a variant of hypersomnia where individuals can sleep deeply at brief and odd intervals and may have hallucinations or difficulty moving.

Review Video: <u>Chronic Insomnia</u>
Visit mometrix.com/academy and enter code: 293232

Review Video: <u>Insomnia Management</u>
Visit mometrix.com/academy and enter code: 666132

PARASOMNIAS

Parasomnias are medical conditions or events that disturb sleep processes, disorders of arousal, or disorders of the sleep-wake transition. **Somnambulism**, or sleepwalking, is the prime example of the latter type of disorder; with somnambulism, the person is awake enough to be active but not really aware of their actions. Interventions include the use of benzodiazepines, such as diazepam, and pre-sleep relaxation. **Frightening dreams or nightmares** during the REM portion of sleep are parasomnias. **Leg problems** include nocturnal leg cramps in healthy middle-aged or elderly individuals, and restless leg syndrome, which are both parasomnias. Restless leg syndrome is a relative misnomer because it can also affect the arms, and it is characterized by increased surface sensitivity in the extremities, which can cause bursts of movement during sleep.

CAUSES OF DISTURBED SLEEP PATTERNS IN THE ELDERLY AND TREATMENT FOR INSOMNIA

About half of adults over age 65 have a **disturbed sleep pattern** primarily resulting in **insomnia**, the inability to fall asleep or remain asleep long enough to feel rested. Insomnia is defined as less than 6 hours of daily sleep, the need for more than 40 minutes to fall asleep, or tenseness upon awaking. The main causes of a disturbed sleep pattern related to aging are urgency to urinate, aging-associated changes such as lower blood flow, a waning of stage 3 sleep (non-REM deep sleep) probably due to morning alterations in core body temperature, disease-related pain, and specific sleep-related pathological conditions. **Behavioral modifications** are preferred over use of sleep medications for treatment of insomnia. These include nighttime denial of fluids, elimination of caffeine-containing foods and drinks, relaxation therapies, and changing behavioral patterns. The latter includes actions such as temporarily getting up if failing to fall asleep within 30 minutes, controlling the number of hours of sleep until return to a normal pattern, and restricting other activities in bed.

INTERVENTIONS FOR OBSTRUCTIVE SLEEP APNEA

Patients with **obstructive sleep apnea** are often treated with positive airway pressure, of which the two major types are continuous positive airway pressure (**CPAP**) and bilevel positive airway pressure (**BiPAP**). Most often in the **home setting** CPAP is used due to cost and simplicity. Patients usually get fitted in a sleep center, where a polysomnography tech can fit the patient for equipment and adjust settings, including pressure. Patients should be taught to report issues with comfort or equipment, or if sleep symptoms worsen with wear. In **rehab settings**, it is important to get equipment that is comfortable for the patient and find out home CPAP settings. For new CPAP users, adherence to CPAP is important to establish. Interventions to make patients more comfortable include adding humidification, choices of interface, and follow-up by an expert to determine if settings need to be adjusted. Educating patients on long-term effects of uncorrected sleep apnea can be beneficial, as well as behavioral therapy.

Functional Health Patterns

The Function of the Rehabilitation Team and Transitions of Care

Collaboration

FACILITATING REFERRALS

The rehabilitation nurse's role related to a patient's discharge after inpatient rehabilitation includes **assessment of the patient's needs** prior to discharge in order to determine who will benefit from outpatient and home health services, and **establishing a plan of care** that includes necessary services and realistic target outcomes. Some services needed may include home health care, PT, OT, speech therapy, or specialized programs, such as outpatient cardiac rehabilitation. The nurse will usually work with the **facility's case manager**, and preauthorization for treatments must be obtained. Care should be **coordinated** to ensure that interventions are carried out in a timely manner and duplication of services is avoided. The nurse should review referral information and assess the patient's and caregiver's learning needs and ensure they receive the education needed. For rehabilitation nurses working in home health or outpatient settings, **referral** often includes social workers, PT, OT, and community-based support groups. The rehabilitation nurse should be familiar with the process for making the referrals and with the types of resources available for patients in the area.

CASE MANAGEMENT

Case management is a multifaceted set of activities that focus on providing client care services. The definition of case management varies according to the field of practice and the organization defining it. The **Case Management Society of America (CMSA)** defines case management as "a collaborative process of assessment, planning, facilitation, and advocacy for options and services that meet an individual's health needs through communication and available resources to promote quality cost-effective outcomes." There are other definitions, such as that espoused by **the American Nurses Credentialing Center (ANCC)**, that list additional purposes such as decreasing fragmentation and repetition of care. The ANCC also sees nursing case management as a process of "assessment, planning, implementation, evaluation, and interaction." Case managers work in a variety of settings, including private practices, insurance companies, health maintenance organizations, and various types of health care facilities.

CRITICAL FUNCTIONS

About 70% of case managers are professional nurses. **Rehabilitation nurses** acting as case managers operate under several standards of practice outlined by the American Nurses Association, the Association of Rehabilitation Nurses, and the CMSA. The initial function of a case manager is the **identification** of appropriate individuals or groups. The case manager then utilizes all available data to **assess the patient's needs** and how they may be met, including information about the person's health status, functional skill levels, psychosocial condition, financial capabilities, and environment. The case manager develops an **individualized plan** based on this data. **Implementation** of the plan involves many aspects such as obtaining authorizations, managing financial issues, and documenting all actions and correspondence. A case manager is a **coordinator**. They synchronize communications, services, and follow-up. The manager is also responsible for **monitoring** the patient's adherence to the arrangements and constantly evaluating the entire process.

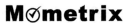

MANAGEMENT AREAS

Typically, a case manager is responsible for coordination of care and management of aspects of quality, cost, and outcomes.

- **Care coordination** involves the synchronization of the work of all team members.
- **Quality management** is a continuous process of providing excellence of care and identifying areas for improvement through monitoring.
- The case manager is also responsible for **cost management** and the achievement of cost-effectiveness through optimal use of available resources.
- **Outcomes management** refers to the systematic evaluation of desired parameters (such as quality of life, goal achievement, or use of available services) and then application of results to health care delivery. There are national agencies that summarize outcomes research, such as the **Agency for Healthcare Research and Quality**.

RELATIONSHIP TO MANAGED CARE

Managed care is basically a process of cost containment in which non-medical administrators such as insurance companies dictate the provision of services and medications. Managed care systems are the dominant configurations for providing health care in today's world. Case management services must deal with the managed care system that controls **payment for services**. The rehabilitation case manager deals with high-risk patients, which means they may need to **advocate** for patients and deal with the managed care service to provide optimal care. However, the two are not diametrically opposed, as both are concerned with cost containment and providing a continuum of care including prevention, wellness, rehabilitation, and various levels of care from acute to hospice settings.

CERTIFICATION AND ACCREDITATION ISSUES

At present, certification for case managers is not obligatory. However, there are two organizations providing certification if desired: the **Commission for Case Manager Certification**, which authorizes a "Certified Case Manager" (CCM) title; and the **ANA's American Nurses Credentialing Center (ANCC)**, which certifies bachelor's degree or higher nurses with 1 year of clinical experience. There are several groups that accredit case management facilities or organizations relevant to rehabilitation: the **Commission on Accreditation of Rehabilitation Facilities (CARF)**; the **Utilization Review Accreditation Commission (URAC)**, which is part of the American Accreditation HealthCare Commission; and the **National Committee for Quality Assurance (NCQA).** URAC sanctions case management services in both healthcare and workers' compensation venues. Certification, accreditation, and maintenance of standards of practice are important for case management because the multifaceted nature of the job makes it susceptible to legal and ethical issues.

The Function of the Rehabilitation Team and Transitions of Care

REHABILITATION TEAM ROLES

ROLES AND NECESSARY SKILL SETS OF THE REHABILITATION NURSE

In the late 1990s, Nolan and Nolan described six **roles** of the rehabilitation nurse and the corresponding knowledge and **skill sets** necessary to perform them.

- One role is the assessment of the patient's **physical condition and delivery of needed care**, which entails knowledge of anatomy, physiology, pathology, therapies, and diagnostic tools.
- The nurse must also be able to **teach and counsel** the patient, which requires the ability to evaluate learning styles and facilitate learning.
- They must be sensitive to and understand how to deal with patient **moods and coping mechanisms** in order to institute psychosocial interventions.
- The nurse also needs to understand **family dynamics** in order to assist the patient in dealing with family.
- A rehabilitation nurse may need to deal with patient issues related to **sexuality** and should be knowledgeable and sensitive.
- Finally, the nurse, particularly in community-based rehabilitation (CBR), serves a health care liaison role and should therefore possess knowledge about **health delivery systems**.

NECESSARY KNOWLEDGE AND SKILL BASE FOR COMMUNITY-BASED REHABILITATION NURSES

A **CBR** nurse is typically a registered nurse with additional specialty training and a background in rehabilitation nursing. The CBR nurse visits a patient in the patient's home or practices in a clinic, school, religious setting, or workplace. The required **knowledge and skill set** for these nurses is large and diverse. They need to understand adult learning principles, anatomy and physiology, health promotion practices, socialization theories, and more. They must act as counselors and educators in addition to providing disability health care. They need to possess good communication skills and knowledge of current research. The **home rehabilitative (sometimes called restorative) nurse** generally carries out programs designed by a physician (and perhaps a physical therapist).

ROLES OF REHABILITATION TEAM MEMBERS

Members of the rehabilitation team can vary depending on the type of facility. Generally, the **rehabilitation nurse** acts as the team coordinator as well as educator, caregiver, client advocate, and possibly other roles. This person should be a registered nurse and licensed as either a certified rehabilitation registered nurse (CRRN) or certified rehabilitation registered nurse–advanced (CRRN-A). There may be a **case manager** who works with the patient and family to optimize care in a cost-effective manner. The **primary physician** manages the medical and/or surgical aspects of care, authorizes referrals, and acts as a consultant. This primary physician may be a physiatrist specializing in physical medicine and rehabilitation. Several **therapists** may be part of the team, including a physical therapist, an occupational therapist, and possibly a recreational or art therapist. Mental health needs of the patient generally dictate that a **psychologist or psychiatrist** as well as a **social worker** be part of the team. If a patient has communication problems, a **speech-language pathologist** is utilized.

REHABILITATION NURSE MANAGER

Nurse managers administer distinct areas of nursing care, report to nurse executives, and forge relationships with other members of the interdisciplinary team. The chief nurse manager role is to provide **leadership** through a vision of the potential capabilities of the unit. The vision is implemented through development of a **tactical plan** incorporating defined and quantifiable goals and actions. A nurse manager should be an agent for **change**. They should also act as a **coach** or **mentor** to inspire the growth and development of other employees through positive reinforcement and promotion from within of better performers. Leadership styles vary, but the most successful leaders are **emotionally intelligent**, which means they are driven by qualities such as empathy, self-awareness, self-control, the desire to achieve, and social adeptness.

SPECIFIC NURSE MANAGER ROLES RELATED TO FISCAL MANAGEMENT

Most nurse managers are responsible for preparation of a **yearly operating budget**. This budget addresses three areas: expected revenue or income, expenses, and projected capital requirements. **Revenue** can be estimated by correlating it to the following: the average daily patient census, the Functional Independence Measure (FIM) of typical patients and the associated case mix group (CMG), the number of patient discharges, and the average length of stay. **Expenses** are business expenditures. In this setting, the major expenses are personnel salaries and fringe benefits. Determination of adequate but cost-effective staffing requirements should reflect patient acuity or severity relative to resources. Additional expenses include supplies and rental of equipment. **Capital requirements** include such things as equipment, furniture, or construction. Fiscal needs can be internally monitored through use of productivity measures, streamlining, and prioritization.

SPECIFIC NURSING PRACTICE AND PATIENT CARE DELIVERY ROLES

The nurse manager is responsible for promoting and disseminating information about the **values and objectives** of the nurses and other team members. The nurse manager works with the nurse executive to identify and implement the **care delivery system** most suited to their unit. There are several possible delivery models, including: a **team nursing approach**, in which an RN is responsible for a large group of patients and other personnel; **primary nursing**, where only registered nurses are utilized to care for a smaller group of patients; and a **modified primary nursing system** integrating various types of nurses. A **patient-focused model** may be incorporated into any of these systems by cross training of other personnel to improve care delivery. The nurse manager is generally responsible for maintaining standards of practice, competency, care, and accreditation.

OTHER RESPONSIBILITIES

A nurse manager is a **human resource manager** for the unit's nursing and support personnel. The rehabilitation nurse manager is usually responsible for recruiting, interviewing, hiring, and keeping personnel. They collaborate with the actual human resource department on issues such as compensation, benefits, and employee relations. Another function of the nurse manager is to act as an **advocate for persons with disabilities** through administration of awareness activities, media campaigns, or legislative work. The nurse manager is also the point person for dissemination of **new research findings** and implementation of **professional practice models** incorporating new nursing theories.

NURSING STAFF DEVELOPMENT

The basis of nursing staff development is further education. The nurse manager should facilitate **staff education** through orientation, in-house training, and continuing education programs. **Implementation** of educational programs requires identification of manpower and resources, prioritization of needs based on the patient mix and other requirements, sorting out specific educational needs, and providing a conducive atmosphere. Professional nurses and other medical professionals must keep up with new advances in order to provide quality care. In addition, staff development opportunities should be presented periodically to **unlicensed assistive personnel** such as nurse's aides and multiskilled workers who perform other technical tasks.

Community Reintegration or Transition to the Next Level of Care

DISCHARGE PLANNING AND COMMUNITY REINTEGRATION OF THE PATIENT

Discharge planning is the process of defining needs and ways to meet those needs after a patient is discharged or released from the hospital or other health care setting. The process should really begin as soon as a patient is **admitted** so that provisions are made prior to discharge. A large part of this planning should be compiling and making available to the patient and family a list of **community resources**. These compilations should include features such as available home health care services, outpatient rehabilitation assistance, assisted living facilities, equipment vendors, and other support services. Prior to discharge, the patient and their subsequent caregiver need to be **educated** about care needs, infection control, emergency procedures, and the

The Function of the Rehabilitation Team and Transitions of Care

like. Eventual **community reintegration,** if possible, encompasses a return to family and community life, independent functioning, reestablishment of contextually normal roles, and reestablishment as a contributor to society.

PRINCIPLES OF COMMUNITY-BASED REHABILITATION MODEL

The World Health Organization has developed a **model for community-based rehabilitation (CBR)**. The basic principles of the model are:

- Use of all available community resources
- Community involvement in aspects of planning, choice, and assessment
- Dissemination of knowledge to persons with disabilities and others
- Maximal utilization of referrals at all levels of involvement

Other tenets of CBR include promotion of functional independence of people with disabilities, empowerment, and cultivation of positive attitudes by others. CBR programs must be specific to the **community** they serve. Exact CBR resources can include actual health care services, transportation, housing facilities, and community buildings. The great majority of CBR is done in a **home-based setting**.

COMMUNITY RESOURCES AND SUPPORT GROUPS

Community resources are a collection of assistance programs or services provided to community members. Such resources may be **organizations** serving a certain geographical area or certain **groups of people**. Typically, the goal of community resources is to positively impact community growth and to improve the quality of life of community members. These resources may be available at no cost or at low cost and may be run by the government, local businesses, or other community members.

A **support group** consists of members that are united because of an illness, disability, cause, or issue. The group is usually **nonprofessional** and may function to provide information, share personal experiences, provide empathy, suggest resources, and lend a listening ear. Support groups may have various aspects to render support and assistance. Some aspects of support groups may include **financial and emotional care**, and may also extend to family members, caregivers, and healthcare providers involved in the patient's care. Some support groups meet in person, while others may be online. Online groups may be more accessible for some patients with disabilities, providing community for the patient even though they are unable to leave home.

COMMUNITY-BASED HOUSING OPTIONS FOR INDIVIDUALS WITH DISABILITIES

Most community-based housing options for individuals with disabilities are residential and differ in the amount of supervision, support services, and amount of individualized care. An **independent living center**, for example, assists the patient with many services that are not centrally located. In a **private or state-run boarding home**, the fairly mobile individual is responsible for their own personal care. **Integrated housing** is really an independent option with access to community services. **Assisted living** means an individual room within a complex that offers services as well as meals. A **residential facility** is a closely knit group of patients sharing support services. More supervised environments include supervised environmental living facilities for the mentally ill with comprehensive services, group homes segregated by disability type, institutions providing individualized care on a constant basis, and congregate care facilities for people who have mobility impairments. Facilities, financial considerations, disability type, and geographical location affect choices for care.

BARRIERS TO COMMUNITY REINTEGRATION OF PATIENTS WITH DISABILITIES OR CHRONIC ILLNESS

Certain patient populations are inherently **difficult to reintegrate** into the community. These include the pediatric and geriatric patient populations as well as those with mental illness. Elderly individuals, for example, may have multiple functional impairments, polypharmacy issues, insufficient financial resources, and/or lack of transportation. **Community transportation issues** have been addressed more aggressively in

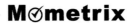

recent years, as in the 1990 Americans with Disabilities Act (ADA) mandating accessible public transportation. **Employment** is another problem; the ADA also bans potential employers from asking questions about disability. **Housing options** for individuals with disabilities may be unavailable or too expensive. Adequate **attendant care** may be unavailable. **Caregivers**, especially if they are family members, often feel overburdened. People with disabilities are also at increased risk for abuse, assault, and substance abuse.

CARE SETTING OPTIONS FOR PEDIATRIC PATIENTS WITH SPECIAL NEEDS

Traditionally, pediatric rehabilitation was primarily supplied in acute inpatient units. In today's healthcare setting, services have shifted more toward use of **outpatient or community-based programs**, particularly **home health care services** provided through an agency. The main role of a pediatric rehabilitation nurse providing home health care is one of an **educator**. As the pediatric rehabilitation nurse will be in the home a limited number of hours, it is important to teach other family members about the child's care. State programs—and to a lesser extent, federal Medicaid programs—are the major sources for **reimbursement** of services. Other care settings for the pediatric patient with special needs include outpatient clinics and therapy units and services performed within the school setting. The **family** must always be included in the rehabilitation process, which means the family has needs as well. One resource is **respite care or temporary residential care** for the patient to give the parents or regular caregivers time off to relax and renew themselves. The federal government does authorize state funding for respite care.

ADAPTIVE EQUIPMENT AND TECHNOLOGY

Voice-activated call systems usually require a base station of some type accompanied by a wearable device (such as a pendant or watch) or small stationary devices in different rooms. The call system is typically activated by code words, such as "Call 911," and then it automatically initiates the call to emergency services. Some devices include fall detection. Others allow voice communication with a call center. Monthly fees vary from about $30 to $80.

Computer-supported prosthetics uses microprocessor technology. There are limb prosthetics with computer-supported knees, feet, hands, and elbows. Microprocessor-enabled prosthetics move and adjust automatically without conscious thought or effort on the part of the wearer. The computerized system in the prosthetics makes all the necessary adjustments according to sensory input that the computer receives. Computer-supported prosthetics tend to be much more expensive than traditional prosthetics and are heavier and have a limited battery life, so they must be recharged periodically. The increased cost may be offset by fewer falls and injuries. Special sensors in some prosthetics are able to detect electrical signals generated by muscle movement through implanted electrodes, and the bionic arm, for example, can even provide a sensation of touch.

SPECIAL CONSIDERATIONS FOR INDIVIDUALS WITH INTELLECTUAL/DEVELOPMENTAL DISABILITIES
NECESSARY KNOWLEDGE WHEN CARING FOR PEOPLE WITH I/DD

Currently the term **intellectual/developmental disability** (I/DD) is generally used to describe a broad variety of mental and/or physical conditions that impede an individual's functionality at an expected developmental level. Most people with these types of disabilities were institutionalized until about the 1970s. A **nursing I/DD specialty** was established in 1997. Nurses caring for people with an I/DD need to understand the physiologic and genetic causes of I/DD, appropriate medications, and the relationship between I/DD and other chronic diseases. They must be cognizant of the **psychosocial aspects** of I/DD, such as difficult behavior, speech processing and other communication problems, lack of social skills, associated mental health issues, and developmental effects. They should understand **family dynamics** and the hardships that patients with I/DD place on caregivers. The I/DD nurse also needs to be knowledgeable about the **community service system** that impacts the nurse's practice.

ISSUES RELEVANT TO PEOPLE WITH DEVELOPMENTAL DISABILITIES

People with developmental disabilities often get inadequate health care, either because of inaccessibility of services or because of behavioral and learning problems that alienate healthcare workers. **Health care**

The Function of the Rehabilitation Team and Transitions of Care

205

consent is often a difficult issue because, legally, adults with I/DD are considered competent unless confirmed otherwise. These individuals are at risk for **sexual abuse**, but they may be unable to verbalize the abuse. When adolescents with developmental disabilities get ready to leave the educational system, a **transition plan** is developed around age 16 under the **individualized education plan (IEP)**, which may allow continued vocational and other training until they are 21 years old. Nevertheless, for people with developmental disabilities, the **unemployment rate** is high after leaving the educational system. As adults with I/DD age, they may face disorder-specific or medication-related **health problems** in addition to problems associated with normal aging. People with I/DD place hardships on their family members, especially during childhood, transition periods, and as they age.

SYSTEM OF SERVICES RELATED TO DEVELOPMENTAL DISABILITIES

On a federal level, the Developmental Disabilities Act is overseen by the **US Administration on Disabilities (AoD)**. In turn, the AoD also regulates funding of certain state organizations such as state Protection and Advocacy agencies and State Councils on Developmental Disabilities, as well as the research-oriented University Centers for Excellence in Developmental Disabilities. At the state level, most services for children and adolescents are **programs** within the school or child welfare system or **early interventional plans**. Most adult forms of assistance are **residential options** such as supervised group homes, adult foster care, or if possible, more independent choices. The latter is termed **supported living** or **comprehensive community-based services**, and a yearly plan for the person is set up by a team of caregivers and medical personnel to address the person's needs. State agencies usually offer employment services as well.

HABILITATION VS. REHABILITATION

Habilitation refers to making the best use of the abilities and maximizing the facility for independent living of a person with developmental disabilities by providing a range of medical, psychological, learning, and family services. **Rehabilitation** implies a re-education process. Many people with I/DD need initial learning or habilitation, but some also have physical problems or losses requiring rehabilitation. People with I/DD, especially children, are at higher risk for falls and other injuries than the population at large. Some have a propensity to develop other diseases. Examples include the increased prevalence of heart disease in adult patients with Down syndrome, and the high frequency of joint problems in older individuals with cerebral palsy due to nervous system degeneration.

PATIENT AND FAMILY EDUCATION
CHALLENGES TO HEALTH EDUCATION OF PATIENT AND FAMILY

One-fifth of the American population is **functionally illiterate**, a definition referring to anyone able to read only at the fifth-grade level or below. Lower literacy skills have been found to equate to **low adherence to treatment instructions**, which results in more time in the hospital and poorer outcomes. This segment of the population needs constant reinforcement of principles in order to learn. The **developmental level** of the learner affects their learning curve. Educational plans for **children** need to account for their developmental and cognitive level, their attention span, and their relationship with the parent; children tend to learn through active involvement. Educational plans for **adolescents** must take into consideration their need for independence and their emphasis on body image. **Elderly individuals** generally need individualized programs because they can have a variety of unique challenges such as impaired cognition, issues with frequency of elimination, or nutritional issues. Information must be presented slowly and repetitively and reinforced through use of methods such as audiovisual aids or support groups. For dealing with **cultural or language barriers**, most facilities can provide translators.

DOCUMENTATION AND EVALUATION OF LEARNING ACTIVITIES

Teaching activities should always be **documented** in terms of patients, content, time and location of the activity, teaching methods used, and mode of assessment. Such documentation serves as **legal evidence** if necessary and is also a basis for **reimbursement**. **Evaluation** of the patient education process is generally measured in terms of patient and family adherence to the desired goals, also known as concordance. **Adherence to a regimen** is the ultimate behavioral change objective. If it is low, it can be improved through a

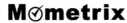

number of strategies to identify reasons and then implement ways to alleviate the problems. For example, if the behavioral change is too complex, it can be simplified and broken down into phases. The nurse should also be aware of and direct patients to community resources upon discharge to reinforce the learning process and adherence.

FAMILY CONFERENCES

If patients with chronic illness or disability lack the mental capacity to make decisions, family members usually become the primary **medical decision-makers** in the absence of a predetermined health care power of attorney. Convening a **family conference** is helpful in cases where there is disagreement among family members regarding the plan of care. Once the family members are updated about the medical status of the patient, a respectful and honest conversation should take place in which each family member's opinions and concerns about what the plan of care should be are elicited. Issues related to long-term care of an individual with disabilities may also be complicated by **financial issues** related to care, especially if other members of the family lived with the individual prior to their injury or illness, and their own housing or finances could be jeopardized by the patient beginning to receive Medicaid or Medicare.

CONFLICT RESOLUTION

Conflict is an almost inevitable product of teamwork, and the leader must assume responsibility for **conflict resolution.** While conflicts can be disruptive, they can produce positive outcomes by opening dialogue and forcing team members to listen to different perspectives. The team should make a plan for dealing with conflict. The best time for conflict resolution is when differences emerge but before open conflict and hardening of positions occur. The leader must pay close attention to the people and problems involved, listen carefully, and reassure those involved that their points of view are understood. Steps to conflict resolution include:

- Allow both sides to present their side of the conflict without bias, maintaining a focus on opinions rather than individuals.
- Encourage cooperation through negotiation and compromise.
- Maintain the focus, providing guidance to keep the discussions on track and avoid arguments.
- Evaluate the need for re-negotiation, formal resolution process, or third-party involvement.
- Utilize humor and empathy to diffuse escalating tensions.
- Summarize the issues, outlining key arguments.
- Avoid forcing resolution if possible.

RESPITE CARE

Respite care is the psychological and physical support provided to caregivers. Respite care takes many forms. Especially in cases involving long-term care, caregivers need to be encouraged to talk with others in similar situations, facing similar challenges, by attending caregiver support groups. To better understand illnesses, **support services** are available for spouses, family, and children/siblings of individuals suffering from long-term illnesses. Respite care may be **placement** of a person with disabilities at an assisted living residence for a weekend, giving the family care providers a "weekend off." Respite care may be someone **residing** in the home of a patient, allowing the family caregivers to take a vacation. Community-based rehab nurses can help by identifying when caregivers need respite care and by supplying **resources** for respite care. Rehabilitation facility nurses can help by providing **information** about respite care to families on or before discharge, so that the family knows what to do when needing a break from the challenges they may face.

Legislative, Economic, Ethical, and Legal Issues

Integration of Legislation and Regulations in Care Management

AMERICANS WITH DISABILITIES ACT

The 1990 Americans with Disabilities Act (ADA) is civil rights legislation that provides individuals with disabilities—including those with mental impairment—access to employment and the community. While employers must make reasonable accommodations for individuals with disabilities, the provisions related to the community apply more directly to **older Americans**. The ADA covers not only obvious disabilities but also disorders such as arthritis, seizure disorders, psychiatric disorders, and cardiovascular and respiratory disorders. Communities must provide transportation services for individuals with disabilities, including accommodation for wheelchairs. Public facilities (schools, museums, physician's offices, post offices, restaurants) must be accessible with ramps and elevators as needed. Telecommunications must also be accessible through devices or accommodations for the deaf and blind. **Compliance** is not yet complete because older buildings are required to provide access that is possible without "undue hardship," but newer construction of public facilities must meet ADA regulations.

INDIVIDUALS WITH DISABILITIES EDUCATION ACT

The latest version of the Individuals with Disabilities Education Act (**IDEA**) was issued in 2004 by US Department of Education. The major points and provisions are as follows:

- Access (from ages 3 to 21) to free and suitable public education in settings with other children
- Schemes to identify children with special education needs
- Individualized education plans (IEPs) for each child
- Procedures for parents to be involved in the process
- Evaluation protocols
- Confidentiality
- Transition services into preschool and out into adulthood
- Processes to correctly classify minority children
- Grants for early intervention services for children under 3 years of age

OSHA AND THE FDA

The US Department of Labor's **Occupational Safety and Health Administration (OSHA)** sets standards for:

- Proper hand washing
- Wearing gloves and other personal protective equipment (PPE)
- Bagging specimens in biohazard bags
- Disposing of needles and lancets in a sharps container
- Cleaning up spills to prevent spread of bloodborne pathogens
- Harmful chemical control
- Safe equipment use
- Adequate work space

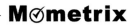

Check for updates regularly at OSHA's website. These updates are required to be adopted as part of the facility's standards of practice.

Review Video: <u>What is OSHA (Occupational Safety and Health Administration)?</u>
Visit mometrix.com/academy and enter code: 913559

The US **Food & Drug Administration (FDA)** is responsible for the following:

- Assigning the official (generic) name for drugs when it approves them
- Reporting recalls and adverse events through MedWatch
- Publishing a free, downloadable "Orange Book" of approved drugs
- Dividing drugs into five schedules, based on their potential for abuse, numbered Schedule I (generally illegal) to Schedule V (generally benign)
- Setting the temperature regulations for dish sanitization

ADULT PROTECTIVE SERVICES

Adult protective services (APS) are available in all states but may be administered differently. APS is most often part of a department of social services. APS provides protective social services to older adults, age 60 or 65 and older. In all but a few states (10%), vulnerable adults, such as those with disabilities, are included under APS. The purpose of APS is to identify and prevent neglect, abandonment, and abuse, which may be psychological, physical, sexual, or financial. Those with disabilities are especially vulnerable to abuse because they may not be able to self-report or protect themselves. Some states allow anonymous reporting, and most provide some sort of protection against civil or criminal liability or professional disciplinary action for those making the report if it is done in good faith. APS carries out investigations, assesses risk and mental abilities, provides counseling, assists the individual in obtaining necessary services, develops a case plan for the individual, and monitors ongoing services.

CHILD PROTECTIVE SERVICES

Child protective services (CPS) are similar to adult protective services in that CPS receives reports of possible abuse or neglect and carries out investigations and interventions to ensure the safety and security of children and adolescents. Children with disabilities are especially at risk of abuse and neglect. CPS is most often part of a department of social services, but this may vary. For example, in Mississippi, the Department of Child Protection Services is an independent agency. When a report is received by CPS, it is investigated by a social worker who can intervene in the event of a crisis, remove a child from the home, and place the child in foster care if necessary. The services that are provided by CPS vary somewhat from one state to another. In most cases of neglect and abuse, the goal is to assist the parents to provide adequate care and, if the child has been removed from the home, reunification. If the child is unable to safely return to the home, CPS may facilitate adoption or permanent placement of some type. CPS may also help to identify resources for children with disabilities so that they can be more safely provided for in the home environment.

VOCATIONAL EDUCATION ACT OF 1963

The intent of the Vocational Education Act of 1963 was to expand job opportunities and to help the states to maintain, modernize, and develop vocational education programs at the secondary and post-secondary levels, as well as to provide funds for part-time employment for young people engaged in vocational education programs full-time. States were allowed to decide which type of vocational programs the funds would be allocated to. Funds were provided to build area facilities for vocational education and training. Money was intended to provide for vocational education programs for occupations that were in demand for the following:

- Secondary students
- High school graduates
- School dropouts
- Those with academic, socioeconomic, or physical handicaps
- Employed people in need of more training or retraining

The Vocational Education Act was instrumental in developing work-study programs and advisory committees to help determine the need and focus of vocational programs. The Act provided grants to colleges and universities to pay for research and training to encourage development of experimental programs aimed at those with handicaps that might interfere with their being successful in more traditional vocational training.

REHABILITATION ACT OF 1973

The Rehabilitation Act of 1973 has several sections that mandate **affirmative action** and nondiscrimination regarding employment in executive branch federal agencies (**Section 501**) and with federal government contractors receiving over $10,000 (**Section 503**). **Section 504** requires compliance with federal standards for physical disability in facilities using federal funds, bans housing discrimination in public accommodations or private housing receiving federal funds, prohibits unfairness in federally funded schools, and prohibits discrimination in privately operated transportation services receiving federal assistance. **Section 508** obliges federal agencies to make electronic and information technology accessible to individuals with disabilities.

DEVELOPMENTAL DISABILITIES ASSISTANCE AND BILL OF RIGHTS ACT OF 2000

The Developmental Disabilities Assistance and Bill of Rights Act of 2000 (**DD Act**) broadly defines the term **developmental disability** as "a severe, chronic disability" of an individual that:

1. is attributable to a mental or physical impairment or combination of mental and physical impairments
2. is manifested before the individual attains age 22
3. is likely to continue indefinitely
4. results in substantial functional limitations in three or more of the following areas of major life activity:
   a. self-care
   b. receptive and expressive language
   c. learning
   d. mobility
   e. self-direction
   f. capacity for independent living
   g. economic self-sufficiency
5. reflects the individual's need for a combination and sequence of special, interdisciplinary, or generic services, individualized supports, or other forms of assistance that are of lifelong or extended duration and are individually planned and coordinated.

The act is meant to be as **inclusive** as possible, and some states have enacted less comprehensive definitions.

AFFORDABLE CARE ACT

The Patient Protection and Affordable Care Act of 2010, also known as Obamacare or simply the Affordable Care Act, allocated money to offset the costs of insurance for those who could not otherwise qualify. Provisions that are relevant to disability and rehabilitation include:

- Expanded coverage
- The right to choose a physician

- Prohibition of discrimination based on disability or chronic health condition
- Improved long-term supports for people with disabilities
- The ability to remain on the parents' insurance plan until age 26
- Elimination of lifetime limits of coverage and restriction of annual limits
- Requirement that insurance companies provide an appeal process
- Sliding scale for payment of insurance
- Requirement that insurance companies provide coverage to any adult age 19 to 64 who applies
- Requirement that pre-existing conditions must be covered and cannot exclude a person from receiving insurance
- Free preventive care

IMPACT ACT OF 2014

The Improving Medicare Post-Acute Care Transformation Act of 2014 (IMPACT Act) amended Title XVII of the Social Security Act and applies to long-term care hospitals, skilled nursing facilities, home health agencies, and inpatient rehabilitation facilities. The IMPACT Act outlines specific requirements and provides reporting tools for the different types of facilities. For example, standardized assessment tools are to be used to collect data. The IMPACT Act requires that these facilities collect and report standardized data in order to improve outcomes for Medicare beneficiaries. The IMPACT Act requires development of standardized patient assessment data elements (SPADEs) for clinical categories:

- Quality measures: Skin, functional status, medication reconciliation, falls, transfers/transitions
- Resource use: Estimated cost per beneficiary, discharge, readmission rates
- Assessment categories: Functional status, cognitive function, special services, medical conditions/comorbidities, impairments

Additionally, the IMPACT Act supports the priority areas of "Meaningful Measures":

- Effective communication/coordination of care
- Effective prevention/treatment of chronic disease
- Promotion of healthy living
- Affordable care
- Safe care
- Strengthening person/family engagement

ADDITIONAL DISABILITY-RELATED LAWS

A multitude of laws have been passed to protect individuals with disabilities. Important disability-related laws include the following:

- **Section 188 of the Workforce Investment Act** bans discrimination against individuals with disabilities in federally funded employment service centers.
- The **Fair Housing Act** prohibits inequities related to any type of housing or housing-related transaction on the basis of disability.
- The **Architectural Barriers Act** mandates adherence to accessibility standards in federally financed housing.
- Education is also addressed through programs such as the **No Child Left Behind program** and the **New Freedom Initiative**.
- The **Air Carrier Access Act** forbids public air carriers with regularly scheduled services from discriminating against individuals with disabilities.
- The **Telecommunications Act, Section 255**, requires telecommunications equipment manufacturers and providers to provide products enhancing accessibility.

Legislative, Economic, Ethical, and Legal Issues

ADDITIONAL LEGISLATION RELEVANT TO REHABILITATION

Over the years, many acts of legislation relevant to rehabilitation have been enacted. Key milestones include the creation of the **Veterans Bureau** and the **Disabled Veterans Rehabilitation Act of 1943**, **Title VII of the 1978 amendments to the Rehabilitation Act of 1973** (which crafted the Comprehensive Services for Independent Living program), and several original inclusions and amendments to the Social Security Act of 1935. Regarding the latter, the initial **Title V of the Social Security Act of 1935** set up a federal-state system for "crippled" children that was later expanded in 1963 to include children at risk for mental illness. **Social Security Disability Insurance (SSDI)** was authorized in 1956 by amendment. Supplemental Security Income (SSI) included people with blindness or other disabilities by amendments enacted in 1972.

HIPAA

HIPAA stands for **Health Insurance Portability and Accountability Act** of 1996. HIPAA's Title I regulates healthcare accessibility, especially in the cases of job change and loss; Title II regulates patient privacy rights.

HIPAA requires the following:

- Every patient's medical record must bear a unique identifier to prevent misidentification.
- Patients must be given access to their protected health information (medical records) at any time, upon request.
- Only relevant health information can be disclosed to authorized parties.
- A record must be kept of every disclosure.
- Every patient, or the patient's parents/guardians, must receive a Notice of Privacy Practices, outlining how the protected health information will be used.
- Physical access to protected health information must be limited (including electronic files via password protection or swipe cards, firewall, and SSL encryption).
- Retired electronic equipment must have all data records wiped clean.

> **Review Video: What is HIPAA?**
> Visit mometrix.com/academy and enter code: 412009

WORKERS' COMPENSATION SYSTEM

The workers' compensation system was developed to reimburse workers for work-related injuries and illnesses. The benefits included in a workers' compensation program include income replacement when a worker is unable to work; support for the worker's dependents in the case of work-related death; hospital, medical, and funeral expenses; and in some cases, travel and parking expenses associated with work-related injury or illness. In most cases, the employer must provide workers' compensation benefits regardless of whether or not an accident was a result of employee neglect. It is important for the employee to understand that if they accept workers' compensation benefits, they are no longer able to seek legal actions against the employer for their injuries.

MEDICARE

Medicare, a federally directed program, was introduced by the Title XIX Social Security Act in 1965. It provides health insurance to elderly patients and to patients with disabilities. The patient who is covered will receive hospital, doctor, and further medical care as needed. The patient's income is not a factor for eligibility. **Original Medicare** consists of **Part A** and **Part B**, and covers the majority of medical care when the patient seeks care at a facility that accepts Medicare. If the patient requires prescription drug assistance, they may opt into **Part D**, which is the Medicare drug plan, or they may opt into the **Medicare Advantage Plan (Part C)**, which bundles Parts A, B and D.

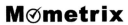

MEDICARE PART A

Medicare Part A covers hospital care (inpatient), care at a skilled nursing facility or nursing home, hospice care, and home health care. Anyone 65 years of age or older that is eligible to receive **Social Security** is automatically enrolled even if still working. Patients are also able to receive Social Security if they or their spouse put money into the system by way of working for at least 40 quarters. If the patient has less than 40 quarters of work, Medicare Part A requires a payment each month. If the patient is not yet 65 but has a complete disability that will remain for the rest of their life, Medicare Part A can be used after receiving Social Security benefits for 2 years. A patient with ongoing renal disease who needs either dialysis or transplant can become eligible for Part A without waiting for 2 years.

MEDICARE PART B

Medicare Part B covers both medically necessary services and preventive services such as doctor visits, physical therapy, occupational therapy, speech therapy, medical equipment, assessments, clinical research, mental health support and wellness visits. The patient has to **pay a monthly premium for Medicare Part B,** which is either directly billed to the patient or deducted from their Social Security or other benefit payment. The program covers 80% of the authorized expense for any medical attention that is required (following a yearly deductible).

MEDICAID

1965 Title XIX Social Security Act introduced **Medicaid** as a federal/state matching plan for low-income individuals supervised by the federal government. Funding comes from federal and state taxes, with no less than 50%, but no more than 83% being funded federally. Each state is able to add optional eligibility criteria on the list, and they may also put restrictions (to a point) on federally directed aid. Patients who receive Medicaid cannot get a bill for the aid, but states are able to require small copayments or deductibles for particular types of help.

Federal regulations require that states support certain individuals or groups of individuals through Medicaid, although not everyone who falls below the federal poverty rate is eligible. **Mandatory eligibility groups** include the following:

- Patients deemed categorically needy by their state, and receive financial support from various federal assistance programs.
- Individuals receiving Federal Supplemental Security income (SSI).
- Patients that are older than 65 that are blind or have complete disability.
- Pregnant women and children younger than 6 years of age who live in families that are up to 133% of the federal poverty level (some states allow for a higher income to meet eligibility in this class).
- Adults under the age of 65 that make less than or equal to 133% of the federal poverty level and are not receiving Medicare.

> **Review Video: Medicare & Medicaid**
> Visit mometrix.com/academy and enter code: 507454

213

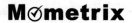

Cost-Effective Patient-Centered Care

COST CONSIDERATIONS IN REHABILITATION NURSING

The rapidly rising costs of health care need to be curtailed; the system is now focusing on attaining better outcomes while controlling costs. Principles of cost containment are as follows:

- Close examination of over- and underutilization of services in health care.
- **Improved coordination and cooperation** over the entire quality of care continuum.
- Placing greater emphasis upon **prevention** by awarding incentives for wellness behaviors in patients as well as stressing early detection of disease.
- Increased usage of **evidence-based guidelines** in the treatment of various diseases, which helps to contain costs.
- **Electronic medical records** and improved information regarding the costs of products and services used by providers and patients; this allows informed decisions about the comparative effectiveness of treatments.

ACCESS TO AND COST OF HEALTH CARE FOR INDIVIDUALS WITH DISABILITIES

The issues of access to and cost of health care for individuals with disabilities are intertwined. Traditionally, rehabilitation services were offered in a fee-for-service environment that emphasized treating the individual without much consideration of cost. In today's circumstances, however, financial and other resources are increasingly given in terms of the likelihood of **achieving a preferred outcome**. For example, a certain minimal length of stay is considered desirable and services are withdrawn at that time or referrals are denied by the payer if the payer deems them unnecessary. Services may be available, but **access** is not granted by insurance plans, Medicaid, or Medicare, often severely impacting individuals with disabilities who have many needs. Alternatively, these people may be denied **affordable health insurance**. Healthcare costs for individuals with disabilities have been documented in various studies to be at least 4 times the amount for other patients. **Cost containment measures** affect quality of care and patient outcomes.

REIMBURSEMENT OPTIONS

REIMBURSEMENT PRACTICES RELEVANT TO HOME HEALTH CARE SERVICES

Managed care insurance programs, Medicare, and Medicaid **reimburse** home health care services based on nursing documentation of homebound status. **Homebound status** means that the patient is unable to easily leave home alone or with assistance, requires skilled care at home, and has no other readily accessible options to address these needs. Since physical, occupational, and speech therapies are reimbursable and often accessible skills, the rehabilitative or restorative nurse may need to aggressively present a **case for reimbursement**. **Home plans** must be established and reviewed by a physician at least every 60 days to obtain reimbursement. An agency providing these services must be **Medicare certified** if applicable. Reimbursement for home care is primarily paid through **Medicare Part A** with limits outlined by the Health Care Financing Administration (HCFA). Home health agencies are accredited through the **Community Health Accreditation Partner** (part of the National League for Nursing), the **Accreditation Commission for Health Care**, or the **Home Care Accreditation program**, associated with the Joint Commission on Accreditation of Healthcare Organizations.

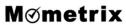

MEDICARE AND INSURANCE REIMBURSEMENT GUIDELINES FOR HOME OXYGEN THERAPY

Prior to discharge, in order to be reimbursed for subsequent home oxygen therapy, a patient must have an **oxygen saturation level of less than 89%** or **oxygen pressure ≤55 mmHg** while resting or walking. If the patient has other cardiopulmonary diseases, a PaO_2 between 55 and 60 mmHg is allowed. These exceptional patients must also demonstrate other evidence of **supplemental defects**. They must have dependent edema indicative of congestive heart failure, an enlarged right ventricle on ECG, or a hematocrit of more than 55%. Alternatively, their proof could be a drop during sleep of $PaCO_2$ to <55 mmHg (or an incremental drop of at least 10 mm) or oxygen saturation to <85%. Another avenue is the same type of drop during exercise. **Home oxygen prescriptions** must be very specific in terms of rate delivered, minimum daily usage, source, delivery method, and whether portability is needed.

UTILIZATION REVIEW

The purpose of utilization review is to determine if services are utilized appropriately and in accordance with evidence-based criteria and provided in a cost-effective manner. CMS requires that all hospitals that it reimburses conduct utilization review, usually done by a utilization review nurse, who reviews the patient's medical records to determine if the patient's treatment and placement (such as in ICU) is appropriate and meets the criteria for medical necessity according to established protocols. Healthcare providers at all levels, including home health agencies, and insurance companies carry out utilization reviews as well. Utilization reviews may be prospective (such as when gaining preauthorization for treatments), concurrent (ongoing review while the patient receives treatment), or retrospective (review of the medical record of treatment). Screening tools that are in common use in inpatient hospitals to prevent over- and under-utilization include Milliman and InterQual criteria. Utilization review for inpatients may include up to 4 steps:

1. The utilization review nurse assesses the patient's need for care and makes recommendations.
2. The nurse consults with the utilization insurance nurse.
3. If the hospital and insurance utilization nurses cannot agree, then the physicians discuss the issue peer-to-peer.
4. If the insurance company denies a claim, an appeal may be filed.

Ethical Considerations and Legal Obligations that Affect Practice

ETHICS

ETHICAL PRINCIPLES

Autonomy is the ethical principle that the individual has the right to make decisions about his or her own care. In the case of children or patients with dementia who cannot make autonomous decisions, parents or family members may serve as the legal decision maker. The nurse must keep the patient and/or family fully informed so that they can exercise their autonomy in informed decision-making.

Justice is the ethical principle that relates to the distribution of the limited resources of healthcare benefits to the members of society. These resources must be distributed fairly. This issue may arise if there is only one bed left and two sick patients. Justice comes into play in deciding which patient should stay and which should be transported or otherwise cared for. The decision should be made according to what is best or most just for the patients and not colored by personal bias.

Beneficence is an ethical principle that involves performing actions that are for the purpose of benefitting another person. In the care of a patient, any procedure or treatment should be done with the ultimate goal of benefitting the patient, and any actions that are not beneficial should be reconsidered. As conditions change, procedures need to be continually reevaluated to determine if they are still of benefit.

Nonmaleficence is an ethical principle that means healthcare workers should provide care in a manner that does not cause direct intentional harm to the patient:

- The actual act must be good or morally neutral.
- The intent must be only for a good effect.
- A bad effect cannot serve as the means to get to a good effect.
- A good effect must have more benefit than a bad effect has harm.

ETHICS COMMITTEES AND OMBUDS

The ombuds and ethical consult teams can be activated at most facilities by anyone with a concern, including nursing staff, rehabilitation staff, patients, family, or community members, usually by simply calling or emailing, but procedures and availability may vary from one institution to another.

An **ombud** is a person charged with advocating for the rights of the patient and for adequate patient care, and with assisting in resolving conflicts. The ombud may visit patients and work with staff to resolve moral distress and ethical conflicts. In many cases, the ombud is a trained volunteer and often serves geriatric patients, those with disabilities, and/or those in long-term care.

An **ethical consult team** is usually composed of interdisciplinary team members who meet on request to assist with solving ethical problems. The team members also often educate other staff members, patients, and community members about ethical issues and provide recommendations and advice.

ETHICAL AND LEGAL PATIENT RIGHTS

One of the most important concepts pertaining to ethical and legal patient rights is **informed consent**, which means that the patient has the right to information about treatments and procedures before they give permission for those actions. This includes information about risks and benefits. Informed consent is absolutely essential before participation in research projects and human experimentation. **Advance directives** are documents that indicate a person's preference and medical treatment plan if they become incapacitated. There is a law called the **Patient Self-Determination Act** that ensures these rights. The Fourteenth Amendment to the United States Constitution, common law, and other precedents also guarantee the right to die and the prerogative to decide and decline medical treatments. In many states, a person can sign a **living will** that defines medical decisions (such as the right to die) in the case that they become incapable of

216

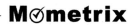

communicating them. A **durable power of attorney** assigns another competent person to act on the patient's behalf if the patient becomes incapacitated. A **guardianship** is a legal relationship in which a court-mandated guardian acts on behalf of a ward who is incapable of functional independence.

ANA's Code of Ethics for Nurses with Interpretive Statements

Currently, there are 9 provisions in the American Nurses Association's *Code of Ethics for Nurses with Interpretive Statements*. **Provisions 1, 2, and 3** essentially say that the nurse should provide services in a manner that respects human dignity, that the nurse's main commitment is to the patients, and that the nurse should act as a patient advocate. **Provision 4** says that the nurse is responsible and accountable for individual nursing decisions and actions. **Provision 5** says that the nurse has a commitment to self as well, in terms of maintenance of integrity and personal and professional growth. The **last 4 provisions** address advancement of the nursing profession and its values, specifically use of individual and collective actions, general contribution to nursing improvement, participation in community and national efforts, and collective assertion of nursing values.

Ethical Theories That Can Impact Decision Making for Rehabilitation Nurses

Ethical theories generally fall into one of four categories: ethics of divine commands, selfishness, duty and respect, or consequences. Decisions built on religious moral beliefs of right and wrong are based on **ethics of divine commands**. Other people will make choices based on the **ethics of selfishness or egoism**, which means that people delineate what is right for them as long as it does not get in the way of the rights of others. Practice based on the **ethics of duty and respect** is more oriented toward what is defined as right in a legal sense; this is a deontological theory, meaning the focus is on what is defined as right and less on the consequences. The **ethics of consequences** is a utilitarian or practical approach concentrating on the outcome perceived to be good for the most people.

Ethical Policies Regarding Assisted Suicide, Euthanasia, and Suicide

Assisted suicide is the act of providing a consenting patient with medication that will induce death under specific criteria (often referred to as physician-assisted suicide or medical aid in dying). It is protected in some states with various versions of death-with-dignity laws. Currently, the following states have versions of death-with-dignity laws: California, Colorado, District of Columbia, Hawaii, Maine, New Jersey, New Mexico, Oregon, Vermont, and Washington. Euthanasia, the painless killing of an individual with an incurable illness or injury, is illegal and not supported by the American Nurses Association. However, patients can refuse to receive medical treatments and pain medications, an action that could contribute to **passive euthanasia**. **Suicide**, deliberately killing oneself, is legal.

Ethical Decision-Making Model

There are many ethical decision-making models. Some general guidelines to apply in using ethical decision-making models could be the following:

- Gather information about the identified problem.
- State reasonable alternatives and solutions to the problem.
- Utilize ethical resources (for example, clergy or ethics committees) to help determine the ethically important elements of each solution or alternative.
- Suggest and attempt possible solutions.
- Choose a solution to the problem.

It is important to always consider the **ethical principles** of autonomy, beneficence, nonmaleficence, justice, and fidelity when attempting to facilitate ethical decision-making with family members, caregivers, and the healthcare team.

NUREMBERG CODE

The Nuremberg Code was established after World War II to address human medical experimentation. It remains the basis for clinical research guidelines such as the National Institutes of Health federal Title 45, Part 46, Protection of Human Subjects. There are 10 basic tenets of the Nuremberg Code. The first is **informed, voluntary consent** of subjects. Several portions address the **study design**, such as the expectation of benefits from the study, design principles based on animal studies or prior knowledge regarding the problem being evaluated, no expected inherent harmful outcomes such as death or disability, the greater probability for potential good than endangerment, the prevention of patient suffering, and the protection of patients. The Code also states that researchers must possess **appropriate qualifications**. Subjects may withdraw from the research at any time, and the study will be terminated if it is in the best interests of the patients.

AMERICAN HOSPITAL ASSOCIATION'S PATIENT'S BILL OF RIGHTS

The AHA originally published "A Patient's Bill of Rights" in 1973 and revised it in 1992. In 2008, the association also issued a simplified pamphlet called "The Patient Care Partnership," which lists the following six patient expectations, rights, and responsibilities:

- High-quality hospital care
- Clean and safe environment
- Patient involvement in their own care
- Protection of patient privacy
- Preparation for the patient/family for leaving the hospital
- Help with billing and filing insurance claims

POLST/MOLST

The **POLST** (Physician Orders for Life-Sustaining Treatment) and **MOLST** (Medical Orders for Life-Sustaining Treatment) are two different names for essentially the same document, which varies somewhat from one state to another; for example, in Iowa, it is called the iPOST (Iowa Physician Orders for Scope of Treatment). The POLST/MOLST document is intended for those who have a serious illness or are near the end of life so that they can give input into the types of treatment they want. The form is usually one page, front and back, with check boxes to indicate preferences. Most are in bright colors so they are easily recognizable. The form should be filled out during consultation with a healthcare professional. For example, individuals can indicate if they want to be taken to the hospital or stay at home, have CPR attempted or not, and be maintained on a ventilator or not. While a POLST/MOLST is not the same as a DNR, it can help to ensure that the person's wishes are respected. To be legally binding, the POLST/MOLST form must be signed by the healthcare professional (varies according to the state) because the POLST/MOLST represents medical orders. In many states, the person to whom it applies or a health proxy must also sign.

ABUSE AND NEGLECT

INDICATORS OF ABUSE THAT MAY BE IDENTIFIED IN THE PATIENT HISTORY

The healthcare provider should always be aware of the presence of any **indicators** that may present a potential for or an actual situation that involves **abuse**. These indicators may present in the **patient's history**. Some examples of indicators concerning their primary complaint may include the following: vague description about the cause of the problem, inconsistencies between physical findings and explanations, minimizing injuries, long period of time between injury and treatment, and over-reactions or under-reactions of family members to injuries. Other important information may be revealed in the family genome, such as family history of violence, time spent in jail or prison, and family history of violent deaths or substance abuse. The patient's health history may include previous injuries, spontaneous abortions, or history of pervious inpatient psychiatric treatment or substance abuse.

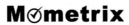

During the collection of the patient history, the financial history, the patient's family values, and the patient's relationships with family members can also reveal actual or potential **abuse indicators**.

- The **financial history** may indicate that the patient has little or no money or that they are not given access to money by a controlling family member. They may also be unemployed or utilizing an elderly family member's income for their own personal expenses.
- **Family values** may indicate strong beliefs in physical punishment, dictatorship within the home, inability to allow different opinions within the home, or lack of trust for anyone outside the family.
- **Relationships** within the family may be dysfunctional. Problems such as lack of affection between family members, co-dependency, frequent arguments, extramarital affairs, or extremely rigid beliefs about roles within the family may be present.

During the collection of the patient history, the sexual, social, and psychological history of the patient should be evaluated for any signs of actual or potential abuse.

- The **sexual history** may reveal problems such as previous sexual abuse, forced sexual acts, sexually transmitted infections (STIs), sexual knowledge beyond normal age-appropriate knowledge, or promiscuity.
- The **social history** may reveal unplanned pregnancies, social isolation as evidenced by lack of friends available to help the patient, unreasonable jealousy of significant other, verbal aggression, belief in physical punishment, or problems in school.
- During the **psychological assessment** the patient may express feelings of helplessness and being trapped. The patient may be unable to describe their future, become tearful, perform self-mutilation, have low self-esteem, and have had previous suicide attempts.

NURSING OBSERVATIONS THAT MAY INDICATE ABUSE

During the initial assessment, observations may also be made by the provider that can provide vital information about actual or potential abuse. **General observations** may include finding that the patient history is far different from what is objectively viewed by the provider or that there is a lack of proper clothing or lack of physical care provided. The home environment may include lack of heat, water, or food. It may also reveal inappropriate sleeping arrangements or lack of an environmentally safe housing situation. Observations concerning **family communications** may reveal that the abuser answers all the questions for the whole family or that others look to the controlling member for approval or seem fearful of others. Family members may frequently argue, interrupt each other, or act out negative nonverbal behaviors while others are speaking. They may avoid talking about certain subjects that they feel are secretive.

INDICATORS OF ABUSE THAT MAY BE EVIDENT DURING THE PHYSICAL ASSESSMENT

During the **physical assessment** the provider should always be aware of any **indicators of abuse**. These indicators may include increased anxiety about being examined or in the presence of the abuser; poor hygiene; looks to abuser to answer questions for them; flinching; over or underweight; presence of bruises, welts, scars or cigarette burns; bald patches on scalp for pulling out of hair; intracranial bleeding; subconjunctival hemorrhages; black eye(s); hearing loss from untreated infection or injury; poor dental hygiene; abdominal injuries; fractures; developmental delays; hyperactive reflexes; genital lacerations or ecchymosis; and presence of STIs, rectal bruising, bleeding, edema, or poor sphincter tone.

IDENTIFYING AND REPORTING NEGLECT OR LACK OF SUPERVISION IN CHILDREN

While some children may not be physically or sexually abused, they may suffer from profound **neglect** or **lack of supervision** that places them at risk. Indicators include the following:

- Appearing dirty and unkempt, sometimes with infestations of lice, and wearing ill-fitting or torn clothes and shoes
- Being tired and sleepy during the daytime

- Having untended medical or dental problems, such as dental caries
- Missing appointments and not receiving proper immunizations
- Being underweight for stage of development

Neglect can be difficult to assess, especially if the nurse is serving a homeless or very poor population. Home visits may be needed to ascertain if adequate food, clothing, or supervision is being provided; this may be beyond the care provided by the nurse, so suspicions should be reported to appropriate authorities, such as child protective services, so that social workers can assess the home environment.

IDENTIFYING AND REPORTING NEGLECT OF THE BASIC NEEDS OF ADULTS

Neglect of the basic needs of adults is a common problem, especially among the elderly, adults with psychiatric or mental health problems, or those who live alone or with reluctant or incapable caregivers. In some cases, **passive neglect** may occur because an elderly or impaired spouse or partner is trying to take care of a patient and is unable to provide the care needed, but in other cases, **active neglect** reflects a lack of caring which may be considered negligence or abuse. Cases of neglect should be reported to the appropriate governmental agency, such as adult protective services. Indications of neglect include the following:

- Lack of assistive devices, such as a cane or walker, needed for mobility
- Misplaced or missing glasses or hearing aids
- Poor dental hygiene and dental care or missing dentures
- Patient left unattended for extended periods of time, sometimes confined to a bed or chair
- Patient left in soiled or urine- and feces-stained clothing
- Inadequate food, fluid, or nutrition, resulting in weight loss
- Inappropriate and unkempt clothing, such as no sweater or coat during the winter and dirty or torn clothing
- A dirty, messy environment

NEGLECT AND ABUSE OF THE ELDERLY AND INDIVIDUALS WITH DISABILITIES

The elderly and individuals with disabilities are at risk for neglect and abuse when they have impaired mental processes or physical deficits that affect ADLs. They are also at risk when there are caregiver problems such as:

- The caregiver is experiencing a high amount of stress.
- The caregiver has a substance abuse problem.
- The caregiver is physically abusive or violent.
- The caregiver is emotionally unstable or has a mental illness.
- The caregiver is dependent on the elderly or disabled individual for money, emotional support, or physical support.

The nurse should act to help a caregiver to cope more effectively to prevent abuse from occurring by providing an outlet for emotions and referring to resources. It's important to ask patients in private whether anyone prevents them from using medical assistive devices or refuses to help them with ADLs. However, many will not admit to abuse. If there are risk factors present or signs of abuse, the nurse must act to preserve the safety of the individual. Most states require the reporting of elder abuse and neglect. Assist the person in accessing resources in the community to improve their living situation.

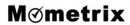

Promoting a Safe Environment

JOINT COMMISSION'S PATIENT SAFETY GOALS

The Joint Commission has a set of **goals that impact patient safety** for each type of healthcare facility. Within the hospital environment, there are several goals that pertain:

- Each facility must have a way to identify patients that will avoid errors of identification.
- Caregivers are to give careful, accurate communications about patients and their care so that mistakes are not made.
- A system to avoid medication errors must be in place.
- Medications must be reconciled when the patient moves from place to place within the hospital or is discharged to other caregivers.
- The risk of infection must be decreased so that patients are at less risk for hospital-related infections.
- The facility must have a fall prevention program and evaluate its effectiveness.

All patients and family must be encouraged to be active in their own care to help to avoid errors. They must also know how to make sure their concerns for safety of care are heard and acted upon.

ASPECTS OF PATIENT SAFETY IN THE HOSPITAL

Deliberate decisions by the health care providers/facility can help create an environment conducive for patient safety. Some of those aspects include:

- **Educating the patient on signaling staff**: The patient must be educated about the use of the call light, and the call light placed within easy reach. If the patient is unable to use the call light, then an alternative means of calling for help, such as a handheld bell, should be available. If the patient is unable to manage any type of signaling system, then the nurse should check on the patient at least every hour.
- **Protecting from falls and electrical hazards**: All clutter should be removed from floors and cords secured away from walkways. All electrical appliances should be checked to ensure they are working properly and have no frayed cords. Patients should be provided assistive devices, such as walkers, if necessary, to improve stability.
- **Making appropriate room assignments**: Patients with the greatest need for supervision should be placed closest to the nursing desk and within the line of sight whenever possible. In environments such as critical care, each nurse should be able to visualize their patient assignment from their nursing station.

MEDICATION ERRORS

There are about 7,000 deaths yearly in the United States attributed to **medication errors.** Studies indicate that there are errors in 1 in 5 doses of medication given to patients in hospitals. Patient safety must be ensured with proper handling and administering of medications:

- **Avoid error-prone abbreviations or symbols**. The Joint Commission has established a list of abbreviations to avoid, but mistakes are frequent with other abbreviations as well. In many cases, abbreviations and symbols should be avoided altogether or restricted to a limited approved list.
- **Prevent errors due to illegible handwriting or unclear verbal orders**. Handwritten orders should be block printed to reduce chance of error; verbal orders should be repeated back to the physician.
- **Institute barcoding and scanners** that allow the patient's wristband and medications to be scanned for verification.
- **Provide lists of similarly-named medications** to educate staff.
- Establish an **institutional policy** for the administration of medications that includes protocols for verification of drug, dosage, and patient, as well as educating the patient about the medications.

Legislative, Economic, Ethical, and Legal Issues

PATIENT DEFICITS THAT IMPEDE SAFETY

Certain patient deficits can inherently impede their safety, including the following:

- **Visual impairment**: Patients are at risk of trips, slips, falls, burn injuries, poisoning (mistaken containers, ingredients), and medication errors because of taking the wrong medication or wrong dosage.
- **Hearing impairment**: Patients are at increased risk of falls and may not hear danger signals, such as fire alarms, smoke detectors, police/fire sirens, and tornado warning sirens, and may, therefore, not be aware that they are in danger. Most smoke detectors emit a high-frequency alarm that cannot always be detected by those with high-frequency hearing loss.
- **Sensory/Perceptual impairment**: Patients (such as those with stroke or brain injury) may exhibit a wide variety of impairments so safety concerns may vary. For example, those with one-sided neglect may have injuries to the neglected side, such as from running into doors or other things. Those with face blindness may easily get lost if away from familiar places or people.

PROMOTION OF PATIENT SAFETY IN REHABILITATION SETTINGS

The first step in promotion of patient safety in rehabilitation settings is to determine the procedures and transitions that present the greatest **risks to safety**. It is then recommended that the facility take a proactive line of attack to address safety risks. Depending on the specific risk, these **strategies** could include actual elimination of the error, tactics to reduce errors or detect them before harm has occurred, the design of protocols to lessen adverse effects if errors do occur, and creation of a work environment that addresses errors and possible changes after their occurrence. It is important to periodically **evaluate safety process outcomes** in terms of the degree and cost of implementation as well as the immediate impact on patients and long-term effectiveness.

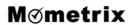

Quality Improvement Processes

QUALITY IN THE HEALTH CARE SETTING

Quality means maintenance of the highest and finest standards. However, the perception of quality depends on many factors, including the perspective from which it is assessed. According to the **National Quality Forum (NQF)**, the major areas of quality concern in a health care setting are medical errors, overtreatment, and undertreatment.

- **Medical errors** or instances of **ill-advised care** occur in up to 30% of hospital settings, and these errors can lead to serious or life-threatening events.
- **Overtreatment**, whether through unnecessary medications or therapies or system duplication, occurs almost as often as medical errors.
- Another major source of quality concern is **undertreatment**. It is estimated that half of the patient population does not receive full care due to lack of accessibility.

HEALTH CARE INDICATORS OF QUALITY

Three of the main regulatory bodies concerned with health care indicators of quality as applied to the rehabilitation setting are the **Centers for Medicare and Medicaid Services (CMS)**, the **Joint Commission (JC)**, and the **Healthcare Facilities Accreditation Program (HFAP)**. Their main roles are standard development and monitoring of programs enrolled in CMS and facility accreditation (JC and HFAP). All of these circulate **standards of care** including highest achievable norms, but they do not specifically outline ways to achieve compliance. There is also a private organization called the Commission on Accreditation of Rehabilitation Facilities (**CARF**) that accredits rehabilitation programs. From a nursing point of view, quality is more about recognition and implementation of best practices. Various research groups have looked at the impact of nursing indicators on patient outcomes, such as the staff mix, nursing care hours a patient receives daily, educational level of nurses, and number of patient falls. The individual consumer views the quality of health care from their own perspective, including information gleaned through websites or other sources.

STANDARDIZED TOOLS TO MEASURE QUALITY

Some standardized tools for measurement of quality are listed below:

1. **Functional Independence Measure (FIM)**: Instituted by the Uniform Data System for Medical Rehabilitation (UDSMR) and used internationally for uniform documentation of frequency and severity of 18 items related to disability
2. **Minimum Data Set (MDS)**: A standardized database linked to Medicare (CMS) reimbursement and long-term care that covers predetermined indicators of quality
3. **Medical Outcomes Trust health status questionnaires**: Patient questionnaires regarding health status and outcomes, available in different forms reflecting a number of questions
4. **Rating scales:** A variety are available to grade outcomes, risk factors, cognitive functioning, etc.
5. **Outcome and Assessment Information Set (OASIS)**: Developed by CMS for assessment of home health care

USE OF QUALITY INDICATORS TO ASSESS REHABILITATION NURSING PRACTICES

There are a number of quality indicators that relate closely to rehabilitation nursing practices. Each can be evaluated in terms of either internal indicators or National Database of Nursing Quality Indicators (NDNQI). One good indicator of rehabilitation nursing practice is the **prevalence of hospital-acquired pressure ulcers** compared to the prevalence in peer institutions (should be lower than others). The successful **prevention of nosocomial infections** is a good indicator. This can be measured relative to two parameters surveyed by the National Nosocomial Infection Surveillance System: the incidence of iatrogenic methicillin-resistant *Staphylococcus aureus* (MRSA) and the incidence of vancomycin-resistant enterococci (VRE). Ideally, the incidence of these diseases should be less than 0.31 or 0.15 per 1000 patient days respectively. It can also be internally monitored in terms of percentage of nurses adhering to hand hygiene policies. Lastly, the NDNQI has data related to the **rate of falls** in various types of units, and the goal is to have less than in peer hospitals.

EXAMINING QUALITY OF CARE

One way of examining quality is to look at certain indicators relative to benchmarks. **Quality reviews** can be done subsequent to events or during them, known as retrospective or prospective respectively. Information about quality of care can be obtained through careful **auditing of facility records**. There are also a number of tools that can be used to gain perspective about processes in the units. Types of **diagrams** that may provide insight include a cause-and-effect or fishbone diagram or a radar or circular diagram. **Charting** is useful. Chart types include flowcharts and another type of chart called the Pareto chart, which plots the percentage of different events contributing to a particular problem. Other useful tools are **brainstorming sessions** and regular use of **check sheets** that enumerate compliance with established procedures.

PERFORMANCE IMPROVEMENT METHODOLOGIES
PDCA/PDSA

The Plan-Do-Check-Act (PDCA), or alternatively the Plan-Do-Study-Act (PDSA), is also known as the Shewhart cycle. It is a method of continuous quality improvement. PDCA is simple and understandable; however, it may be difficult to maintain this cycle consistently because of lack of focus and commitment. PDCA may be more suited to solving specific problems than organization-wide problems.

- **Plan**: Identifying, analyzing, and clearly defining the problem, setting goals, and establishing a process that coordinates with leadership. Extensive brainstorming, including fishbone diagrams, identifies problematic processes and lists current process steps. Data are collected and analyzed, and root cause analysis is completed.
- **Do**: Generating solutions from which to select one or more and then implementing the solution on a trial basis.
- **Check** (or Study, in PDSA): Gathering and analyzing data to determine the effectiveness of the solution. If effective, then continue to Act; if not, return to Plan and pick a different solution.
- **Act**: Identifying changes that need to be made to fully implement the solution; adopting the solution and continuing to monitor results while picking another improvement project.

SIX SIGMA

Six Sigma is a performance improvement model developed by Motorola to improve business practices and increase profits. This model has been adapted to many types of businesses, including health care. Six Sigma is a data-driven performance model that aims to eliminate "defects" in processes that involve products or services. The goal is to achieve Six Sigma, meaning no more than 3.4 defects per 1 million opportunities. This program focuses on continuous improvement with the customer's perception as key, so that the customer defines that which is "critical to quality" (CTQ). Two different types of improvement projects may be employed: DMAIC (define, measure, analyze, improve, control), for existing processes or products that need improvement, and DMADV (define, measure, analyze, design, verify), for development of new high-quality processes or products. Both DMAIC and DMADV utilize trained personnel to execute the plans. These personnel use martial arts titles: green belts, black belts (execute programs), and master black belts (supervise programs).

SIX SIGMA DMAIC

The first model for **Six Sigma** is DMAIC. It is used when existing processes or products need improvement, and it is used in healthcare quality:

- **Define** costs and benefits that will be achieved when changes are instituted. Develop a list of customer needs based on complaints and requests.
- **Measure** values at the input and output of a process as well as at any relevant interim process stages. Collect baseline data, establish costs, perform analysis, and calculate sigma rating.

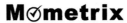

- **Analyze** root or other causes of current defects, use data to confirm, and uncover steps in processes that are counterproductive.
- **Improve** by creating potential solutions, develop and pilot plans, implement, and measure results, determining cost savings and other benefits to customers.
- **Control** includes standardizing work processes and monitoring the system by linking performance measures to a balanced scorecard, creating processes for updating procedures, disseminating reports, and recommending future processes.

LEAN SIX SIGMA

Lean Six Sigma, a method that combines Six Sigma with concepts of "lean" thinking, is a method of focusing process improvement on strategic goals rather than on a project-by-project basis. This type of program is driven by strong senior leadership that outlines long-term goals and strategies. Physicians are an important part of the process and must be included and engaged. The basis of this program is to reduce error and waste within the organization through continuous learning and rapid change. There are four characteristics:

- Long-term goals with strategies in place for 1- to 3-year periods
- Performance improvement as the underlying belief system
- Cost reduction through quality increase, supported by statistics evaluating the cost of inefficiency
- Incorporation of improvement methodology, such as DMAIC, PDCA, or other methods

CRRN Practice Test #1

Want to take this practice test in an online interactive format?
Check out the bonus page, which includes interactive practice questions and
much more: **mometrix.com/bonus948/crrn**

1. When conducting the 10-meter walk test for a patient with an incomplete spinal cord injury, what does a flying start refer to?

  a. Not counting the first 2 meters walked
  b. Urging the patient to walk as fast as possible
  c. Using assistive devices to increase speed
  d. Walking faster at the beginning than at the end

2. How much liquid should a patient who performs self-catheterization take in each day?

  a. 8 ounces
  b. 16 ounces
  c. 2 quarts
  d. 1 gallon

3. Nursing interventions to help decrease insomnia include all of the following EXCEPT:

  a. Engaging the patient in activities during the day to decrease napping
  b. Administering prn sleeping medications if the patient is having difficulty falling asleep
  c. Limiting caffeine-containing beverages in the afternoon and evening
  d. Allowing the patient to rest during the day so they do not become overfatigued

4. A 57-year-old man with diabetes mellitus type 2 has developed neuropathy, and his wife tells the nurse he is experiencing erectile dysfunction. Using the PLISSIT model for assessing sexuality, which of the following should the nurse do FIRST when speaking to the patient?

  a. Ask permission to discuss sexual function.
  b. Provide limited information about sexual function.
  c. Provide suggestions for dealing with erectile dysfunction.
  d. Suggest intensive therapy.

5. The spinal nerves at which level are responsible for a man to have an erection?

  a. Sacral nerves 2–4
  b. Lumbar nerves 3–5
  c. Thoracic nerves 10–12
  d. Thoracic nerves 6–9

6. Under Medicare's prospective payment system, how are payment rates set?

  a. In advance and based on various criteria
  b. Applied on an individual basis
  c. Based on a national standard
  d. Based on actual costs

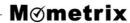

7. What affect does an adequate amount of REM sleep have on stroke patients?

a. It delays recovery of muscle function.
b. It decreases cognitive function.
c. It turns short-term memory of muscle movements into long-term memories.
d. It increases symptoms of depression.

8. The Rehabilitation Act (1973, amended 1998) established the Rehabilitation Services Administration. What is the function of this agency?

a. To enforce provisions of the Rehabilitation Act
b. To provide financial assistance to those with disabilities
c. To fund and oversee state vocational rehabilitation agencies
d. To assess eligibility for vocational services

9. The best way to test muscle tone of the external anal sphincter is to:

a. Check an anal reflex by tapping around the anus.
b. Check a bulbocavernosus reflex by lightly circling the anus with a finger.
c. Check an anocutaneous reflex with pinpricks around the anus.
d. Conduct a digital rectal exam.

10. When teaching tracheostomy care at home, it is important the caregivers understand:

a. Cleaning and changing the trach tube must be done under sterile conditions.
b. The trach tube can be reused after it has been cleaned properly.
c. The trach tube can only be changed by a Respiratory Therapist who will come to the home.
d. A new, sterile trach tube must be used each day.

11. To comply with Occupational Safety and Health Administration (OSHA) guidelines for a safe working environment after some staff members experienced musculoskeletal injuries, a rehabilitation center is developing a formal ergonomics program. Which one of the following should be the first step in developing the program?

a. Identify units at high risk.
b. Identify tasks that carry high risk.
c. Carry out direct observations.
d. Collect baseline injury data.

12. The caregiver for an 80-year-old woman with advanced Alzheimer disease states that she frequently chokes on food. Which of the following foods served by the caregiver is LEAST likely to cause choking?

a. A cup of coffee
b. Moderately thick split pea soup
c. Soft white bread
d. Finger foods, such as hot dogs

13. BiPAP therapy can be considered for those patients with sleep apnea who:

a. Cannot afford CPAP
b. Have difficulty exhaling against positive pressure
c. Find a CPAP mask to be uncomfortable
d. Have insurance that will not cover a CPAP machine

14. Constraint-induced movement therapy (CIMT) for those with stroke or traumatic brain injury (TBI) includes constraint of the uninvolved upper extremity and which of the following other measure(s)?

    a.   Forced use of weakened limbs for 90 minutes daily

    b.   Massed practice

    c.   Forced use of weakened limbs for 90% of waking hours and massed practice

    d.   Doing progressively more difficult tasks in small steps for 90 minutes daily with positive reinforcement

15. The CRRN is administering the Digit Span Test to a patient with evidence of dementia. How many digits can an individual with normal intelligence and ability to comprehend and respond usually remember and repeat?

    a.   2–3

    b.   3–5

    c.   5–7

    d.   8–10

16. Difficulty in carrying out tasks or movements when asked is:

    a.   Parkinsonism

    b.   Ataxia

    c.   Apraxia

    d.   Dysphagia

17. A 22-year-old male with a T2 spinal cord injury attends a football game, sitting in the shade in his wheelchair for 3 hours in 92-degree weather at 85% humidity. Which of the following is the primary concern?

    a.   Hyperthermia

    b.   Dehydration

    c.   Pressure sore

    d.   Bladder distention

18. You are caring for a 47-year-old male who has suffered a traumatic brain injury affecting the brain stem. The most accurate way in which to monitor the effectiveness of the patient's ventilations is by:

    a.   Pulse oximetry

    b.   Continuous arterial blood gas monitoring

    c.   Intrathecal monitoring

    d.   Capnography

19. You are caring for a patient with a stage 1 pressure ulcer. The most important nursing intervention to prevent worsening of his ulcer is:

    a.   Assess skin temperature each shift.

    b.   Turn and reposition the patient every 2 hours and prevent pressure on the ulcer site.

    c.   Monitor the patient's skin care practices and make note of the type of soap or lotions used.

    d.   Assess the patient's nutritional status.

20. Which of the following is NOT required for Medicare coverage of treatment in an inpatient rehabilitation facility (IRF)?

    a.   The patient had at least 3 days of acute hospitalization within 30 days prior to admission to an IRF.

    b.   The patient needs and is prescribed at least 2 different types of therapy.

    c.   The patient needs and is prescribed at least 3 hours of therapy daily.

    d.   Treatment can continue as long as the patient requires the qualifying level of treatment.

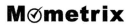

21. All of the following are common bladder irritants EXCEPT:

    a. Water
    b. Caffeinated beverages
    c. Honey
    d. Sugar and artificial sweeteners

22. A rehabilitation center is seeking accreditation from the Commission on Accreditation of Rehabilitation Facilities (CARF) and has undergone an evaluation but is awaiting a survey. How long must the rehabilitation center be in conformance with CARF standards before the survey can be carried out?

    a. 30 days
    b. 3 months
    c. 6 months
    d. 12 months

23. As part of a mobile rehabilitation service, the rehabilitation nurse makes a post-discharge evaluation visit to the home of a 48-year-old man recovering from burn injuries. The man answers the door and appears intoxicated; he smells of alcohol, slurs words, and swears at the nurse. Which is the MOST appropriate nursing action?

    a. Ask if there is someone else at home with whom the nurse could speak.
    b. Call the physician for guidance.
    c. Reschedule the visit and leave without entering the home.
    d. Remain supportive, not responding to hostile words, and complete evaluation.

24. In what year did the Americans with Disabilities Act go into effect?

    a. 1989
    b. 1990
    c. 1991
    d. 1992

25. A method of reimbursement used by Medicare to provide a fixed reimbursement amount for specific services is:

    a. HIPAA
    b. PPS
    c. The Affordable Care Act
    d. CARF certification

26. The organization responsible for providing accreditation to thousands of health care organizations in the United States is:

    a. The National Hospital Review Board
    b. The Commission on Accreditation and Review
    c. The U.S. Food and Drug Administration
    d. The Joint Commission

27. The daughter of a patient who has had a stroke feels that her mother has been neglected by some of the nursing aides. Her concerns should be brought to the attention of:

    a. Medicare
    b. Her congressman
    c. The state ombudsman
    d. The local television station

28. A 40-year-old patient sustained a TBI and is in a vegetative state, maintained on life support. Prior to the accident, the patient was estranged and lived separately from her husband, who has a health care power of attorney for her. A decision regarding continuation of life support must be made, but the family members cannot agree. Who of the following has the LEGAL right to make the decision?

    a. The patient's mother
    b. The patient's 18-year-old daughter
    c. The patient's estranged husband
    d. The facility's ethics committee

29. The nursing model that views nursing as both a science and an art is:

    a. The King theory of nursing
    b. The Neuman theory of nursing
    c. The Rogers theory of nursing
    d. The Liberal theory of nursing

30. A 38-year-old man, deaf in the right ear, works in the computing department at a county hospital, which receives Medicare payments. He has a brain tumor removed but suffers 80% residual hearing deficit in the left ear. The hospital administrator demotes him because of his hearing impairment. Which of the following laws protects this individual from denial of employment opportunities, such as promotions, because of his disability?

    a. HIPAA
    b. Section 504 of the Rehabilitation Act of 1973
    c. OSHA
    d. Workers' compensation

31. A 35-year-old patient with a history of a traumatic brain injury has had increased insomnia with his depression. He has taken Benadryl in the past to help with sleep but was sensitive to the anticholinergic side effects. Which of the following medications would be the most likely to also have anticholinergic side effects?

    a. Melatonin
    b. Ambien
    c. Seroquel
    d. Sonata

32. What is the goal of medication therapy with bowel incontinence?

    a. To avoid any episodes of incontinence by performing digital evacuation of stool on a regular schedule
    b. To reduce stool frequency and improve stool consistency
    c. To try to control bowel and bladder incontinence with medications alone
    d. To loosen stools in preparation for colostomy placement

33. What is the mechanism of action of an impedance threshold device?

    a. Increase intrathoracic pressure and decrease venous return to the heart.
    b. Decrease intrathoracic pressure and increase venous return to the heart.
    c. Increase intrathoracic pressure and increase venous return to the heart.
    d. Decrease intrathoracic pressure and decrease venous return to the heart.

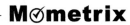

34. You are caring for an 18-year-old female who suffered a complete spinal cord injury in a drunk driving accident. She tells you that she enjoyed reality TV shows before her accident, but that she has no desire to watch any now. You know this can be a symptom of:

a. Anxiety
b. PTSD
c. Bipolar disorder
d. Schizophrenia

35. A patient's ability to identify their needs and express their needs to others is:

a. Self-actualization
b. Psychomotor analysis
c. Self-advocacy
d. Receptive aphasia

36. A 21-year-old woman who has never been employed was involved in a traffic accident at age 19 and suffered a severe head injury, leaving her unable to work because of cognitive impairment. She had lived since infancy with her grandmother, who has legal custody and received Social Security payments after retirement. Upon the grandmother's death, the patient is without income but received $15,000 in life insurance. Which of the following statements is MOST accurate?

a. She is not eligible for Social Security disability benefits because she has not been employed.
b. She is eligible for Social Security disability benefits because her grandmother received Social Security payments prior to her death.
c. She is eligible for Social Security payments because she has a disability.
d. She is eligible for state welfare assistance and Supplemental Security Income (SSI) only.

Refer to the following for questions 37–41:

> A 62-year-old man with stage III COPD lives alone and is enrolled in a pulmonary rehabilitation program. His skin is dry and urine concentrated. He is chronically short of breath and breathes rapidly at a 1:1 ratio of inspiration to expiration, has a chronic cough, and sputum is very thick and difficult to expectorate. His resting PaO_2 is 72 mmHg. He complains of poor appetite but eats 75% of meals (total about 1,400 calories) but drinks only 1–2 glasses of water daily. He states he still smokes 1 pack of cigarettes daily. He drinks 2–3 glasses of wine daily and admits to smoking marijuana 3–4 times monthly. His medications include salmeterol (*Serevent Diskus*) and ipratropium bromide (*Atrovent*) as well as an inhaled corticosteroid (*Pulmicort Respules*) because of repeated exacerbations.

37. The first breathing exercises the patient learns are pursed-lip breathing and diaphragmatic breathing. What should be the goal for the ratio of inhalation to exhalation for pursed-lip breathing exercises?

a. Inhalation and exhalation should be equal in duration but slowed.
b. Exhalation should be double the duration of inhalation.
c. Inhalation should be double the duration of exhalation.
d. Exhalation should be 3 times the duration of inhalation.

38. As part of this patient's pulmonary rehabilitation, several programs may be indicated. Which of the following programs is MOST essential to slow the progression of the patient's COPD?

a. Smoking cessation
b. Alcoholics Anonymous
c. Drug rehabilitation
d. Diet and nutritional counseling

231

39. The COPD patient has a gait assessment to determine if he has mobility issues that may limit his independence in the community because of increased risk of falls. Assessment findings include:

- Gait speed for 5 meters: 0.3 m/second
- Timed Up and Go (TUG): 17 seconds
- Performance-Oriented Mobility Assessment (POMA): 0–1 in all categories

Considering these results, which is the BEST description of his risk for falls?
- a. The patient is at no risk for falls. He can ambulate freely.
- b. The patient is at mild risk for falls. He may need to use an assistive device, such as a cane.
- c. The patient is at moderate risk for falls. He should use a walker and may need assistance.
- d. The patient is at severe risk for falls. He probably requires assistive devices, supervision, and assistance.

40. Which of the following interventions is MOST likely to provide relief of the patient's current symptoms?
- a. Increasing fluid intake to at least 8 (8 ounce) glasses daily
- b. Increasing food intake to 2,000 calories daily
- c. Providing low-flow oxygen during sleep and exercise
- d. Switching from an inhaled to long-term oral corticosteroid

41. The patient complains that he has difficulty doing routine self-care because he gets so tired. Which of the following patient statements MOST indicates a need for education?
- a. "I use my walker when I stand at the sink so that I have support if I need it."
- b. "I keep the temperature at 70° because I feel cold a lot."
- c. "I have ordered meals from Meals on Wheels."
- d. "I try to rush and bathe, dress, cook, and clean first thing in the morning and rest afterward."

42. Which gland is responsible for secreting the hormone that is responsible for the "fight or flight" response in a stressful situation?
- a. Adrenal
- b. Thyroid
- c. Pancreas
- d. Thymus

43. The legal statute put into place to ensure that patient care is delivered based on what the patient needs is:
- a. Medicare
- b. The IMPACT Act
- c. The Affordable Care Act
- d. The Americans with Disabilities Act

44. In developing evidence-based guidelines to reduce urinary tract infections in patients with indwelling catheters, which of the following should carry the MOST weight in developing new policies?
- a. Best practices identified through literature review
- b. Nursing staff preferences
- c. Physician preference
- d. Cost-effectiveness

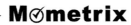

45. A 70-year-old man with stage III Parkinson disease lives alone and is wearing soiled and stained clothing on admission. He is unshaven, and his hair is long and uncombed. He apologizes for his appearance. Which of the following is the MOST appropriate nursing diagnosis?

    a. Neglect, unilateral
    b. Self-esteem, chronic low
    c. Self-care deficit, toileting
    d. Self-care deficit, dressing/grooming

46. A patient with macular degeneration is a project manager whose job is computer-based. The patient has recently experienced a sudden irreversible loss of central vision, rendering the patient legally blind. What accommodation can the patient expect at the workplace in accordance with the Americans with Disabilities Act?

    a. Assignment of essential job duties to other staff members
    b. Assistive technology for the computer such as screen readers
    c. Provision of a personal assistant to help with job duties
    d. Reassignment to a lesser position that requires no accommodations

47. What is the definition of a cultural encounter?

    a. A negative interaction between a healthcare provider and someone who is of a different cultural background
    b. The process of encouraging medical professionals to interact with those of a different cultural background from their own
    c. A coordinated effort between two cultural groups to gather and work through their differences
    d. The egocentric behaviors of a set of individuals who are intolerant of those from a different culture

48. Which step in the nursing process involves applying the nursing interventions identified to help with a specific diagnosis?

    a. Assessing
    b. Planning
    c. Implementation
    d. Evaluating

49. An operating philosophy and method that creates a maximum value for patients while reducing waste is:

    a. Plan, Do, Check Act
    b. IRF-PAI
    c. The Lean approach
    d. Quality measure analysis

50. The medical service that is covered under Medicare Part A is:

    a. Laboratory tests
    b. Appointments with a primary care provider
    c. Appointments with a specialist
    d. Prescription drug coverage

51. A patient with a spinal cord injury has developed a stage II pressure ulcer (4 cm in diameter) on the medial aspect of the right knee. In addition to relieving pressure, which of the following is the MOST appropriate treatment?

    a. Cleanse with antiseptic and expose to the air.
    b. Apply wet-to-dry saline dressings.
    c. Cleanse with normal saline and apply a hydrocolloid dressing.
    d. Apply a heat lamp to the area 3 times daily.

52. Which of the following is a VIOLATION of the American Medical Association's guidelines for informed consent?

    a. Description of risks and benefits of treatment
    b. Presentation of only the three most cost-effective treatment options
    c. Review of the nature and purpose of treatment
    d. Comparison of success rates for similar treatment at different facilities

53. The pain theory that states that pain is an emotion that occurs when a stimulus is stronger than usual is the:

    a. Specificity theory
    b. Gate control theory
    c. Intensive theory
    d. Pattern theory

54. The pain theory that states that signals are sent to a specialized "pain center" in the brain is the:

    a. Intensive theory
    b. Specificity theory
    c. Gate control theory
    d. Pattern theory

55. You are caring for a patient who sustained a stroke that has affected his speech. Based on the residual effects of his stroke, you know the stroke has affected:

    a. The pituitary gland
    b. The right side of his brain
    c. The left side of his brain
    d. The brain stem

56. A tool used to assess a child's performance in self-care, mobility, and cognition is:

    a. WeeFIM
    b. PeeWee
    c. TOT Stats
    d. INFAcare

57. The legal statute in place that mandates specific health care insurance companies to provide health insurance to all people and charge the same rates despite pre-existing conditions is called:

    a. Medicare
    b. Medicaid
    c. The Affordable Care Act
    d. The IMPACT Act

58. Which of the following lab tests is MOST accurate to evaluate long-term protein deficiency?

    a. Total protein
    b. Albumin
    c. Prealbumin
    d. Transferrin

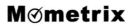

59. A busy outpatient rehabilitation medicine practice is reviewing their patient satisfaction scores regarding wait time to see a provider. They have set a goal of having patients wait no more than 30 minutes. The actual wait time has been 40–45 minutes. This evaluation is known as a:

- a. Clinical practice guideline
- b. Sensitivity level
- c. Specificity level
- d. Gap analysis

60. All of the following are side effects of vasopressors EXCEPT:

- a. Peripheral cyanosis
- b. Dysrhythmias
- c. Hypertension
- d. Hypotension

61. The most effective treatment for a patient with sleep apnea is:

- a. BiPAP (bi-level positive airway pressure)
- b. CPAP (continuous positive airway pressure)
- c. Capnography
- d. An impedance threshold device

62. General guidelines for a renal diet are:

- a. Low sodium, low phosphorous, and low protein
- b. Low sodium, high phosphorous, and high protein
- c. Low sodium, low phosphorous, and high protein
- d. High sodium, high phosphorous, and high protein

63. Which of the following medications may be injected into the bladder wall to help with the symptoms of neurogenic bladder?

- a. Botulinum toxin
- b. Baclofen
- c. Viagra
- d. Nitric oxide

64. A 45-year-old woman states that she sometimes leaks a small amount of urine when she coughs or sneezes. Which of the following control methods is MOST appropriate?

- a. Using a urethral plug
- b. Taking an anticholinergic agent daily
- c. Wearing protective incontinence pads
- d. Using the "knack" to prevent incontinence

65. A setting in which you would expect to see a Certified Rehabilitation Registered Nurse is:

- a. A long-term care facility
- b. An acute care clinic
- c. An intensive care unit at a local hospital
- d. A renal dialysis center

66. You are at a social event when an acquaintance asks about their friend's mother who had been at the facility where you work while she was rehabilitating after brain surgery. Your best response is to:

- a. Tell the patient is doing well and will be undergoing extensive rehabilitation.
- b. Explain to her that you are not able to discuss the care or prognosis of any patients.
- c. Deny having seen the patient.
- d. Tell her the patient is at your facility, but that you cannot discuss her care.

235

67. A patient with a traumatic brain injury who has seizures has been identified as a candidate who may benefit from having a service animal. He has a cat that has been trained to identify the changes in him just before he has a seizure. He is inquiring how to go about having the cat certified as a service animal. Your best response is:

    a. You will provide him with the online resources that explain how to certify the cat.
    b. Only dogs are allowed to be certified service animals.
    c. There is no specific training or certification that needs to be done and the cat will just need to wear one of the harnesses identifying him as a service animal.
    d. It is impossible for a cat to predict when a seizure may occur.

68. A sentinel event is:

    a. A sudden decline in patient satisfaction scores
    b. A local national disaster that requires implementation of the hospital's emergency management plan
    c. A situation within a healthcare facility that places the employees and patients in a position of danger
    d. An unplanned incident within a healthcare facility that results in death or psychological damage to a patient

69. You are caring for a patient with a traumatic brain injury. He has had Parkinsonism symptoms from his injury and is suffering from insomnia as a result of the uncontrollable tremors and movements. The most appropriate sleeping medication for him to use is:

    a. Benadryl
    b. A dopamine agonist
    c. Remeron
    d. Amitriptyline

70. The CRRN is assisting a patient with multiple sclerosis with an exercise regimen. Which one of the following should the CRRN carefully monitor to avoid exacerbating neurological symptoms?

    a. Fatigue
    b. Strength
    c. Overheating
    d. Pain

71. What is the average length of a full sleep cycle?

    a. 3 hours
    b. 2 hours
    c. 90 minutes
    d. 60 minutes

72. A 38-year-old male who sustained a spinal cord injury is concerned about remaining sexually active with his wife. Your best answer is:

    a. That it is unlikely he will be able to achieve an erection due to his injury
    b. That he will require a surgical procedure for a penile implant in order to be sexually active
    c. There are medications available that may help him to function sexually
    d. That he should have no problem with having a healthy sex life with his wife

73. For the Inpatient Rehabilitation Facility Patient Quality Reporting Program, a facility that does not meet reporting requirements is subject to what percentage of reduction to its annual increase factor?

    a. 1%
    b. 2%
    c. 4%
    d. 5%

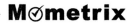

74. A patient using crutches for 2-point ambulation without weight bearing must be able to ascend and descend the stairs to his front door before discharge. Which of the following is the correct procedure for ascending stairs?

    a. Hold onto the railing and hop from step to step using a single crutch.
    b. Place crutches first on the higher step, then the well foot and the injured foot.
    c. Place the well foot first on the higher step, then the crutches and injured foot.
    d. Lift the injured foot and place the well foot on the higher step before the crutches.

75. Which of the following laws requires that communities provide transportation services for persons with disabilities, including accommodations for wheelchairs?

    a. Emergency Medical Treatment and Active Labor Act (EMTALA)
    b. Older Americans Act (OAA)
    c. Omnibus Budget Reconciliation Act (OBRA)
    d. Americans with Disabilities Act (ADA)

76. Which of the following is the BEST description of naturopathy?

    a. A system that focuses on strengthening the body's defense mechanisms rather than trying to heal particular disease symptoms
    b. A system that involves balancing qi (vital energy) by inserting tiny needles into specific sites referred to as acupoints
    c. A system that involves applying pressure or electric stimulation at acupoints to promote healing
    d. A system that involves various manipulations of muscles and joints and alignment of the spine to maintain health

77. During mealtime, when assisting a patient with dysphagia, you should:

    a. Have their upper body elevated 45-degrees.
    b. Give small bites of foods that are difficult to chew and swallow, but large bites of soft foods.
    c. Offer liquids after each to bite help move food down.
    d. Discourage talking while eating.

78. You are the CRRN caring for a patient who has had a CVA. He is scheduled to go to Physical Therapy and you are assessing him before he leaves the unit. A contraindication to him participating in physical therapy would be:

    a. An oxygen saturation level of 93% via pulse oximeter
    b. A non-fasting blood sugar level of 128
    c. A resting heart rate of 49 bpm
    d. A blood pressure of 126/84 mmHg

79. A patient received a back injury in a work-related incident and is unable to return to work because of an inability to stand for prolonged periods. What can the person expect from workers' compensation?

    a. Vocational retraining
    b. Permanent disability payment
    c. Alternative treatments, such as acupuncture
    d. Compensation for pain and suffering

80. Which of the following effects does alcohol have on the sleep cycle?

    a. Increases the length of REM sleep
    b. Decreases the length of REM sleep
    c. Prolongs the length of time it takes to fall asleep
    d. Provides deeper, more restful sleep

81. When the Centers for Medicare and Medicaid Services (CMS) conducts an on-site inspection of an inpatient rehabilitation facility (IRF), which one of the following should the CRRN expect that the auditors will survey in detail?

    a. Clinical staffing levels
    b. Financial management
    c. Advertising/Marketing
    d. Maintenance staff

82. A 27-year-old female has a complete spinal cord injury as a result of a motorcycle accident. You are evaluating her level of or motor and sensory function using the ASIA scale. On assessment, you find that she has no motor or sensory function at the sacral segments S4–5. This would give her an ASIA scale rating of:

    a. ASIA A
    b. ASIA B
    c. ASIA C
    d. ASIA D

83. The pain theory that states that there are small fibers controlled by larger fibers which are responsible for communicating signals to the spinal cord is called the:

    a. Gate control theory
    b. Intensive theory
    c. Pattern theory
    d. Specificity theory

84. Which of the following patients would not be a candidate to receive a baclofen pump?

    a. 55-year-old with spasticity due to a spinal cord injury that does not respond to oral baclofen
    b. 39-year-old who sustained a traumatic brain injury 3 months ago
    c. 69-year-old who has painful spasms of the limbs interfering with performing ADLs
    d. 23-year-old with an incomplete spinal cord injury causing spasticity, not responding to any oral antispasmodics

85. What relationship is seen between diet and sleep?

    a. Lack of sleep causes an increased appetite
    b. Lack of sleep causes a decreased appetite
    c. Oversleeping causes an increased appetite
    d. Oversleeping causes a decreased appetite

86. A patient with severe chronic migraines wishes to reduce dependence on medications to control pain. Which of the following alternative treatments is MOST likely to reduce migraine pain?

    a. Biofeedback
    b. Massage
    c. Exercise program
    d. Low-fat diet

87. The organization that provides accreditation to rehabilitation facilities that meet their requirements is:

    a. JCAHO
    b. Medicare
    c. Medicaid
    d. CARF

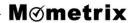

88. What is the first step in performing a bedside dysphagia assessment on the patient who has suffered a stroke?

a. Swallowing regular water
b. Swallowing thickened water
c. Swallowing saliva
d. Eating pureed foods

89. Stiffening in a muscle, joint, or the skin that results in reduced range of motion is:

a. Paralysis
b. Arthritis
c. A contracture
d. Dystrophy

90. A 47-year-old female with an incomplete spinal cord injury has a prn order for hydrocodone for leg pain to use when her antispasmodics are not as effective. She took a dose of this medication 30 minutes ago. She has complaints of low back pain following a rigorous physical therapy session and is requesting something else to take for that pain. Your best response is:

a. You will ask her physician for another prn order for an opioid analgesic.
b. The medication that was given for her leg pain should also help with her back pain.
c. She will have to wait until she is due for another dose of hydrocodone.
d. You will contact the physical therapist and see if they can work with her more to help relieve the pain.

91. Which of the following BEST describes the necessary elements of a cardiac rehabilitation program?

a. Medications, evaluation, and exercise
b. Evaluation, exercise, education, and counseling
c. Education, occupational therapy, and exercise
d. Diet, exercise, and education

92. A 72-year-old female has sustained a stroke which has caused her to have right-sided hemiplegia. She has speech problems with forming words, problems with dressing and bathing due to the hemiplegia, and is developing contractures in her right hand. Considering the problems she now has with day-to-day life, which of the following would be considered a problem with performing instrumental ADLs?

a. Dressing
b. Bathing
c. Housekeeping
d. Brushing teeth

93. Which of the following theories suggests that one must look at the person in terms of his/her family unit because the members of a family have different roles and behavioral patterns, so a change in one person's behavior will affect the others in the family?

a. Theory of Planned Behavior (Ajzen)
b. Theory of Reasoned Action (Fishbein and Ajzen)
c. Family Systems Theory (Bowen)
d. Theory of Human Caring (Watson)

94. The class of drugs whose goal is to decrease muscle excitability is:

a. Skeletal muscle relaxants
b. Smooth muscle relaxants
c. Cardiac muscle relaxants
d. Parasympathetic muscle relaxants

Refer to the following for questions 95–96:

> A patient had a stroke of the left hemisphere and is nonfluent in speech and has poor ability to repeat words or attempt words but her comprehension and hearing are intact. She is able to produce some intelligible words when trying to sing songs with which she was familiar with during an activity program. The patient is cooperative and is able to focus attention fairly well.

95. Which of the following speech therapies for aphasia may BEST benefit this patient?
- a. Stimulation-facilitation therapy
- b. Melodic intonation therapy
- c. Cognitive linguistic therapy
- d. Promoting Aphasic's Communicative Effectiveness (PACE)

96. Which other problems are MOST likely to also occur with this patient because of the location of her stroke?
- a. Right visual field deficit, tendency toward depression, slow, cautious behavior, and difficulty with mathematics
- b. Spatial and perceptual deficits and impairment of fine motor skills with impulsivity and "left-sided neglect"
- c. Easily distractible and difficulty with basic directions (up or down, front or back)
- d. Left hemiparesis and short-term memory loss and lack of awareness of disability

97. An intervention that may be helpful to the stroke patient to reduce their urge bladder incontinence symptoms is to:
- a. Invest in adaptive clothing that can be changed from a seated position.
- b. Use washable absorbent pads on the furniture and bed.
- c. Practice Kegel exercises.
- d. Carry an extra set of clean clothing with them.

98. The goal of the Quality and Safety Education for Nurses initiative is to:
- a. Provide extensive education for nurses so they can go on to assist in meeting quality measures and meaningful use goals.
- b. Prepare nurses so they can go forth and improve the quality and safety of the healthcare system in which they work.
- c. Establish specific protocols within a healthcare setting that can be used to improve patient safety.
- d. Ensure the nursing staff within a healthcare setting has completed annual continuing education course requirements.

99. A patient is being discharged home on an anti-seizure medication. His wife calls shortly after they leave to say the medication is not covered by insurance and it is very expensive. Your most appropriate response is:
- a. Unfortunately, there is no other option than to treat the infection with that particular medication.
- b. She should try to contact the pharmaceutical company to see if they can get approved for their patient assistance program.
- c. Ask the prescribing provider if a less expensive medication can be called in to the pharmacy.
- d. The insurance should be contacted to see if a prior authorization or another process can be completed to get drug coverage.

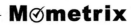

100. Which of the following clinical scenarios would be included within the Certified Rehabilitation Registered Nurse scope of practice?

    a. Performing a visual screening exam for an adolescent child's sports physical

    b. Administering immunizations to a 2-year-old patient who is being seen for a well-child visit

    c. Assisting in a code situation, following ACLS protocol, in the emergency room

    d. Educating a paraplegic patient on the proper technique for self-catheterization

101. When teaching a patient how to use a suppository to stimulate a bowel movement, it is important that they know:

    a. That even if the suppository causes diarrhea, it is important to still insert one daily

    b. Not to insert the suppository into stool in the rectum; remove the stool manually first

    c. That fluids should be limited 2–4 hours before inserting a suppository

    d. That the suppository can be taken orally to help lubricate the GI tract

102. Which of the following should be the FIRST step in conflict resolution?

    a. Utilize humor and empathy to diffuse escalating tensions.

    b. Summarize the issues, outlining key arguments.

    c. Force a resolution.

    d. Allow both sides to present their side of the conflict without bias.

103. An elderly patient with moderate dementia tends to wander at night and sleep throughout the daytime. Which is the BEST approach to dealing with this problem?

    a. Use sleep medication to induce sleep.

    b. Keep patient awake and engaged during daytime hours.

    c. Use side-rails and restraints to keep the patient in bed.

    d. Place alarms and/or safety gates and allow the person to stay up at night.

104. The third step in the nursing process is:

    a. Assessing and gathering data on the patient

    b. Planning how to meet patient goals

    c. Formulating a list of nursing diagnoses

    d. Implementing nursing interventions to achieve patient goals

105. When completing the Inpatient Rehabilitation Facility Patient Assessment Instrument (IRF-PAI) for a patient with traumatic bilateral amputations of parts of both lower limbs for admission to a rehabilitation center, how does the CRRN measure and/or record the patient's height?

    a. Upper body length plus the length of the longest limb

    b. Upper body length plus 35% for below-knee and 25% for above-knee amputations

    c. Patient's reported height prior to the amputations

    d. Estimated height based on the percentages of amputation

106. Which of the following best describes a case mix group as defined by the Health Insurance Prospective Payment System (HIPPS)?

    a. A classification system based on utilization of resources

    b. A dataset containing elements to review for a comprehensive assessment of patient function

    c. A classification system based on clinical characteristics of patients

    d. A dataset used by home health agencies to measure outcomes and risk factors

107. A 25-year-old man suffered a complete spinal cord injury at level T8 during a snowmobiling accident and has been admitted to a rehabilitation center. His records show that he barely spoke in the acute hospital and seemed quite detached, but now he is hostile toward staff, throws things, refuses to cooperate with therapy, and has told his family and friends to stop visiting. What is the MOST likely cause of this behavior?

    a. Pain
    b. Brain injury
    c. Medication reaction
    d. Grief

108. A patient who has persistent, dull pain is receiving stimuli to which type of pain receptor?

    a. Mechanical
    b. Thermal
    c. Chemical
    d. Polymodal

109. Parents of a child with cerebral palsy who is now wheelchair-bound express their concerns about his ability to go to school. You advise them that:

    a. There are laws in place to ensure he has equal access to an education or special education despite his disabilities.
    b. They may want to hire private tutors for him to be educated at home.
    c. Most children with cerebral palsy stop going to school once they are in a wheelchair.
    d. There are inpatient facilities similar to boarding schools where he will have to go to earn a full education.

110. When planning a diet for the spinal cord injury patient who has had issues with constipation due to a neurogenic bowel, it is important to include:

    a. A limited amount of fluid, generally <1 L daily
    b. Extra servings of foods such as cabbage, cauliflower, and carrots
    c. Limited servings of fiber-rich foods
    d. Foods high in fiber, such as whole grains and fresh fruits and vegetables

111. An injury at which level of the spinal cord may allow the patient to operate a motorized wheelchair on their own?

    a. C4
    b. C5
    c. C3
    d. C2

112. A 2-year-old is being discharged from the hospital after treatment for a respiratory illness. While in-patient, testing was completed, and the child was diagnosed with cystic fibrosis. The family is going to need extensive services at home, along with education about the illness. What is the most appropriate step to take next?

    a. Contact the Case Manager or Social Worker who handles discharges so that all necessary home care can be coordinated.
    b. Call the home health service and let the family know they will set up an appointment to meet with them at home to go over the information they will need.
    c. Advise the parents to schedule an appointment with the patient's doctor so that this can be reviewed in the office.
    d. Provide written material on the disease process, along with special care that will be necessary, so the parents can read this when they can relax at home.

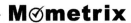

113. The medication that has shown the most success in helping patients with an acute spinal cord injury is:

    a. Dopamine
    b. Anticoagulant therapy with IV heparin
    c. Baclofen
    d. Methylprednisolone

114. One of the positive benefits of the team nursing model is that:

    a. The nurse is responsible for the duties being performed without performing them personally.
    b. The staff's competency level may not meet the level of the patient's needs.
    c. The strengths of all involved healthcare workers are used to provide the best care possible.
    d. All members of the team must be focused on the patient and his or her needs.

115. Which of the following is the responsibility of the referring provider in a consultation?

    a. Explain to the patient the purpose for a consultation and the name of the consulting provider.
    b. Contact the patient's insurance carrier to request a peer-to-peer review for any future treatments.
    c. Inform the patient that they will need to seek the services of a provider within a certain specialty on their own.
    d. Wait for a request for records and any diagnostic testing that has been completed.

116. In order to align and perfect the fit and function of a prosthetic limb, the prosthetics specialist may use:

    a. A Smart Glove
    b. A computer-supported prosthetic
    c. A personal response system
    d. A TENS unit

117. How does rehabilitation care differ from acute care?

    a. With acute care, the primary focus is on the patient's survival, while rehabilitation focuses on teaching self-care.
    b. With acute care, the patient is only seen outpatient, while rehabilitation is typically done on an in-patient basis.
    c. Acute care focuses on acute illnesses, not chronic medical conditions, while rehabilitation focuses only on mobility issues following an illness.
    d. Acute care is handled by the primary care physician, while rehabilitation is carried out with a team of specialists.

118. Which of the following is the FIRST step in doing a cultural assessment?

    a. Explain the purpose of a cultural assessment.
    b. Ask permission to do a cultural assessment.
    c. Take thorough notes during communication.
    d. Establish trust.

119. Which diagnostic test measures residual urine in the bladder?

    a. Cystoscopy
    b. Cystogram
    c. Bladder scan
    d. Pelvic CT scan

120. The stage of sleep in which the brain becomes more active is:

    a.   Alpha wave sleep
    b.   Non-REM sleep
    c.   Delta wave sleep
    d.   REM sleep

121. Besides sleep apnea, a sleep study can also be used to diagnose:

    a.   Parkinson's disease
    b.   Metabolic syndrome
    c.   REM sleep behavior disorders
    d.   Epilepsy

122. A patient who has had a stroke is left with right hemiplegia. She says that she would really like to learn to feed herself again. This is an example of a(n):

    a.   Patient-centered goal
    b.   Institution goal
    c.   Joint Commission directive
    d.   Self-actualization goal

123. The wife of a spinal cord injury patient is asking if there are any natural remedies that could help with her husband's muscle spasms rather than relying on conventional medications. Your best response is:

    a.   Any oral supplement she can find at the local health food store should work.
    b.   There are a few, but you should ask his doctor before trying any alternative medications.
    c.   There are no known natural remedies for muscle cramps.
    d.   Try loading up on potassium-rich foods and supplements to decrease cramping.

124. Orem's theory of self-care states that the goal of nursing is to serve patients and assist them to provide self-care. According to this theory, which of the following comprise the three categories of needs?

    a.   Psychological, physiological, and social
    b.   Universal, developmental, and health
    c.   Food, air, and water
    d.   Psychological, spiritual, and physical

125. A patient is placed on an SSRI antidepressant for her mild to moderate depressive symptoms. She has been trying to increase her activity level and she asks if she can continue with her same exercise routine while on the medication. Your best response is:

    a.   She should continue with her current routine, but she may find that she is more easily fatigued initially.
    b.   She should continue with her current routine, and she should notice a higher endurance level.
    c.   She should steadily increase her activity level as the medication builds in her system.
    d.   She should decrease her activity level by half until the drug levels stabilize.

126. A 56-year-old arthritic patient is chair bound with a total score on the Braden Scale of 16 based on the following: sensory perception, 4 (no impairment); moisture, 3; activity, 2; mobility, 3; usual nutrition pattern, 2; and friction and shear, 2. Which is the MOST accurate description of this patient's risk of developing a pressure sore?

    a.   Very minimal risk
    b.   Breakpoint for risk (moderate)
    c.   Small chance of developing a sore
    d.   Strong likelihood of developing a pressure sore

127. The main difference between a power of attorney and a healthcare proxy is:

a. A power of attorney makes all decisions for you when you are unable to and a healthcare proxy serves as a backup if that person is not available.

b. A power of attorney gives a facility the power to make decisions for you and a healthcare proxy gives your physician the power to make decisions for you.

c. A power of attorney gives a family member the power to take over your finances and a healthcare proxy assigns someone to ensure they are making good decisions.

d. A power of attorney makes financial decisions for you when you are unable to and a healthcare proxy is a document that assigns someone to make medical decisions for you.

128. What are nursing quality indicators?

a. Evaluation results gathered from employee reviews regarding nursing performance

b. Information released quarterly and annually regarding the quality of nursing care at the unit level

c. A reward system utilized by organizations to recognize those nurses who have high evaluation scores

d. A tool used for evaluating potential employees to ensure they have received good reviews in the past

129. According to WHO's International Classification of Impairments, Disabilities, and Handicaps (ICIDH), which of the following terms is used to describe limitations and disadvantages that interfere with social functioning?

a. Pathology

b. Impairment

c. Disability

d. Handicap

130. Which of the following groups of medications may slow rehabilitation in brain injury patients?

a. Antispasmodics

b. Anticholinergics

c. Beta blockers

d. Dopamine agonists

131. According to Centers for Medicare and Medicaid Services (CMS) guidelines, the Inpatient Rehabilitation Facility Patient Assessment Instrument (IRF-PAI) initial discharge report must be completed by when?

a. Day of discharge

b. Day 5 after discharge (including discharge day)

c. Day 17 after discharge (including discharge day)

d. Day 27 after discharge (including discharge day)

132. The document that outlines the conversation between a medical provider and patient outlining the specific treatments the patient agrees to when faced with a life-threatening emergency is called:

a. A POLST

b. An advanced directive

c. A medical healthcare proxy

d. A medical power of attorney

245

133. Capacity, as it refers to medical issues, is defined as:

    a. The assessment of a person's ability to understand and interpret information in order to make decisions, as determined by a medical evaluation

    b. A legal term that defines whether a person has the mental competence to make legal decisions

    c. The amount of information a person can interpret at one time to be an informed decision-maker in their health care

    d. The approved amount of medical services a person can receive within a given time period as determined by their insurance carrier

134. A medication frequently given to patients with a decreased level of consciousness during the acute phase (<1 month) after a traumatic brain injury is:

    a. Amitriptyline

    b. Bromocriptine

    c. Levodopa

    d. Methylphenidate

135. Which of the following patients would be most likely to show impairment on the Mini Mental Status Exam?

    a. A 54-year-old female attorney with mild short-term memory impairment

    b. A 62-year-old male college professor with moderate short-term memory impairment

    c. A 67-year-old male, educated through grade 6, with moderate short-term memory impairment

    d. A 57-year-old male engineer with very mild short-term memory impairment

136. The tool used to describe the activity level of a person with a brain injury is:

    a. The Braden scale

    b. The Harris-Benedict scale

    c. Glasgow's hierarchy

    d. The Ranchos Los Amigos scale

137. A 15-month-old child is being evaluated for hearing deficit. Which of the following is a NORMAL hearing response for a 15-month-old child?

    a. Coos and gurgles and looks in direction of sound

    b. Comforts at sound of parent's voice and tries to emulate sounds

    c. Begins first words, imitates sounds, follows directions, and points to objects

    d. Knows about 20–50 words, and points to body parts or familiar objects when asked

138. Which grief theory identifies grief as a fluid, ever-changing process rather than a linear process?

    a. Freud's Model of Bereavement

    b. Kubler-Ross Grief Cycle

    c. Bowlby's Attachment Theory

    d. Parkes' Four Phases and Four Tasks of Grief

139. A medication to help with symptoms of neurogenic bladder, with the least amount of anticholinergic side effects, is:

    a. Oxybutynin

    b. Tolterodine

    c. Propiverine

    d. Solifenacin

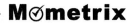

140. The Certified Rehabilitation Registered Nurse functions as a patient advocate by:

a. Reporting any medication errors that occur involving the patient
b. Following the Clinical Pathway for the patient's diagnosis
c. Not sharing any personal information the patient has told you
d. Protecting the health, safety, and rights of the patient

141. The type of urinary catheter that would be most appropriate for the patient with a neurogenic bladder is:

a. Protective undergarments, rather than catheterization
b. Indwelling catheter
c. Condom catheter
d. Short-term, or intermittent catheter

142. Which one of the following is included in the Lawton Instrumental Activities of Daily Living Scale?

a. Toileting
b. Dressing
c. Family support system
d. Transportation availability

143. You are helping a patient and her family with the discharge planning process. She will need PT to help with her multiple sclerosis symptoms, but she lives in a rural area where PT is not readily available. She has Medicare for her primary insurance. She is inquiring about having PT via a telehealth service. Your best response is that:

a. You will request the physician order this, and that it can be set up for her.
b. A Physical Therapist can come to her home and perform the services there.
c. She will have to return to the rehabilitation facility for PT services.
d. PT services are rarely available via telehealth, but it is hoped they will be in the future.

144. In order to improve the quality and effectiveness of healthcare, the government established:

a. The Agency for Healthcare Research and Quality
b. Joint Commission
c. CARF
d. HIPAA

145. The purpose of quality improvement is to:

a. Improve employee satisfaction.
b. Monitor the leadership skills of the administration of a healthcare facility.
c. Implement specific changes in healthcare that have a measurable improvement for a group of patients.
d. Provide specific training and education opportunities to employees to ensure the quality of the care provided is reaching high standards.

146. For stroke patients, success of the early supported discharge model of care especially depends on which one of the following?

a. Patient motivation
b. Linking to community services
c. Family support
d. Reimbursement

147. Which one of the following types of data must be reported according to provisions of the Improving Medicare Post-Acute Care Transformation Act of 2014?

a. Cost-effectiveness of care
b. Detailed information regarding diagnostic tests
c. Standardized patient assessment data
d. Comprehensive psychosocial assessment

148. The nursing theory that involves unfreezing, changing, and refreezing in order to promote change is called:

a. Erikson's stages of development
b. Paget's hypothesis
c. Lewin's change theory
d. Maslow's hierarchy

149. A 17-year-old adolescent is recovering from surgical evacuation of a subdural hematoma, diagnosed 2 weeks after a car accident. His total score on the Glasgow Coma Scale (GCS) is 10:

- Eye opening: 3, responds to verbal stimuli
- Verbal: 3, uses inappropriate words
- Motor: 4, withdraws in response to pain

Based on these scores, which of the following BEST describes his condition?

a. Coma
b. Severe head injury
c. Moderate head injury
d. Mild head injury

150. Which of the following is a LONG-TERM goal of cardiac rehabilitation?

a. Reversing or stabilizing atherosclerosis
b. Reducing risk of reinfarction
c. Managing/controlling symptoms
d. Reducing psychological stress

151. The theory that specific acts are judged based on the intention of the action and not its outcome is called:

a. Autonomy
b. Malfeasance
c. Deontology
d. Paternalism

152. You are helping a female patient and her husband formulate a meal plan based on a diabetic diet. Following those guidelines, the amount of grain and starch she should have daily is:

a. Unlimited servings
b. 6–11 servings
c. 3–5 servings
d. 1–2 servings

153. A tool used to implement change in an organization is:

a. A gap analysis
b. The Plan, Do, Check, Act cycle
c. A competency redistribution
d. A quality measure analysis

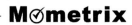

154. A 21-year-old complete spinal cord injury patient is apprehensive about attending a support group for those who have suffered this type of injury. You are explaining some of the positive benefits of participating, one of which is:

    a. Finding who he can blame for his situation
    b. Meeting members of the opposite sex
    c. Finding solutions to problems he is having from those who have gone through the same process
    d. Verbalizing his feelings when he is asked to do so during that portion of the meeting

155. As part of a bowel-training program, the patient has daily scheduled defecation. What is the BEST time to schedule a bowel movement?

    a. First thing in the morning after arising
    b. At bedtime
    c. 2 hours after a meal
    d. 20–30 minutes after a meal

156. Which of the following can be used to prevent a DVT?

    a. Beta blockers
    b. Intermittent pneumatic compression device
    c. Antispasmodics
    d. Smart Glove

157. The Harris-Benedict formula is used to:

    a. Predict fall risk in the hospitalized patient.
    b. Predict risk of skin breakdown in the hospitalized patient.
    c. Predict calorie requirements in the hospitalized patient.
    d. Predict risk of sepsis in the hospitalized patient.

158. Which of the following interventions is the BEST method to prevent joint fusion from heterotopic ossification after a spinal cord injury?

    a. Using a standing frame/table
    b. Careful handling of limbs
    c. Passive range of motion exercises
    d. Braces to support joints

159. A device that can help stroke rehabilitation patients to improve range of motion and function in the hands is:

    a. A finger contracture orthotic
    b. A Smart Glove
    c. A resting hand splint
    d. A terry cloth hand cone

160. Which of the following can be a sign of excessive stress in the work environment?

    a. Good working relationships with co-workers
    b. Insomnia
    c. Having an alcoholic drink twice a month during a social outing
    d. Using all of your allotted vacation days each year

161. A patient with a spinal cord injury develops signs of autonomic dysreflexia (sweating and flushing above injury, severe headache, nasal congestion, anxiety, nausea). He first does a pressure release and checks his indwelling catheter, which is in place and draining freely. What should he do next?

    a. Perform digital stimulation to stimulate a bowel movement.
    b. Lie down flat.
    c. Call 911.
    d. Take nifedipine or nitroglycerine sublingually.

162. An example of a third-party payer is:

    a. The patient
    b. The patient's employer
    c. A health insurance company
    d. A worker's compensation coverage company

163. A 65-year-old woman has recovered well from a stroke but has become increasingly withdrawn and states she does not want to see friends or family because she looks "old and unattractive" and is afraid of dying. According to Erikson's Stages of Development for older adults, for which of the following tasks does the patient show a NEGATIVE outcome?

    a. Body transcendence vs. body preoccupation
    b. Ego transcendence vs. ego preoccupation
    c. Socializing vs. sexualizing
    d. Ego differentiation vs. work role preoccupation

164. A 19-year-old man with an above-knee right amputation is depressed and refuses to see his parents. The parents ask the rehabilitation nurse for an update on their son's condition. Which of the following is MOST appropriate in accordance with HIPAA regulations?

    a. Advise the parents that information regarding the patient's condition is private.
    b. Provide a brief general update, without specific details
    c. Refer the parents to the physician to get information.
    d. Tell the patient he should speak to his parents.

165. A 3-year-old boy has a presumptive diagnosis of autism. Which of the following behaviors is MOST supportive of this diagnosis?

    a. The child insists of keeping a favorite toy with him at all times.
    b. The child throws temper tantrums when he is thwarted or tired.
    c. The child occasionally sits and rocks back and forth and bangs his head against the wall.
    d. The child does not make eye contact, resists being held, and speaks less than previously.

166. Which type of dysphagia is not caused by a stroke?

    a. Oral dysphagia
    b. Pharyngeal dysphagia
    c. Epiglottis dysphagia
    d. Esophageal dysphagia

167. A role model in nursing is different than a preceptor or mentor in that the role model:

    a. Is looked up to for their professionalism and clinical skills without holding a formal responsibility to educate others
    b. Has a more hands-on approach to providing training to nursing students
    c. Has more responsibility in regard to making hiring decisions
    d. Is responsible for providing all of the professional constructive criticism to new nurses

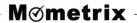

168. A 48-year-old woman with diabetes mellitus type 1 has developed almost constant dribbling of urine. Which of the following types of incontinence MOST corresponds to this symptom?

a. Urge
b. Induced
c. Overflow
d. Functional

169. Of the following interventions, which is the most sensitive for assessing for a fluid volume deficit?

a. Measuring and recording urine output
b. Performing daily weights
c. Assessing skin turgor
d. Evaluating for an elevated heart rate

170. A patient with an incomplete spinal cord injury who suffers from chronic pain may benefit from:

a. A personal response system
b. Continuous arterial blood gas monitoring
c. Biofeedback therapy
d. A Smart Glove

171. The diagnosis of bipolar disorder can be made when a person has at least one episode of a manic or hypomanic state. One of the criteria for a manic state is:

a. Being quiet or withdrawn
b. Depressed mood
c. Suicidal ideation
d. Inflated self-esteem

172. A 20-year-old woman with cerebral palsy has flexion contractions of the hips and knees with moderate spasticity and very limited abduction as well as occasional stress incontinence. She plans to marry and asks advice about positioning for sexual activity. Which of the following positions is MOST likely to allow successful intercourse?

a. Prone position flat in bed
b. Supine position flat in bed
c. Sitting or wheelchair position
d. Side-lying with bolster between knees

173. Trouble with having the motor ability to correctly form and speak words is called:

a. Dysarthria
b. Aphasia
c. Apraxia
d. Ataxia

174. You are assessing a 13-year-old girl with a spinal cord tumor who will be going through intensive occupational and physical therapy to help improve strength and independence with her ADLs. You notice several scattered bruises on her back and upper arms, and you strongly suspect these may be due to child abuse. What is the most appropriate next step?

a. Ask the child's parent or guardian if the child is in an abusive position at home.
b. Try to get the child alone and ask her if someone has been hurting her.
c. Report the suspected case of abuse to the appropriate agency.
d. Make a mental note of the patient's name and occasionally check her chart to see if she continues to have bruises or injuries documented.

175. Following a TBI, a 57-year-old woman has a Functional Independence Measure (FIM) score of 40 on admission and 63 on discharge, with discharge scores in all areas ranging from 3–4. What level of independence or care in the home is MOST indicated by these scores?

    a. Complete independence in care
    b. Modified independence, including use of assistive devices and activity modification
    c. Supervision only (stand by without physically assisting)
    d. Minimal to moderate contact assistance (physically assisting)

Answer Key and Explanations for Test#1

1. A: The 10-meter walk test is used to assess a patient's speed in walking 10 meters. During the test, the patient can use any assistive devices or assistance normally used. The length that is marked is actually 14 meters, but only the middle 10 meters are counted. The "flying start" refers to the first 2 meters of the distance. These 2 meters are not counted in the time but allow the patient to gain some momentum. Likewise, the last 2 meters (often used for turning if more than one length is to be walked) are not counted. Normal values are typically greater than 1 meter per second until age 80.

2. C: Patients performing self-catheterization should drink at least 2 quarts of liquids daily but should try to drink most of this in the first half of the day. They should drink primarily water and try to avoid citrus juices as they make the urine more alkaline, which is conducive to growing bacteria. Approximately 7 ounces of cranberry juice should be drunk each day to make the urine more acidic to decrease bacterial growth.

3. D: Allowing the patient to rest during the day will increase their difficulties with sleeping at night. Limiting caffeine, using prn sleep medications, and having the patient engaged in activities during the day can all help to promote a healthy sleep cycle. Educating the patient on a healthy sleep pattern with waking and sleeping at the same time every day can also help to promote a normal sleep cycle.

4. A: Because patients may be embarrassed and uncomfortable discussing sexual functioning (especially with someone of the opposite gender), the PLISSIT model begins with asking the patient's permission to discuss sexual function. If the patient agrees, then the nurse can go to the next steps:

- P: Ask permission.
- LI: Provide limited information about sexual function.
- SS: Provide specific suggestions for dealing with sexual dysfunction.
- IT: Refer to a specialist in sex therapy for intensive therapy.

If the patient declines, the nurse should tell the patient they can discuss it later if he changes his mind and ask if there is someone else with whom the patient would feel more comfortable discussing the issue.

5. A: Damage to the 2nd-4th sacral nerves can result in a man being unable to attain a reflex erection. Difficult or impaired physical sexual response can occur with any spinal cord injury that occurs at T11–12 and below. The degree of dysfunction is dependent upon their sexual function before the injury and the extent of the sustained injury.

6. A: With Medicare's prospective payment system, payment rates are set in advance and are based on various criteria, such as the diagnosis and type of service, rather than on the actual costs of care. This system aims to control the costs of care by encouraging efficient care. Patients are classified according to the type of facility:

- Inpatient: Diagnosis-related groups.
- Skilled nursing facility: Resource utilization groups.
- Home health agency: Home health prospective payment system.
- Rehabilitation Center: Inpatient Rehabilitation Facility Patient Assessment Instrument (IRF-PAI).

7. C: During REM sleep, the brain converts the short-term memories of muscle movements into long-term memories. This helps with forming "muscle memory" and is essential for patients undergoing rehabilitation for a disorder that has affected muscle function. Following a stroke, patients are often very tired and seem to sleep a lot, which is normal and very healthy for the recovery process.

8. C: The Rehabilitation Services Administration of the Department of Education funds and oversees state vocational rehabilitation agencies. This agency carries out annual reviews and periodic on-site monitoring and publishes these reviews. It also supports a number of different programs, including the Payback Information Management System job board and the Rehabilitation Long-Term Training grant program as well as providing grants for underserved populations.

9. D: The best way to assess the external anal sphincter is with a digital rectal exam. This muscular ring usually has a puckered appearance but can be flattened or scalloped with a lower motor neuron injury. A loss of sensation during a digital rectal exam indicates an injury above the level of L3.

10. B: Tracheostomy care can be taught to caregivers so this can be performed at home without having a Respiratory Therapist come to the home each day. The trach tube can be reused at home once it has been cleaned with soap and water and once mucus inside the tube has been cleaned out. In the hospital setting, trach care is done using aseptic technique to prevent contamination, but it is done under "clean" conditions at home.

11. D: When developing an ergonomics program, the first step is to collect baseline injury data from incident reports and Occupational Safety and Health Administration (OSHA) logs. Data should include the type of activity that brought about the injury (such as lifting a patient), the cause, the type of injury and the body part affected, the location of the injury, and the date as well as the days of work lost or days with modified workload. These data can then be used to identify high-risk units, to make observations in these units, to carry out a risk analysis, and to formulate injury prevention recommendations.

12. B: Moderately thickened liquids, such as split pea soup, are less likely to cause choking in Alzheimer patients than thin liquids, such as coffee. Products such as *Thick-It* are available to add to thin liquids, but infant rice cereal and yogurt may also be used. Foods that are sticky, such as white bread and thick oatmeal, may cause an obstructive plug to form. Finger foods, such as carrot sticks and hot dogs, may cause choking if not chewed properly. The patient should be seated in an upright position while eating and should use a straw or sippy cup for liquids.

13. B: BiPAP is very similar to CPAP in that both devices provide positive airway pressure to assist patients with breathing during sleep. The difference with BiPAP is that the amount of pressure can be adjusted to different levels for inhalation and expiration. BiPAP is usually used for those patients who have difficulty exhaling against the pressure setting on a CPAP machine. It is more expensive than traditional CPAP therapy and not all insurance carriers will cover this expense.

14. C: CIMT is characterized by constraint of an uninvolved upper extremity (usually through use of a mitt or sling), forced use of weakened limbs for 90% of waking hours, and massed practice exercises for at least 6 hours (with a 1-hour break), 5 days per week, usually for 2 or 3 weeks. Exercises typically involve functional activities performed repeatedly over 15–20 minutes. Massed practice for the lower limbs includes treadmill walking, climbing steps, and sit-and-stand exercises. Shaping, doing progressively more difficult tasks in small steps for 90 minutes daily with positive reinforcement, may be combined with CIMT.

15. C: The Digit Span Test is done to assess attention and recall. For the test, the CRRN begins by stating two random numbers, such as 8 and 15, and asks the patient to repeat the numbers. If the patient can do this correctly, the CRRN then starts over and states three different numbers and so on, adding a number each time until the patient makes mistakes. If the patient scores less than 5, this is an indication of impaired attention. People can normally remember 7 (plus or minus 2) digits.

16. C: Apraxia is the condition in which people have difficulty carrying out specific tasks when asked to do so. This can be something like the inability to perform a specific ADL. Apraxia can be caused by damage to the posterior parietal complex of the brain and occurs due to stroke, an acquired brain injury, or dementia. Physical and occupational therapy is the treatment for apraxia to help relearn how to perform the tasks, which have become difficult.

17. A: Because of autonomic nervous system dysfunction, thermoregulation (including sweating) is impaired, so hyperthermia is of great concern in high temperatures. Body temperature fluctuates according to ambient temperature, even in the shade. Patients with injuries higher than T6 are especially at risk. The patient may readily develop signs of heat stress or even heat stroke, so patients should be advised to keep a cool, damp cloth around the neck, mist the face and neck with cool water, remain hydrated, and wear light, unconstricting clothing.

18. D: Of these choices, capnography is the most accurate way to measure the effectiveness of a patient's ability to ventilate. Pulse oximetry measures a patient's oxygen saturation level but does not monitor the amount of carbon dioxide that is being expelled through respirations. Capnography provides a measurement of the expired or end-tidal carbon dioxide concentrations. This provides real time readings of the exchange of air in the patient's lungs and the atmosphere. The monitoring device can be adapted for use with a nasal cannula or oxygen mask.

19. B: While all of these interventions are important for the patient with a pressure ulcer, regardless of the stage, the most important is to reposition the patient frequently. The primary cause of pressure ulcers is excessive pressure applied to the bony protuberances. By relieving that pressure, the root cause of the problem is addressed. This is especially important when the ulcer is classified as a stage 1 and the skin is still intact.

20. A: A prior period of at least 3 days of acute hospitalization is not required for treatment in an IRF but is required for treatment in a skilled nursing facility (SNF). The IRF patient must need and be prescribed at least 3 hours of rehabilitation therapy daily and must need and be prescribed at least 2 different types of therapy, such as speech therapy, physical therapy, and occupational therapy. In a SNF, Medicare covers treatment only while the patient shows improvement. In an IRF, treatment can continue as long as the patient requires the qualifying level of treatment.

21. A: Water is the best beverage to drink to decrease irritation of the bladder. The other answers listed are known to cause bladder irritation. Other irritants include tea, milk and milk products, carbonated beverages, coffee, spicy foods, tomatoes and tomato juice, citrus juice and fruits, and corn syrup.

22. C: Gaining accreditation from the Commission on Accreditation of Rehabilitation Facilities (CARF) is a lengthy process. An organization must first conduct an evaluation to determine if it conforms to CARF standards and must align its practices with these standards. The organization can request an on-site survey 3 months in advance of the desired survey date, but the organization must be in conformance with CARF standards for 6 months prior to the survey. Once the survey is completed, CARF issues a ruling regarding accreditation. When accredited, the organization must complete a quality improvement plan.

23. C: When visiting a patient in the home environment, safety is always the most important issue, so if a patient is hostile, drugged, and/or intoxicated, the nurse should reschedule the visit and leave. Other safeguards include:

- Visit during daytime hours
- Carry a preprogrammed (police, 911, agency) cellular phone
- Wear inexpensive clothing, jewelry, and watch
- Carry identification (agency, organization)
- Avoid visiting high-crime areas alone
- Report observed abuse after leaving home
- Provide others with the schedule of visits
- Enter a home only on invitation

24. B: The Americans with Disabilities Act became a law in 1990. It prohibits discrimination against anyone who has a disability in all areas of public life. The purpose of the law is to ensure all people with disabilities have the same rights and opportunities as everyone else. Amendments to the Act were signed into law in 2009 to further clarify the definition of disability.

25. B: The Prospective Payment System (PPS) is a method of reimbursement established by Medicare to provide a predetermined, fixed amount of payment to facilities and organization offering specific services. The patient's classification is determined using the IRF-PAI tool to classify patients in a specific category that identifies which services they will need while undergoing skilled or rehabilitative nursing care. The fee for these services varies depending on the type of facility offering the services, but it ensures that specific services will be reimbursed appropriately.

26. D: The Joint Commission was established in 1951 with the primary goal of ensuring that health care organizations are providing the safest and highest quality of care available. Organizations must undergo on-site reviews and analysis of policies and procedures that are used to ensure this care is being provided effectively. The on-site surveys are performed every three years, or more frequently if necessary.

27. C: The Ombudsman is an official whose sole responsibility is to investigate accusations of mistreatment or complaints against administration in positions in which there is an imbalance of power. This includes residents of a nursing home or rehabilitation facility in which there are concerns about treatment. The person in this role will go to the facility and investigate all of the allegations to determine whether there was wrongdoing on the part of the facility. This could result in a recommendation for an investigation from the state licensing body to determine whether a corrective action is necessary to improve care.

28. C: The patient's estranged husband has been given health care power of attorney, which gives him the right to make decisions if the patient is unable to do so. While divorce may automatically revoke the health care power of attorney in some states, the patient and her husband are not divorced. The legal document takes precedence over family ties, such as those of the mother and daughter. This is not a decision rendered by ethics committees. If family members want to challenge the husband, their recourse is to take the matter to court.

29. C: The Rogers Theory of Unitary Human Beings views nursing as a science and an art. It provides a way to view the unitary human being, who is integral with the universe. This theory states that nursing focuses on people and the human-environmental process. A change of pattern or organization of these fields are transmitted by waves. This theory is based on the belief that, by identifying this pattern, there can be a better understanding of human experience.

30. B: Section 504 of the Rehabilitation Act of 1973 prevents discrimination based on disabilities and applies to all employers and organizations receiving federal financial assistance or payments, such as Medicare or Medicaid. The law defines a disability as a physical or mental impairment that limits one or more major life activities (hearing, seeing, walking, talking, performing tasks, learning). Employers/organizations must make reasonable accommodations that do not cause undue hardship. Those with disabilities must have access to federal programs, services, and benefits, and cannot be denied access because of physical barriers or be denied opportunities, such as promotion, in employment.

31. C: Seroquel can also have noticeable anticholinergic side effects. These include dry mouth, constipation, urinary retention, impaired concentration, confusion, and memory impairment. These occur due to the blockage of acetylcholine, which impairs the function of the parasympathetic nervous system. The parasympathetic nervous system controls involuntary movement, such as smooth muscle in the bowel, which can cause these side effects.

32. B: The goal of medication therapy with bowel incontinence is to reduce stool frequency and improve stool consistency. A regular bowel regimen needs to be established with the patient to try to establish a pattern of bowel elimination. For patients who have infrequent, low volume stools (constipation), a bulking agent may be necessary. Patients who have more loose stools, or diarrhea, may require medication to slow the peristaltic action in the gut, like Imodium.

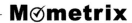

33. B: An impedance threshold device is a valve used in CPR. Its function is to decrease intrathoracic pressure and increase venous return to the heart. The valve is part of a mask or endotracheal tube that may open at high or low pressure. Studies have shown that the device can improve the chances for a return of spontaneous circulation and improvement after cardiac arrest.

34. B: Having little or no interest in activities that used to be pleasurable is a symptom of PTSD. Other symptoms include nightmares, reliving the trauma that occurred, hypervigilance, agitation, and hostility, to name a few. PTSD is usually treated with a SSRI antidepressant and therapy. PTSD symptoms can last for many years and the condition may be very difficult to manage. Most patients will have triggers that continue to bring the flashback of the traumatic event back in their mind for many years after it occurred.

35. C: Self-advocacy is a person's ability to express their needs or goals in order to perform a certain task. This can be hard for some individuals who have been strongly independent all of their lives. For example, a patient who has had a stroke may have difficulty performing some of their ADLs. By self-advocating, they make their needs known in order to better themselves. This also includes the patient in identifying their areas of weakness that may require additional therapy or training to raise their independence level.

36. B: A patient at least 18 years old who becomes disabled before age 22 can receive the "child's" benefit based on a parent's or other legal guardian's (such as grandmother's) Social Security record if the parent/guardian dies or receives Social Security retirement or Social Security disability benefits. In this case, the adult child does not need a record of earnings, although she may legally have earnings of $1,000/month or less and still be eligible for Social Security disability. She is not eligible for SSI because she has resources (life insurance) worth more than $2,000. Welfare requirements vary by state but have similar resource limitations.

37. B: Because air becomes trapped with COPD, the purpose of pursed-lip breathing is to extend the duration of exhalation to double that of inhalation, increasing airway pressure and reducing trapped air by preventing collapse of small airways. The patient breathes through the nose to a slow count of 3 and then exhales through pursed lips while tightening abdominal muscles and attempts to prolong exhalation to a count of 6 or 7. During ambulation, the goal is 2 steps for inhalation and 4–5 steps for exhalation. Pursed-lip breathing is often combined with diaphragmatic breathing.

38. A: Smoking is the greatest risk factor for developing COPD, and smoking cessation is the most essential for slowing the progression of the disease. There is some evidence that combining tobacco and marijuana use has an additive effect on the lungs. Therefore, smoking cessation should include stopping marijuana use, although using marijuana only 3–4 times monthly is not an indication for drug rehabilitation. Guidelines for drinking suggest 1–2 alcoholic beverages per day for males, so this patient is near that limit and probably not drinking enough to need AA. Diet and nutrition are important, but 1,400 calories is probably adequate and smoking cessation may increase appetite.

39. D: This patient is at severe risk for falls. Gait assessment includes:

- Gait speed in 5 meters with slow gait (less than 0.6 m/second) is predictive of functional limitations.
- TUG: patient stands from chair with armrests, walks 3 meters, and turns and sits back down; those requiring at least 14 seconds are at risk for falls (normal: 7–10 seconds)
- POMA tests mobility and gait under different conditions

In this case, the POMA score 0 indicates marked limitation and 1 moderate limitation. A score of 2 indicates no limitations, but this patient showed limitations in all activities associated with sitting, standing, walking, and maintaining balance.

40. A: Rapid breathing, smoking (cigarettes and marijuana), and low fluid intake all lead to dehydration, which is consistent with dry skin, concentrated urine, poor appetite, and thick sputum, so increasing fluid intake may help to alleviate some of these symptoms and improve appetite. Providing low-flow oxygen is usually restricted to those in stage IV COPD with resting PaO_2 of less than 60 mmHg or for those who have marked hypoxemia during exercise. Continuous low-flow oxygen is usually given at PaO_2 less than 55 mmHg. Long-term oral corticosteroid use is not recommended for COPD as it may lead to steroid myopathy, decreased function, and respiratory failure.

41. D: Trying to rush to do many things upon arising is a poor strategy because secretions pool during the night, increasing shortness of breath and intolerance to activity first thing in the morning. Delaying activities for an hour or so after arising and taking medications may increase tolerance. The patient should be taught to pace activities with periods of rest in between rather than exhausting himself by doing them in sequence without rest. Using assistive devices, such as a walker, keeping room temperature at a comfortable level, and utilizing Meals on Wheels are good strategies.

42. A: The adrenal medulla secretes adrenaline, which is responsible for the "fight or flight" response. When the body feels threatened or there is an immense stressor on someone, signals are sent to the brain. The brain, in turn, stimulates the adrenal gland to secrete adrenaline from the adrenal medulla. This causes the heart rate and respiratory rate to increase. This is due to activation of the sympathetic nervous system and suppression of the parasympathetic nervous system.

43. B: The Improving Medicare Post-Acute Care Transformation (IMPACT) Act was signed into law in 2014. It standardized assessments in skilled nursing facilities, long-term care facilities, rehabilitation facilities, and home health agencies. This helps to streamline the identification of the individual needs of patients, thereby eliminating the cost of unnecessary services and improving individualized patient care.

44. A: While all of these elements are important, best practices identified through literature review should carry the most weight when developing evidence-based guidelines. Preferences are often based on subjective rather than objective observations and may relate to familiarity and ease of use. Cost-effectiveness is always an issue and must be considered, but it should not be the primary concern. In some cases, spending more to prevent a problem initially may save money in terms of morbidity and extended medical care in the long term.

45. D: This patient is exhibiting a self-care deficit in dressing and grooming, exemplified by his dirty clothing and failure to shave or comb his hair. Other types of self-care deficits include deficits in bathing and hygiene, feeding, and toileting. If a self-care deficit in one area occurs, the patient should be evaluated for other self-care deficits because more than one deficit is common. Neglect is probably not an issue here, as the patient lives alone. Additionally, his apology suggests that he is concerned about his appearance, which does not usually correlate with low self-esteem.

46. B: The Americans with Disabilities Act requires employers with 15 or more employees or government entities to make reasonable accommodations for disabled individuals, such as being legally blind. These accommodations can include assistive technology, such as screen readers and speech recognition software or magnification devices. Employers do not need to provide accommodations to employees who cannot carry out essential job duties, provide a personal assistant, or reassign the person to another position.

47. B: Cultural encounter is the process of encouraging medical staff to interact with those patients who are from a different cultural background. It has been found that the more a person interacts with those from different cultures, the more their beliefs and practices can be understood. Communities have become very diverse and the medical professional needs to be prepared to address the individual needs and practices of those from different cultures.

48. C: The implementation phase of the nursing process involves applying the nursing interventions identified for a specific patient for their specific diagnosis. The desired outcomes should be achievable. The actions in the implementation phase may entail monitoring the patient for any signs of change, performing specific medical tasks, or educating the patient on a specific process. This phase of the nursing process may take place over hours, days, or even months.

49. C: The Lean approach in healthcare is a set of methods used to maximize the value of healthcare received by the patient by minimizing waste and time. It allows a healthcare organization to analyze a specific component of the services offered to a patient and implement a change that will better that service. This can result in decreased cost to the organization and patient, a streamlined approach to a specific process, and improved patient satisfaction in the process.

50. A: Medicare Part A covers the services available outside of a physician's office. This includes hospitalization, skilled nursing home care for the first 100 days after a 3-day hospital stay, hospice care, home care, and laboratory tests. Medicare Part B covers the care provided within the physician's office.

51. C: A stage II pressure ulcer, characterized by broken skin, is best treated by cleansing with normal saline and applying a moist environment for healing, such as with a hydrocolloid dressing or semipermeable occlusive dressings. Wet-to-dry dressings are no longer advised for wound care because the dry dressing may damage the new tissue when it is removed. Antiseptics and heat treatments should be avoided as they may damage healthy tissue around the wound and delay overall healing. Further pressure to the area or friction and shear must be avoided to prevent further injury.

52. B: Presentation of only the three most cost-effective treatment options is a violation of guidelines regarding informed consent, which include:

- Explanation of diagnosis
- Nature of, and reason for, treatment or procedure
- Risks and benefits
- Alternative options (regardless of cost or insurance coverage)
- Risks and benefits of alternative options
- Risks and benefits of not having a treatment or procedure
- Providing informed consent is a requirement of all states

While providing comparison information is not required, doing so does not violate informed consent.

53. C: The intensive theory is based on Aristotle's theory that pain resulted from excessive stimulation of the sensation of touch. Pain can be induced from intense light, pressure, or temperature. It is thought that repeated stimulation to peripheral nerve fibers can have an accumulating effect to produce the perception of pain.

54. B: The specificity theory of pain states that there is a "pain center" within the brain that interprets pain signals. This theory considers pain as an independent perception with specialized sensory receptors that transmit signals along nerve fibers to the brain. The brain then processes these signals as the sensation of pain.

55. C: A stroke affecting the left side of the brain may cause speech and language problems. Broca's area, near the frontal lobe of the left side of the brain, is responsible for interpreting language and putting together speech patterns. It also has control of the motor function of speech with forming words.

56. A: The WeeFIM is the Functional Independence Measure used to assess a child's performance level in activities related to self-care, mobility, and cognition. It can be used in children from 6 months up to 21 years and it measures the consistent performance in specific skills. These performances are then categorized into Dependent or Independent tasks. It helps to identify specific areas in which a deficiency is occurring to better target specialized therapies and/or treatments to increase independence.

57. C: The Affordable Care Act was signed into place in 2011 by President Barack Obama. The program's goal was to provide a market of insurance carriers that would be required to provide equal rates to everyone seeking health insurance despite pre-existing medical conditions. It has been a very controversial program and has continuously undergone changes and plans for re-organization.

58. B: Albumin (half-life, 18–20 days) is more sensitive to long-term protein deficiencies than to short-term deficiencies (normal values, 3.5–5.5 g/dL). Total protein levels can be influenced by many factors, including stress and infection, but it may be monitored as part of an overall nutritional assessment (normal values, 6–8 g/dL). Prealbumin (half-life, 2–3 days) is most commonly monitored for acute changes in nutritional status (normal values, 16–40 mg/dL). Transferrin (half-life, 8–10 days) is sometimes used as a measure of nutritional status; however, transferrin levels are sensitive to many different things, so transferrin levels alone are not always reliable measurements of nutritional status (normal values, 200–400 mg/dL).

59. D: A gap analysis examines the difference between what is actually being accomplished versus the desired outcome. It identifies specific items that may need to be approached differently in order to achieve the set goal. It can also be helpful in identifying those goals that may not be attainable using the current process in place.

60. D: Vasopressors are used during medical emergencies to treat extremely low blood pressure in order to prevent end organ failure. Their mechanism of action is to cause constriction within the peripheral blood vessels in order to raise blood pressure and increase blood flow to the organs. Examples include epinephrine, norepinephrine, and dopamine. All of these answers can be possible side effects of vasopressors except for hypotension, which is the opposite effect of the medications.

61. B: CPAP has been recognized as the gold standard in treating sleep apnea. It consists of a device worn by the patient with sleep apnea while they are sleeping to increase pressure within the airway to prevent periods of sleep apnea during sleep. It differs from BiPAP therapy in that there is one constant level of pressure for inhalation and expiration, whereas BiPAP has one pressure setting for inhalation and a different one for exhalation.

62. A: Renal recommendations include guidelines for a low sodium, low phosphorous, and low protein diet. For some patients, there may also be fluid restrictions to prevent fluids retention. Excess sodium in the diet also causes fluids retention and can cause an increase in blood pressure and heart failure. With renal disease, the kidneys are not able to excrete potassium adequately, so potassium should be limited in the diet. The kidneys also excrete excess phosphorous, which they are not able to do if they are not functioning properly. This can lead to calcium being pulled from the bones, causing the development of osteopenia or osteoporosis.

63. A: If oral medications are not helpful, botulinum toxin can be used to calm the detrusor muscle and increase bladder capacity. The injection is made into the bladder wall to temporarily paralyze the external sphincter of the bladder to help with emptying. The injection generally lasts 3–9 months.

64. D: The knack maneuver is a use of Kegel exercises for prevention of urinary incontinence. Women are taught to contract the pelvic floor muscles right before and during events that usually cause stress incontinence. For example, if a woman feels a cough or sneeze coming, she immediately contracts the pelvic floor muscles and holds until the stress event is over. This contraction augments support of the proximal urethra, reducing the amount of displacement that usually takes place with compromised muscle support, thereby preventing incontinence. It is particularly useful if used before and during stress events, such as coughing, sneezing, lifting, standing, swinging a golf club, or laughing.

65. A: The Certified Rehabilitation Registered Nurse can work in several patient care environments. They are most commonly employed by long-term care facilities, rehabilitation facilities, sub-acute units, home health or community agencies, or educational institutions to instruct nursing students. The patient population they are most likely to provide care for are those who have chronic medical problems that have led to an alteration in functional ability.

66. B: HIPAA regulations state that the care of a patient cannot be discussed with anyone without appropriate permission. This includes confirming or denying that the patient was seen at a specific healthcare facility. Most people understand this once it is explained to them.

67. B: At this time, only dogs are allowed to be certified service animals. Service dogs have been used to help people who are blind or deaf, by pulling a wheelchair, reminding people to take medications, calming and soothing people with PTSD, and alerting or protecting someone with a seizure disorder. Service dogs have been trained to pick up on the warning signs of an impending seizure to allow the person time to place themselves in a safe position. They also can help during the seizure to make sure the person is kept safe and to notify emergency personnel if necessary.

68. D: A sentinel event is defined by The Joint Commission as any event that occurs in a healthcare setting that results in the death or significant psychological damage of a patient. A root cause analysis is performed when a sentinel event takes place to identify the cause of the incident, as well as put forth measures to help prevent this from happening again.

69. C: Medications that have a high anticholinergic side effect profile may increase the symptoms of Parkinsonism syndrome. Remeron is an antidepressant that promotes sleep but does not have a high anticholinergic side effect profile. Benadryl, an antihistamine, and amitriptyline, a tricyclic antidepressant, have a high likelihood of having anticholinergic side effects. The class of dopamine agonist medications may cause severe nightmares or interference with the REM stage of sleep.

70. C: When assisting a patient with multiple sclerosis or other demyelinating disorders with an exercise regimen, the CRRN should monitor the patient for signs of overheating because an elevated core temperature may trigger Uhthoff's phenomenon—a temporary exacerbation of neurological symptoms. As well as exercise, hot weather, hot tubs, saunas, and fever may also increase risk. The symptoms with multiple sclerosis most commonly affected are visual, but overheating can also affect balance, urinary continence, and other bodily functions.

71. A: The average full sleep cycle is approximately 3 hours. REM sleep, which is essential for providing a truly restful period of sleep, occurs 90 minutes after a person falls asleep. In order to feel fully rested from sleep, the body must go through the full REM cycle. Sleeping in 3-hour intervals will make a person feel more rested since they have achieved at least one full cycle of REM sleep.

72. C: Oral medications, such as Viagra and Cialis, have been proven to help most men with a spinal cord injury to achieve and sustain an erection. There are also injectable medications, such as Caverject, that are injected into the spongy tissue of the penis to help with achieving an erection. If medications fail, a vacuum pump or placement of a penile implant may help.

73. B: In order to meet Medicare requirements, IRFs must meet specific compliance requirements and report them through the Inpatient Rehabilitation Facility Patient Quality Reporting Program. On October 1 of each year, CMS publishes the quality measures that must be reported for the next fiscal year. If an IRF does not meet the reporting requirements, then it is subject to a 2% reduction of its annual increase factor, the amount of annual increase or decrease in payment rates.

74. C: When ascending stairs with crutches, the patient should place the well foot first on the higher step, then the crutches and injured foot. When descending, he should place crutches first on the lower step, then the well foot and the injured foot. Patients should be cautioned NOT to hop from step to step as this may result in injury and/or falls. Crutches should be properly fitted before patient attempts ambulation. Correct crutch height is one hand-width below axillae with handgrips adjusted so the patient supports the body weight comfortably with elbows slightly flexed and crutches tight against the chest wall. Bearing weight under the axillae can cause nerve damage.

75. D: ADA provides persons with disabilities, including those with mental impairment, access to employment and the community. Communities must provide transportation services for persons with disabilities, including accommodation for wheelchairs. Public facilities (schools, museums, physician's offices, post offices, restaurants) must be accessible with ramps and elevators as needed. EMTALA prevents "dumping" from emergency departments. OAA provides improved access to services for older adults and Native Americans, including community services (meals, transportation, home health care, adult day care, legal assistance, and home repair). OBRA provides guidelines for nursing facilities, such as long-term care facilities.

76. A: Naturopathy focuses on strengthening the body's defense mechanisms, rather than trying to heal particular disease symptoms, by various modalities, such as diet, herbs, hydrotherapy, acupuncture, physical therapy, counseling, and homeopathy. Naturopathy stresses that natural approaches to healing are preferable to surgery or medications, but it does not preclude the use of traditional medical treatment. Acupuncture uses needles inserted into acupoints to balance vital energy (qi) while acupressure applies pressure or electric stimulation to acupoints. Chiropractic therapy uses various manipulations of muscles and joints to relieve discomfort and pressure on nerves. Practitioners believe that aligning the spine is critical to maintenance of health.

77. D: The dysphagia patient should be at upright, or as close to a 90-degree incline as possible while eating. Small bites of all types of food should be given, usually 0.5–1.0 teaspoon at a time. Liquids should not be given with each bite to "wash it down" unless the Speech Therapist has instructed this to be done. There is an increased risk of choking while talking and eating at the same time, so talking should be discouraged.

78. C: A resting heart rate of 50 bpm or less is a contraindication to performing exercise or physical activity. Medications, such as beta-blockers, can cause this decrease in heart rate. A primary cardiac cause of the bradycardia, such as an AV block or sick sinus syndrome, can also contribute. Further work up should be done by the patient's physician or a cardiologist to determine whether there is an acute problem.

79. A: If a person has a worksite injury and is unable to return to the same job because of the injury, such as a back injury, then workers' compensation will provide vocational retraining through vocational rehabilitation services. A person cannot receive permanent disability status only because of the inability to carry out a previous job, and workers' compensation typically does not pay for alternative or experimental treatments or provide compensation for pain and suffering. Workers' compensation is administered by each state, so programs may differ.

80. B: Alcohol may induce sleep, and help people sleep more deeply for a while, but it decreases the length of much needed REM sleep. This leaves people feeling poorly rested when they awaken. Alcohol can also cause respiratory depression, which may cause periods of sleep apnea and lead to less restful sleep.

81. A: CMS conducts audits of IRFs to ensure they are meeting safety and quality standards. An on-site inspection is carried out by auditors who review various aspects of service, such as the physical environment, clinical staffing levels, infection control policies, patient care processes, respect for patient's rights, and medication management. Auditors review documentation to ensure that it supports the need for inpatient care and promotes quality improvement. Interviews and observations are also carried out with clinical healthcare providers.

82. A: The ASIA (American Spinal Injury Association) scale is used to classify the degree of impairment that is present due to a spinal cord injury. It documents sensory and motor impairments based on neurological responses, touch, and pinprick, along with motor strength from muscles on each side of the body. Each side of the body is graded independently. Scores can range from an ASIA A with a complete spinal cord injury up to an ASIA E where no deficits are present, but they were in the past.

83. A: The gate control theory of pain outlines the idea that small fibers carry signals to the spinal cord where they can then be transmitted to the brain. These signals can be weak and pass on without any interference, or they can be controlled by larger fibers that act as a gate to control the transmission. If a signal is strong enough, as with intense pain, the larger fibers are not able to control the transmission of the signal.

84. B: The patient with a traumatic brain injury would not be a candidate for an implanted baclofen pump because of the length of their injury. Candidates must be at least 1-year post injury to be considered for the

262

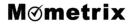

pump. All of the other candidates are ideal for this method of baclofen delivery. If the pump is effective, it will decrease spasticity, which can decrease pain and improve function.

85. A: A lack of sleep can result in an increased appetite and increased calorie consumption. This is due to a fall in leptin levels with sleep deprivation. Leptin is a hormone that regulates appetite. When levels are low, the appetite is stimulated which results in people eating more calories than are really needed. Leptin levels normalize when people have an adequate amount of sleep.

86. A: Biofeedback has proven successful for some patients in reducing the incidence and pain of migraines. Typically, a machine sensor is attached to the body, and the patient concentrates on particular actions, such as increasing blood flow and warmth to the hands, while receiving feedback in various methods (sounds, graphs, lines). Thermal biofeedback requires a thermistor be applied to the hands to measure temperature. As the patient relaxes, reducing stress, vasodilation occurs and the temperature of the hands increases, in turn reducing the headache. Massage and exercise may help reduce overall stress but may not be effective for pain control. While food triggers may cause a migraine, no one diet approach has proven successful.

87. D: The Commission on Accreditation of Rehabilitation Facilities (CARF) was founded in 1966. It provides accreditation and certification to facilities offering services in rehabilitation, opioid treatment plans, behavioral health, aging services, and others. There are currently over 50,000 programs and services accredited by CARF.

88. C: The preliminary step in a bedside dysphagia assessment is a saliva swallowing test. If this test is performed without difficulty, the direct swallowing test is performed. This entails giving the patient thickened water, approximately one-third to one-half teaspoon, followed by 5 more half-teaspoons. If this is performed without difficulty, 3 mL of water is given to the patient. If successful, 5, 10, and 20 mL amounts are given. This is followed by 50 mL to be drunk as fast as possible. If the patient is successful with this, a small piece of dry bread is given and repeated 5 times. The patient should swallow this within 10 seconds to successfully pass the test.

89. C: A contracture causes stiffness and reduced range of motion of muscle, a joint, or skin. When a muscle contracture occurs, there is shortening and stiffening of the muscle fibers. A contracture can occur within a joint capsule due to limited movement. With severe burns, the skin can contract due to scarring which will result in decreased movement. Any condition that causes decreased movement can result in contractures. Losing the ability to move from paralysis can also result in contractures.

90. B: It is a common misconception that if a pain medication is ordered for a specific type of pain, such as leg pain, it is only going to work on the leg pain and not any other discomfort the patient is having. The mechanism of action of opioid analgesics is to attach to the mu and kappa receptors in the spinal cord. This blocks the pain "message" to the brain, which blocks the sensation that there is pain present. This causes a decrease in pain systemically, not just in one specific location in the body.

91. B: According to the United States Public Health Service, evaluation, exercise, education, and counseling are the essential elements of a cardiovascular rehabilitation program. Evaluation includes complete medical assessment and diagnosis. Exercise programs are individually designed and based on diagnosis and exercise testing. Initially, continuous ECG monitoring may be used during exercise. Education should be continuous with the goal of self-care and improved outcomes. Counseling is critical to helping the patient cope with physical and emotional stress and life changes.

92. C: Instrumental ADLs are those activities of daily living that are not essential to providing basic hygiene or self-care. They add quality to life, but are not essential for daily living. These include housekeeping, shopping, managing money, and managing medications. Limitations with instrumental ADLs may come from a physical deficit that prevents a person from performing them, or a cognitive deficit that makes it difficult for them to follow the steps or understand these activities.

93. C: Bowen's Family Systems Theory considers the interrelationship among those in a family unit and comprises a number of concepts, including:

- Triangle theory: two people comprise a basic unit, but when conflict occurs, a third person is drawn into the unit for stability with the resulting dynamic of two supporting one or two opposing one
- Self-differentiation: people vary in need for external approval
- Nuclear family patterns: marital conflict, one spouse dysfunctional, one or more children impaired, and emotional distance
- Projection within a family: problems (emotional) passed from parent to child
- Emotional isolation: reducing or eliminating family contact

94. A: Skeletal muscle relaxants function to decrease muscle excitability, thereby decreasing pain and improving function. They work at the level of the spinal cord, brainstem, and cerebrum. There are two main categories of muscle relaxants: antispasmodic and antispasticity drugs. Antispasmodics treat muscle spasms that occur with peripheral musculoskeletal conditions. Antispasticity drugs decrease increased muscle tone or contractions of muscle from upper motor neuron disorders, such as multiple sclerosis or spinal cord injuries.

95. B: Because the speech center is located in the left hemisphere, and the right part of the brain is dominant for music, this patient may benefit from melodic intonation therapy, which incorporates singing, rhythmic tapping, rhyming, chanting, rapping, and creating songs. The patient begins singing and gradually transitions to speech. Stimulation-facilitation therapy focuses on repetition. Cognitive linguistic therapy helps patients improve comprehension. PACE uses conversation and visual images (pictures, drawings) to help identify the patient's preferred communication style and to promote language use.

96. A: A stroke in the left hemisphere is associated with right visual field deficit, tendency toward depression, slow, cautious behavior, and difficulty with mathematics. Other characteristics may include right paralysis or paresis, the need for frequent reinstruction and reinforcement. Intellectual ability may be altered, and the patient may have difficulty learning new material and may have short-term memory loss. Reading and writing impairment is common. Patients may have expressive, receptive, or global aphasia. The location of the stroke within the hemisphere impacts the outcome. A stroke in the frontal lobe is associated with increased loss of memory and difficulty learning.

97. C: Kegel exercises are intended to strengthen the pelvic floor muscles, which helps to prevent bladder incontinence. It allows the patient to be able to hold their urine until they get to a bathroom. The other interventions listed are important for the patient, but they do not actually help to improve the symptoms of urge bladder incontinence.

98. B: The Quality and Safety Education for Nurses initiative was started in 2005 with the objective to prepare future nurses for the challenge of improving the healthcare settings in which they work. It provides these nurses with the knowledge, skills, and attitudes (KSAs) needed to accomplish this goal.

99. C: There are many different anti-seizure medications available on the market, many of them generic, that are lower priced. The first step should be to ask the prescribing provider if a less expensive version of the medication can be called into the pharmacy. If not, and if this prescription is a long-term medication, it would be worthwhile to contact the pharmaceutical company to inquire about any programs that could help with the cost of the medication. Often, prior authorization can be completed if this medication cannot be replaced with something else.

100. D: Rehabilitation nursing is a specialty field of nursing. It involves providing care and treatment for those patients who have health problems that result in altered functional ability and an altered lifestyle. This field of nursing focuses on providing preventative care to avoid potential health problems that may occur as a result of a change in functional ability. It also has a strong focus on patient education to help with adjusting to the

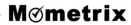

change in functional status they have acquired, along with self-care to prevent possible complications that may arise.

101. B: If a suppository is inserted into the rectum and stool is present, it should not be left in the stool. This will not allow the medication within the suppository to be absorbed in the mucous membranes of the rectum. If stool is present, the patient should be taught to gently remove the stool from the rectal vault before inserting the suppository. Those patients with autonomic dysreflexia may experience pain when a suppository is inserted. A topical anesthetic, such as xylocaine or lidocaine jelly, should be inserted into the rectum first to numb the area.

102. D: Conflict resolution should begin by allowing both sides to present their side of the conflict without bias, focusing on opinions rather than individuals. Other steps (not necessarily in order) include:

- Encourage cooperation through negotiation and compromise
- Maintain the focus, providing guidance to keep the discussions on track and avoid arguments
- Evaluate the need for renegotiation, formal resolution process, or third-party
- Utilize humor and empathy to diffuse escalating tensions
- Summarize the issues, outlining key arguments
- Avoid forcing resolution if possible

103. B: Keeping the patient awake and engaged during daytime hours and preventing or limiting daytime sleeping may help to reestablish a more normal awake-sleep pattern. Adjusting light (brighter in the daytime and lower at night) and placing clocks where the patient can see them or reminding the patient of the time may also help. However, despite these efforts, some people with dementia may be persistent in wandering at night. In this case, safety is a concern, and appropriate alarms and safety gates should be used. Side rails and restraints should be avoided as they may cause injury when the patient climbs over the rails or resists restraints.

104. B: The nursing process is a five-step process. The first step is assessing the patient and gathering data. The second step is formulating a list of nursing diagnoses based on the information gathered during the assessment phase. The third step is the planning phase in which the diagnoses are prioritized and the necessary nursing interventions are identified. The fourth step is the implementation phase in which the nursing interventions are put into place. The fifth step is evaluating the outcome and identifying if the interventions were sufficient to improve the patient outcome.

105. A: The Inpatient Rehabilitation Facility Patient Assessment Instrument (IRF-PAI) is the standardized assessment tool used for patients on admission to inpatient rehabilitation services in order to gather data on the patient's clinical condition and functional status. The IRF-PAI helps determine reimbursement rates; therefore, accuracy is very important. Direct measurement of height and weight must be done. For double amputees, the actual height (upper body plus the longest limb) is recorded, not the patient's height prior to the amputation.

106. C: A case mix group (CMG) is a classification system based on clinical characteristics of patients. Resource Utilization Group (RUG) is a classification system based on utilization of resources, with reimbursement tied to RUG level. The Outcome and Assessment Information Set (OASIS) is a dataset used by home health agencies (HHA) to measure outcomes and risk factors within a specified time frame. Minimum Data Set (MDS) contains elements to review for a comprehensive assessment of patient function. The MDS currently in use is MDS 3.0.

107. D: According to the Kübler-Ross model, known as the five stages of grief, this patient experienced initial denial, during which he remained detached. A stunned reaction after loss is typical as people try to grasp reality. As reality becomes clear, the patient may react with anger directed both inward and outward, sometimes exhibited as hostility, especially in men. During the bargaining stage, people may try to alter the outcome through prayer, promises to God, or changing physicians. Depression may cause withdrawal, sadness,

265

and requests to be left alone. The final stage, acceptance, may occur later as the person accepts the new reality and loses preoccupation with loss.

108. D: Pain receptors, or nociceptors, receive stimuli that send a signal to the brain that interpret these stimuli as pain. Polymodal receptors are responsible for sharp, intense pain and persistent, dull pain. Other types of nociceptors include mechanical, for pain from strong pressure and sharp objects; thermal, for pain caused by burns; and chemical, for pain from pH extremes and environmental irritants.

109. A: The Individuals with Disabilities Education Act (IDEA) was signed into law to ensure that all children have access to an appropriate education despite their disabilities. It also ensures that special education services are available to children. This was originally known as the Education of Handicapped Children Act, which was put into place in 1975. It was updated, amended, and the name changed to IDEA in 1990.

110. D: A patient with constipation issues due to a neurogenic bowel should follow a diet that has at least 15–30 grams of fiber daily (a high-fiber diet). High-fiber foods include whole grains, fresh fruits and vegetables, beans, and plain popcorn. As long as there are not any fluid restrictions due to other medical problems, such as renal disease or unstable heart failure, at least 1.5 L of fluid should be consumed to keep stool soft. Gas-producing foods, such as cabbage, cauliflower, and carrots, should be limited.

111. B: Patients with an injury at the C5 level will require assistance with most of the activities of daily living. With training, though, they should be able to operate a power wheelchair on their own. These patients will have partial or total paralysis of the wrists, hands, trunk, and legs, but may be able to raise their arms and bend their elbows. Breathing may be weakened, but they are still able to speak and use the diaphragm.

112. A: In a complex situation such as this, many care providers will be involved in the ongoing management of this patient with CF. The Case Manager or Social Work services available for discharge planning are a wonderful asset to have to coordinate all of the care necessary. Organizing a care meeting with the services that will be necessary at home can also be very helpful.

113. D: Methylprednisolone has been shown to improve neurologic function up to one year past an acute spinal cord injury. It is most successful if administered within 8 hours of the injury with a starting bolus dose of 30 mg/kg administered over 15 minutes. This is followed by an infusion of 5.4 mg/kg/hour administered over the following 23 hours. If the initiation of therapy is delayed, the maintenance infusion should be given for 48 hours. This has shown to provide the most improvement in neurologic function and significant improvement in motor function.

114. C: The team nursing model consists of a charge nurse or team leader, nurses, and nurse's aides or technicians. The charge nurse assigns patients to specific nurses and the nurses then delegate patient care responsibilities to the aides or technicians, within their scope of practice. It individualizes care for the patient depending on their specific needs, but it depends on everyone doing their part and providing the best care they can.

115. A: The referring provider should be open with the patient regarding the need for a specialty consultation. The reason for the consultation, along with the names of appropriate providers should be discussed. Once the patient agrees to be referred, all pertinent records should be sent to the consultant so that he or she is adequately informed of the patient's history.

116. B: Computer-supported prosthetics use a device that monitors the fit and function of a prosthetic limb. For example, a computer-supported prosthetic leg will send feedback to a computer identifying specific adjustments that need to be made to the limb in order for the patient to have a more accurate gait. In the past, minute adjustments needed to be made to the prosthesis by hand and these were not always completely accurate.

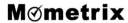

117. A: Acute care occurs following an injury or medical event and the main priority is patient survival while they are recuperating back to their baseline level before the event occurred. Following the acute care phase of treatment, rehabilitation occurs to focus on re-teaching patients how to perform their everyday self-care needs with the changes that have occurred. Of course, patient safety and survival are always the top priorities, but they are not the presenting challenges during rehabilitation.

118. D: The first step in a cultural assessment is to establish trust by respecting ethnic and cultural values and traditions, being a good listener, and making careful observations. Because a cultural assessment is part of an overall evaluation, asking permission or explaining the purpose of the cultural assessment specifically is usually not necessary. In some cultures, taking notes while talking is considered rude, so the nurse should explain the purpose and take brief notes, keeping the focus on the patient and family instead of the paperwork.

119. C: A bladder scan is a type of ultrasound that can be done in the office to measure the amount of residual urine in a patient's bladder. The patient is instructed to void and that amount of urine is measured. The bladder scan is then conducted and the amount of post-void residual urine in the bladder is measured. This should not be more than 100 mL. The patient could be catheterized and the urine measured, but the bladder scan is much more comfortable.

120. D: During REM sleep, the body relaxes and becomes more immobile, but the brain becomes more active. This is the stage of sleep in which most dreaming occurs and is characterized by an increase in respiratory rate and rapid eye movements. REM sleep usually occurs 90 minutes after sleep starts and the first REM cycle is usually the shortest. Periods of REM sleep gradually increase in length the longer a person sleeps.

121. C: A sleep study, or polysomnography, involves monitoring a patient during all phases of the sleep cycle. It can identify if there is an interruption in the sleep cycle that affects a person's ability to get deep, restful sleep. While commonly used to diagnose sleep apnea, a sleep study can also be used to diagnose REM sleep behavior disorders that occur when a person is acting out their dreams during sleep. It can also be used to diagnose narcolepsy, unexplained chronic insomnia, or a periodic limb movement disorder.

122. A: Patient-centered goals are those goals that are established by the patient as important to them. They reflect the patient's desire to gain more functionality and independence in a specific part of their life. For this patient, being able to feed herself so that she is not dependent on others to do this for her is important. Patient-centered goals need to be realistic and attainable. There may be one overall goal the patient wishes to achieve, but this may need to be broken down into smaller goals to gradually be achieved in order to complete the task.

123. B: Before taking any alternative medications, the patient's wife should first discuss this option with his physician. Though usually safe, some alternative medications can interfere with the prescribed medications he is taking, or they may be unsafe for him to take with his specific condition. The physician would do a full medication review in combination with researching natural remedies appropriate to his condition.

124. B: Orem's theory of self-care states there are two agents, the self-care agent (individual) and dependent-care agent (other caregiver), and three categories of needs: universal needs (food, air), developmental needs (from maturation or events), and health needs (from illness, injury). Orem believed the goal of nursing was to serve patients and assist them to provide self-care through identifying the reason a patient needs care, planning for delivery of care, and managing care. A self-care deficit occurs if the self-care agent cannot provide for his/her own care. Nursing assists by providing care, guiding, instructing, supporting, and adjusting the environment to aid patient in self-care.

125. A: Exercise has been proven to help patients suffering from depression by producing a release of endorphins, which can improve mood. The SSRI class of antidepressants cause an increase in serotonin levels within the brain. It has been found that a higher level of serotonin compared to dopamine within the brain can result in increased fatigue or lethargy. This is not noticeable in some patients but may be bothersome to others. Patients should be advised to continue with their current activity and exercise regimen and monitor for any side effects.

Answer Key and Explanations for Test #1

126. B: The Braden Scale (a risk assessment tool) predicts the patient's risk of developing pressure sores at the breakpoint for risk. The scale scores 6 different areas with 1–4 points:

- 23 (best score): excellent prognosis, very minimal risk
- ≤16: breakpoint for risk of pressure ulcer (will vary somewhat for different populations)
- 6 (worst score): prognosis is very poor, strong likelihood of developing pressure ulcers

A score of 2 in usual nutritional pattern is of concern because the patient is eating only about half of her food.

127. D: A power of attorney is someone that is assigned by the patient to have the legal authority to make financial decisions on their behalf when they are unable to. The healthcare proxy is a legal document that assigns all healthcare decision-making to a person when the patient is unable to. These can be the same person or two different people. It is ideal to have two people in these roles that can communicate and work well together, as their decision-making can affect the care that a patient receives.

128. B: Nursing quality indicators are part of a national database that is updated quarterly and annually. This reports the structure, process, and outcome indicators used to evaluate nursing care. These are measures that are considered nursing-sensitive because they are dependent upon the quality of nursing care. Nursing job satisfaction is also considered to be an indicator.

129. D: WHO's ICIDH defines handicap as those limitations and disadvantages that interfere with social functioning and ability to fulfill normal roles (such as the inability to be employed). Pathology is the underlying disorder (such as severing of the spinal cord). Impairment is the loss of function or structure related to physiology, anatomy, or psychology and is observable as signs and symptoms (such as right hemiparesis). Disability is the limit on function imposed by the pathology and impairment (such as the inability to walk unassisted).

130. B: Anticholinergics have been shown to slow rehabilitation in brain injury patients. These medications have been used to treat bladder incontinence and depression. They are also associated with cognitive impairment, dizziness, and confusion. Researchers have found a statistically significant increase in the length of patient hospitalization with the use of anticholinergics on a regular basis.

131. B: The IRF-PAI must be completed by day 5 post-discharge (including day of discharge). Submission of reports in a timely manner is critical for reimbursement. IRF-PAIs submitted by at least day 17 post-discharge are late, and those submitted by at least day 27 post-discharge incur a 25% penalty of the submitted claim. Other important dates include the completion of assessment of patient function by day 3 of admission, with information entered on data collection forms by day 4, and encoding per software by day 10.

132. A: Provider Orders for Life-Sustaining Treatment (POLST) is a document that outlines the specific medical treatments to be carried out by healthcare professionals in the event of a life-threatening crisis. It differs from an advanced directive in that it is identifiable through a community. It is a single-sheet, brightly colored paper and will often include specific treatments that can be carried out by emergency medical personnel before transporting to a medical facility. Use of the POLST was originally started in Oregon in 1991.

133. A: Capacity is often mistaken to mean the same thing as competency. Capacity is determined by a physician, often a psychiatrist, after a series of mental status tests are performed. Once the evaluation is completed, the physician can make a determination whether a person has the capacity to make important legal decisions.

134. B: Bromocriptine is a dopamine receptor agonist that has been helpful for those patients in a vegetative state or those with minimal consciousness. Amitriptyline and methylphenidate are usually given for agitation during the chronic phase (>1 month) following a traumatic brain injury. Levodopa, when combined with carbidopa, is often given for those patients in a vegetative state, but primarily during the chronic phase following a traumatic brain injury.

135. C: The MMSE is used as a preliminary screening tool for determining whether a patient has some cognitive impairment, however, it does have its limitations. Patients over the age of 60 and those with a low education level have been shown to score lower on the test than others. Further testing and work-up is indicated in order to make the diagnosis of dementia, and this should not be relied upon alone.

136. D: The Ranchos Los Amigos scale is used to describe the activity level of a person with a brain injury. It assesses the patient based on 8 levels of activity, ranging from no activity level up to a purposeful/appropriate level of activity. Patients may transition from one level to another without actually entering the level of activity at each individual level. Some patients may plateau at one level without ever reaching the highest level.

137. C: At 12–18 months, a child should begin first words, imitate sounds, follow vocal directions, and point to familiar items when asked. Normal hearing responses:

- ≤ 3 months: positive Moro (startle) reflex to sound, noise disturbs sleep, and reacts to sounds by opening eyes or blinking
- 3–6 months: comforts at sound of parent's voice and tries to emulate sounds; looks in the direction of sound
- 6–12 months: begins to vocalize more with cooing and gurgling with different inflections, responds to name and simple words, and looks in the direction of sound
- 18–24 months: more verbal with about half of vocabulary understandable and knows about 20–50 words; points to body parts or familiar objects when asked

138. B: Kubler-Ross identified 5 phases that a person will go through during the grieving process. These are denial, anger, bargaining, depression, and acceptance. A person does not pass through these phases during the grieving process on a step-by-step basis. They may drift in and out of one phase and into another very fluidly. They may also go back to phases they experienced and go through them again.

139. B: Tolterodine is highly specific to receptors within the bladder, so it is least likely to have systemic anticholinergic side effects. Most of the medications for neurogenic bladder work by blocking the neurotransmitter acetylcholine, which causes muscles to contract. By blocking this neurotransmitter, the detrusor muscle at the bladder neck can relax, which allows it to empty.

140. D: The nurse functions as a patient advocate through many different actions, but the overall goal is to keep the patient safe and ensure they are receiving the highest quality of care possible. This can involve providing necessary education about a disease state or coordinating efforts with many providers for the patient to receive all of the necessary care they need.

141. D: A neurogenic bladder is a condition in which there is no neurologic control of the bladder. These patients usually have urinary retention and do not have the ability to relax the muscles around the bladder neck to express urine. A short-term, or intermittent, catheter should be used for these patients to empty their bladder. They should be trained to perform self-catheterization using a clean technique so that the bladder can be emptied on a regular schedule.

142. D: The Lawton Instrumental Activities of Daily Living Scale is valuable for determining baseline functional ability on admission and progress during treatment as well as the need for supportive services. It assesses eight abilities:

- Telephone use: look up numbers and/or call numbers
- Shopping: food, clothes, or needed items
- Food preparation: plan diet and prepare food
- Housekeeping: perform all or part of household duties
- Laundry: wash all or some personal clothes and linen
- Transportation availability: ability to drive or use public transportation

- Medication: responsible for managing prescriptions and taking medications
- Financial responsibility: keep track of finances, pay bills, and budget correctly

143. D: Physical Therapy is not currently able to bill Medicare for telehealth services. There are currently no telehealth-specific CPT codes available for billing for PT services. Rarely, some private insurance policies will cover telehealth PT services, but this is not a standard service covered and patients will need to contact their insurance company to inquire about coverage. Medicaid does reimburse for telehealth services and has since 2002, but not in all 50 states.

144. A: The Agency for Healthcare Research and Quality was established in 1989 to increase the quality and effectiveness of healthcare by supporting research projects, developing guidelines, and releasing information on healthcare services and delivery systems. It has come under some scrutiny at times and there are plans to merge this agency with the National Institutes of Health.

145. C: The purpose of quality improvement is to implement specific changes in healthcare that have a measurable improvement for a group of patients. Quality improvement is instrumental in improving the way healthcare services are provided, while continually measuring the effect those changes have on the health status of the patients served. This is often measured through patient satisfaction information.

146. B: All of these elements (patient motivation, family support, and reimbursement) are important; however, linking to community services is essential to the success of the early supported discharge model of care. Community services may include meal delivery service and home health agency care. This model decreases the duration of inpatient care but is most appropriate for those with mild disabilities because those with more severe disabilities may need inpatient care and regular contact with physicians.

147. C: The Improving Medicare Post-Acute Care Transformation Act (IMPACT Act) of 2014 requires reporting of standardized patient assessment data elements by long-term care facilities, skilled nursing facilities, home health agencies, and inpatient rehabilitation facilities (IRFs) for Medicare beneficiaries. Quality measure domains include skin integrity/change in skin integrity, functional status and cognitive status, medication reconciliation, incidence of major falls, and transfer of health information and care preferences during transitions.

148. C: Kurt Lewin was considered the father of social psychology. He developed a change theory for nursing that consisted of unfreezing, changing, and refreezing. The unfreezing stage involved examining the old way a patient would perform specific tasks. The changing stage involved teaching the new way to do things and ensuring the patient understood how a specific task would need to be done. The refreezing stage made the new process the standard of how a specific task would be performed from that point forward.

149. C: The Glasgow Coma Scale (GCS) measures the depth and duration of coma or impaired level of consciousness and is used for postoperative assessment. A score of 10 is consistent with a moderate head injury. The GCS measures 3 parameters: best eye response (1–4), best verbal response (1–5), and best motor response (1–6), with a total possible score that ranges from 3–15. Injuries/conditions are classified according to the total score: 3–8, coma; 8 or less, severe head injury; 9–12, moderate head injury; 13–15, mild head injury.

150. A: Cardiac rehabilitation includes both short-term goals and long-term goals. Long-term goals include reversing or stabilizing atherosclerosis, usually through medications, diet, and exercise programs. Other long-term goals include identifying and treating associated risk factors to prevent further cardiovascular disease and promoting healthy psychological functioning. Short-term goals may include reducing risk of reinfarction, managing/controlling symptoms, improving patient's physical conditioning, and reducing psychological stress related to cardiac disease and treatment.

151. C: The ethical theory of deontology was originated from Immanuel Kant. It states that actions should not be judged on their outcome, but rather on their intent. If an action is performed with good and honest intentions, it should be assessed based on that intent rather than a possible poor outcome. This theory asks that the intended moral worth of the action be examined. This can be applied to nursing actions when providing patient care. It is also used as a basis for many religious traditions.

152. B: Current guidelines following the diabetic food pyramid suggest 6–11 servings of grains and starches daily. This category includes complex grains such as oats and rye, but it also includes starchy vegetables. A serving of starchy vegetables, such as potatoes or corn, contain about as many carbohydrates as a slice of bread. Most people do not eat a full 11 servings of grains and starches daily and tend to lean toward the lower end of this range.

153. B: The Plan, Do, Check, Act cycle is used to implement change, solve problems, and continuously improve a process. It starts with planning the elements of change, putting them in place on a small scale in order to test the change, checking the effectiveness of this change, and then acting on putting the change in place on a broader scale. It is a continuous cycle that allows for alterations in the plan until the change is deemed effective.

154. C: Support groups allow a person to feel like they are not alone in their situation. They are a resource where someone can find ways to work through a specific problem or disability by learning from others who have gone through the same process. A person is not required to speak and tell their own story, but it is often helpful to do so. The support group provides an opportunity to gain insight into a problem and learn how others have succeeded in adapting to that problem. Support group meetings should not be complaining or blaming sessions, but rather, a therapeutic environment for people to share, learn, and gain comfort.

155. D: The best time for scheduled evacuation is 20–30 minutes after a meal because eating stimulates motility. The scheduled time (usually daily but may be 3–4 times weekly, depending on individual habits) should be at the same time each day, so work hours or activities should be considered. Stimulation may include drinking hot liquid or rectal stimulation (inserting a gloved, lubricated finger into the anus and running it around the rim of the sphincters). The best position for defecation is upright and leaning forward with knees elevated slightly. The patient should massage the abdomen, strain, and attempt to tighten abdominal muscles and relax sphincters if possible.

156. B: Intermittent pneumatic compression devices are useful in preventing DVT's in those with high risk (immobility, coagulation disorders, status post-operative, etc.) Pneumatic compression stockings should be fit appropriately for the patient. They come in various styles to provide foot, calf, or full leg compression intermittently in order to cause rhythmic compression of the blood vessels and promote blood circulation. They should not be used when there is a known DVT present as this can increase the risk for an embolism.

157. C: The Harris-Benedict formula has been considered the standard guideline for estimating calorie requirements for the acutely ill, hospitalized patient. It uses the basal energy expenditure, activity factor, and injury factor to make this estimation. The activity factor is a number given based on activity level, from sedentary to extra active. The injury factor is based on the type of trauma the patient has sustained, for example, infection, burns, or trauma.

158. C: Heterotropic ossification (development of bony tissue outside of the skeleton, especially near the hip and knee joints) with fusion of the joint or stiffening is best prevented by passive range of motion exercises, although excessive stretching should be avoided and range of motion withheld if inflammation is present. Another problem common to spinal cord injury is osteoporosis, and using a standing frame or braces to facilitate weight bearing may slow development of osteoporosis. Careful handling of limbs can help prevent inadvertent fractures.

159. B: The Smart Glove is a technological assistive device that is worn by a patient during rehabilitation from a stroke or other condition that has affected their ability to achieve hand and finger mobility. It is operated through a Bluetooth connection to record the range of motion a person has while performing specific tasks,

271

usually in a game format. The tasks can be individualized based on a patient's progress with achieving basic range of motion activities up to more advanced fine motor skills.

160. B: Stress in a person's work environment is normal to a certain degree. When the stress is excessive, though, it begins to affect our everyday lives and is exhibited by being short-tempered, not sleeping well, withdrawing, feeling overwhelmed, or self-medicating with alcohol or drugs. It is important to recognize these signs of stress so that they can be addressed when they occur and steps can be taken to decrease stress within the work environment. Prolonged stress can increase the risk for hypertension, heart disease, and diabetes.

161. A: Since the most common causes of autonomic dysreflexia are bladder distention and bowel distention (feces and/or gas), he should do a digital exam to promote a bowel movement. He may use an anesthetic ointment to prevent further stimulation. Because BP rises and heart rate falls, the patient should sit up in order to decrease BP and reduce risk of stroke. The patient should also loosen clothes and check for sores (such as on the feet) or ingrown toenails. Calling 911 for treatment in an emergency department is necessary only if other methods are unsuccessful. Medications may be indicated if trigger cannot be identified and remedied.

162. C: A third-party payer is an organization that pays for the medical expenses of a person. This is usually a health insurance company such as Medicare, Medicaid, or private health insurance. The patient is the first-party payer who purchases the health insurance policy.

163. A: Body transcendence versus body preoccupation is a task of older adulthood and a negative outcome can result in failure to accept the physical/functional changes of aging, leading to despair and fear of death. Other tasks of older adulthood include ego transcendence versus ego preoccupation and ego differentiation versus work role preoccupation. A positive outcome for all tasks of older adulthood leads to meaningful life after retirement, acceptance of bodily/functional changes, acceptance of death, and feeling that life has been good.

164. A: The nurse should advise the parents that information regarding the patient's condition is private because he is an adult. The Health Insurance Portability and Accountability Act (HIPAA) states that health care providers must not release any information or documentation about a patient's condition or treatment without consent, as the individual has the right to determine who has access to personal information. Personal information about the patient is considered protected health information (PHI) and consists of any identifying or personal information about the patient, such as health history, condition, or treatments in any form, and any documentation, including electronic, verbal, or written. Telling patients what they "should" do is inappropriate.

165. D: Early indications of autism include avoiding eye contact, resisting being held, and regressing in language skills. While focusing on a single item or toy, throwing temper tantrums, and repetitive behavior such as rocking back and forth and banging the head against a wall are also common with autism, these behaviors frequently occur in non-autistic 2- or 3-year-olds. Other behavioral indications of autism include development of ritual behavior, sensitivity to light and sound, insensitivity to pain, and constant activity.

166. D: Esophageal dysphagia is due to a blockage within the esophagus that prevents a bolus of food from passing down to the stomach. This usually requires surgery to correct. Oral, epiglottis, and pharyngeal dysphagia occur when there is weakness in the tongue or a neurological problem interfering with pharyngeal motility. These are usually caused by a stroke.

167. A: The role model in nursing is someone that is looked up to because of their day-to-day interactions with patients and the way in which they perform their job responsibilities. The role model is the nursing professional that other nurses, or nursing students, strive to emulate. This is not necessarily a formal position with set responsibilities in educating others, though others can learn how to provide compassionate care from this person.

168. C: Constant dribbling of urine is an indication of overflow incontinence, which can result from diabetic nerve damage that causes a loss of sensation so that urinary retention and bladder distension occurs. Induced incontinence may result from surgical procedures (hysterectomy, prostatectomy, rectal surgery) that damage nerves or muscles that control urination. Urge incontinence is an urgency to urinate as soon as the bladder feels full, so a person may urinate on the way to the toilet or in bed during the night. Functional incontinence is caused by physical or mental impairment, such as dementia, and may also relate to environmental barriers, such as no accessible bathroom.

169. A: Measuring urine output is the most sensitive of these interventions to determine if a fluid volume deficit is occurring. On average, a person should urinate approx. 30 mL/hour. For instance, if 210 mL of urine is measured over a 6-hour period, you know that they have urinated 35 mL/hour on average, which is appropriate. The other interventions are additional ways in which fluid volume status can be assessed, but a change in daily weight can often be a later sign of an abnormality. Skin turgor assessment is not just sensitive to fluid volume, nor is an elevation in heart rate.

170. C: Biofeedback therapy involves undergoing electronic monitoring of certain bodily functions in order to gain willful control of them. Biofeedback can help with chronic pain by helping them to focus on changing the perception of pain they are experiencing. It can also be used to try to control heart rate, blood pressure, migraine headaches, and incontinence.

171. D: Features of a manic state include inflated self-esteem, excessive talking or pressured speech, psychomotor agitation, decreased need for sleep and insomnia, and excessive involvement in pleasurable activities that can have negative consequences. These symptoms interfere with daily life, employment, and maintaining healthy relationships and do not occur as a result of drug abuse.

172. D: The side-lying position with rear entry is usually the most successful to allow intercourse for a woman with flexion contractures from cerebral palsy (or arthritis). Placing a bolster between the legs may help to reduce spasticity and scissoring of the legs. To reduce the chance of stress incontinence during coitus, the patient should be advised to reduce fluid intake for about 3 hours prior to intercourse and to urinate immediately before to ensure that the bladder is empty. If her partner also has disabilities, further accommodations may be needed.

173. A: Dysarthria results from damage to the motor neurons responsible for lip, tongue, and vocal cord control. It is the inability to correctly form words that can be understood. It does not involve any impairment in understanding speech, which is aphasia. Apraxia is the inability to perform specific functions or movements due to paralysis. Ataxia also refers to a loss of control of body movements, especially when ambulating.

174. C: In most states, nurses, other healthcare workers, teachers, and other professionals that provide services to children, have a legal responsibility to report suspected abuse to the appropriate authorities. Failure to report your suspicions could result in disciplinary action by your state nursing licensing board. Be sure to know your state laws pertaining to your responsibilities to report suspected abuse.

175. D: FIM scores range from 18 (total dependence) to 126 (total independence), and a score of 63 comprised of 3 or 4 in each of 18 categories suggests the need for minimal to moderate contact assistance. The patient will require an aide to assist with ambulation and other activities. Lower FIM scores on admission correlate with longer need for inpatient rehabilitation. FIM scores are included as part of the Inpatient Rehabilitation Facility Patient Assessment Instrument required by Medicare for reimbursement for care.

CRRN Practice Test #2

To take this additional practice test, visit our bonus page:
mometrix.com/bonus948/crrn

How to Overcome Test Anxiety

Just the thought of taking a test is enough to make most people a little nervous. A test is an important event that can have a long-term impact on your future, so it's important to take it seriously and it's natural to feel anxious about performing well. But just because anxiety is normal, that doesn't mean that it's helpful in test taking, or that you should simply accept it as part of your life. Anxiety can have a variety of effects. These effects can be mild, like making you feel slightly nervous, or severe, like blocking your ability to focus or remember even a simple detail.

If you experience test anxiety—whether severe or mild—it's important to know how to beat it. To discover this, first you need to understand what causes test anxiety.

Causes of Test Anxiety

While we often think of anxiety as an uncontrollable emotional state, it can actually be caused by simple, practical things. One of the most common causes of test anxiety is that a person does not feel adequately prepared for their test. This feeling can be the result of many different issues such as poor study habits or lack of organization, but the most common culprit is time management. Starting to study too late, failing to organize your study time to cover all of the material, or being distracted while you study will mean that you're not well prepared for the test. This may lead to cramming the night before, which will cause you to be physically and mentally exhausted for the test. Poor time management also contributes to feelings of stress, fear, and hopelessness as you realize you are not well prepared but don't know what to do about it.

Other times, test anxiety is not related to your preparation for the test but comes from unresolved fear. This may be a past failure on a test, or poor performance on tests in general. It may come from comparing yourself to others who seem to be performing better or from the stress of living up to expectations. Anxiety may be driven by fears of the future—how failure on this test would affect your educational and career goals. These fears are often completely irrational, but they can still negatively impact your test performance.

Elements of Test Anxiety

As mentioned earlier, test anxiety is considered to be an emotional state, but it has physical and mental components as well. Sometimes you may not even realize that you are suffering from test anxiety until you notice the physical symptoms. These can include trembling hands, rapid heartbeat, sweating, nausea, and tense muscles. Extreme anxiety may lead to fainting or vomiting. Obviously, any of these symptoms can have a negative impact on testing. It is important to recognize them as soon as they begin to occur so that you can address the problem before it damages your performance.

The mental components of test anxiety include trouble focusing and inability to remember learned information. During a test, your mind is on high alert, which can help you recall information and stay focused for an extended period of time. However, anxiety interferes with your mind's natural processes, causing you to blank out, even on the questions you know well. The strain of testing during anxiety makes it difficult to stay focused, especially on a test that may take several hours. Extreme anxiety can take a huge mental toll, making it difficult not only to recall test information but even to understand the test questions or pull your thoughts together.

Effects of Test Anxiety

Test anxiety is like a disease—if left untreated, it will get progressively worse. Anxiety leads to poor performance, and this reinforces the feelings of fear and failure, which in turn lead to poor performances on subsequent tests. It can grow from a mild nervousness to a crippling condition. If allowed to progress, test anxiety can have a big impact on your schooling, and consequently on your future.

Test anxiety can spread to other parts of your life. Anxiety on tests can become anxiety in any stressful situation, and blanking on a test can turn into panicking in a job situation. But fortunately, you don't have to let anxiety rule your testing and determine your grades. There are a number of relatively simple steps you can take to move past anxiety and function normally on a test and in the rest of life.

Physical Steps for Beating Test Anxiety

While test anxiety is a serious problem, the good news is that it can be overcome. It doesn't have to control your ability to think and remember information. While it may take time, you can begin taking steps today to beat anxiety.

Just as your first hint that you may be struggling with anxiety comes from the physical symptoms, the first step to treating it is also physical. Rest is crucial for having a clear, strong mind. If you are tired, it is much easier to give in to anxiety. But if you establish good sleep habits, your body and mind will be ready to perform optimally, without the strain of exhaustion. Additionally, sleeping well helps you to retain information better, so you're more likely to recall the answers when you see the test questions.

Getting good sleep means more than going to bed on time. It's important to allow your brain time to relax. Take study breaks from time to time so it doesn't get overworked, and don't study right before bed. Take time to rest your mind before trying to rest your body, or you may find it difficult to fall asleep.

Along with sleep, other aspects of physical health are important in preparing for a test. Good nutrition is vital for good brain function. Sugary foods and drinks may give a burst of energy but this burst is followed by a crash, both physically and emotionally. Instead, fuel your body with protein and vitamin-rich foods.

Also, drink plenty of water. Dehydration can lead to headaches and exhaustion, especially if your brain is already under stress from the rigors of the test. Particularly if your test is a long one, drink water during the breaks. And if possible, take an energy-boosting snack to eat between sections.

Along with sleep and diet, a third important part of physical health is exercise. Maintaining a steady workout schedule is helpful, but even taking 5-minute study breaks to walk can help get your blood pumping faster and clear your head. Exercise also releases endorphins, which contribute to a positive feeling and can help combat test anxiety.

When you nurture your physical health, you are also contributing to your mental health. If your body is healthy, your mind is much more likely to be healthy as well. So take time to rest, nourish your body with healthy food and water, and get moving as much as possible. Taking these physical steps will make you stronger and more able to take the mental steps necessary to overcome test anxiety.

Mental Steps for Beating Test Anxiety

Working on the mental side of test anxiety can be more challenging, but as with the physical side, there are clear steps you can take to overcome it. As mentioned earlier, test anxiety often stems from lack of preparation, so the obvious solution is to prepare for the test. Effective studying may be the most important weapon you have for beating test anxiety, but you can and should employ several other mental tools to combat fear.

First, boost your confidence by reminding yourself of past success—tests or projects that you aced. If you're putting as much effort into preparing for this test as you did for those, there's no reason you should expect to fail here. Work hard to prepare; then trust your preparation.

Second, surround yourself with encouraging people. It can be helpful to find a study group, but be sure that the people you're around will encourage a positive attitude. If you spend time with others who are anxious or cynical, this will only contribute to your own anxiety. Look for others who are motivated to study hard from a desire to succeed, not from a fear of failure.

Third, reward yourself. A test is physically and mentally tiring, even without anxiety, and it can be helpful to have something to look forward to. Plan an activity following the test, regardless of the outcome, such as going to a movie or getting ice cream.

When you are taking the test, if you find yourself beginning to feel anxious, remind yourself that you know the material. Visualize successfully completing the test. Then take a few deep, relaxing breaths and return to it. Work through the questions carefully but with confidence, knowing that you are capable of succeeding.

Developing a healthy mental approach to test taking will also aid in other areas of life. Test anxiety affects more than just the actual test—it can be damaging to your mental health and even contribute to depression. It's important to beat test anxiety before it becomes a problem for more than testing.

Study Strategy

Being prepared for the test is necessary to combat anxiety, but what does being prepared look like? You may study for hours on end and still not feel prepared. What you need is a strategy for test prep. The next few pages outline our recommended steps to help you plan out and conquer the challenge of preparation.

STEP 1: SCOPE OUT THE TEST

Learn everything you can about the format (multiple choice, essay, etc.) and what will be on the test. Gather any study materials, course outlines, or sample exams that may be available. Not only will this help you to prepare, but knowing what to expect can help to alleviate test anxiety.

STEP 2: MAP OUT THE MATERIAL

Look through the textbook or study guide and make note of how many chapters or sections it has. Then divide these over the time you have. For example, if a book has 15 chapters and you have five days to study, you need to cover three chapters each day. Even better, if you have the time, leave an extra day at the end for overall review after you have gone through the material in depth.

If time is limited, you may need to prioritize the material. Look through it and make note of which sections you think you already have a good grasp on, and which need review. While you are studying, skim quickly through the familiar sections and take more time on the challenging parts. Write out your plan so you don't get lost as you go. Having a written plan also helps you feel more in control of the study, so anxiety is less likely to arise from feeling overwhelmed at the amount to cover.

STEP 3: GATHER YOUR TOOLS

Decide what study method works best for you. Do you prefer to highlight in the book as you study and then go back over the highlighted portions? Or do you type out notes of the important information? Or is it helpful to make flashcards that you can carry with you? Assemble the pens, index cards, highlighters, post-it notes, and any other materials you may need so you won't be distracted by getting up to find things while you study.

If you're having a hard time retaining the information or organizing your notes, experiment with different methods. For example, try color-coding by subject with colored pens, highlighters, or post-it notes. If you learn better by hearing, try recording yourself reading your notes so you can listen while in the car, working out, or simply sitting at your desk. Ask a friend to quiz you from your flashcards, or try teaching someone the material to solidify it in your mind.

STEP 4: CREATE YOUR ENVIRONMENT

It's important to avoid distractions while you study. This includes both the obvious distractions like visitors and the subtle distractions like an uncomfortable chair (or a too-comfortable couch that makes you want to fall asleep). Set up the best study environment possible: good lighting and a comfortable work area. If background music helps you focus, you may want to turn it on, but otherwise keep the room quiet. If you are using a computer to take notes, be sure you don't have any other windows open, especially applications like social media, games, or anything else that could distract you. Silence your phone and turn off notifications. Be sure to keep water close by so you stay hydrated while you study (but avoid unhealthy drinks and snacks).

Also, take into account the best time of day to study. Are you freshest first thing in the morning? Try to set aside some time then to work through the material. Is your mind clearer in the afternoon or evening? Schedule your study session then. Another method is to study at the same time of day that you will take the test, so that your brain gets used to working on the material at that time and will be ready to focus at test time.

STEP 5: STUDY!

Once you have done all the study preparation, it's time to settle into the actual studying. Sit down, take a few moments to settle your mind so you can focus, and begin to follow your study plan. Don't give in to distractions or let yourself procrastinate. This is your time to prepare so you'll be ready to fearlessly approach the test. Make the most of the time and stay focused.

Of course, you don't want to burn out. If you study too long you may find that you're not retaining the information very well. Take regular study breaks. For example, taking five minutes out of every hour to walk briskly, breathing deeply and swinging your arms, can help your mind stay fresh.

As you get to the end of each chapter or section, it's a good idea to do a quick review. Remind yourself of what you learned and work on any difficult parts. When you feel that you've mastered the material, move on to the next part. At the end of your study session, briefly skim through your notes again.

But while review is helpful, cramming last minute is NOT. If at all possible, work ahead so that you won't need to fit all your study into the last day. Cramming overloads your brain with more information than it can process and retain, and your tired mind may struggle to recall even previously learned information when it is overwhelmed with last-minute study. Also, the urgent nature of cramming and the stress placed on your brain contribute to anxiety. You'll be more likely to go to the test feeling unprepared and having trouble thinking clearly.

So don't cram, and don't stay up late before the test, even just to review your notes at a leisurely pace. Your brain needs rest more than it needs to go over the information again. In fact, plan to finish your studies by noon or early afternoon the day before the test. Give your brain the rest of the day to relax or focus on other things, and get a good night's sleep. Then you will be fresh for the test and better able to recall what you've studied.

STEP 6: TAKE A PRACTICE TEST

Many courses offer sample tests, either online or in the study materials. This is an excellent resource to check whether you have mastered the material, as well as to prepare for the test format and environment.

Check the test format ahead of time: the number of questions, the type (multiple choice, free response, etc.), and the time limit. Then create a plan for working through them. For example, if you have 30 minutes to take a 60-question test, your limit is 30 seconds per question. Spend less time on the questions you know well so that you can take more time on the difficult ones.

If you have time to take several practice tests, take the first one open book, with no time limit. Work through the questions at your own pace and make sure you fully understand them. Gradually work up to taking a test under test conditions: sit at a desk with all study materials put away and set a timer. Pace yourself to make sure you finish the test with time to spare and go back to check your answers if you have time.

After each test, check your answers. On the questions you missed, be sure you understand why you missed them. Did you misread the question (tests can use tricky wording)? Did you forget the information? Or was it something you hadn't learned? Go back and study any shaky areas that the practice tests reveal.

Taking these tests not only helps with your grade, but also aids in combating test anxiety. If you're already used to the test conditions, you're less likely to worry about it, and working through tests until you're scoring well gives you a confidence boost. Go through the practice tests until you feel comfortable, and then you can go into the test knowing that you're ready for it.

Test Tips

On test day, you should be confident, knowing that you've prepared well and are ready to answer the questions. But aside from preparation, there are several test day strategies you can employ to maximize your performance.

First, as stated before, get a good night's sleep the night before the test (and for several nights before that, if possible). Go into the test with a fresh, alert mind rather than staying up late to study.

Try not to change too much about your normal routine on the day of the test. It's important to eat a nutritious breakfast, but if you normally don't eat breakfast at all, consider eating just a protein bar. If you're a coffee drinker, go ahead and have your normal coffee. Just make sure you time it so that the caffeine doesn't wear off right in the middle of your test. Avoid sugary beverages, and drink enough water to stay hydrated but not so much that you need a restroom break 10 minutes into the test. If your test isn't first thing in the morning, consider going for a walk or doing a light workout before the test to get your blood flowing.

Allow yourself enough time to get ready, and leave for the test with plenty of time to spare so you won't have the anxiety of scrambling to arrive in time. Another reason to be early is to select a good seat. It's helpful to sit away from doors and windows, which can be distracting. Find a good seat, get out your supplies, and settle your mind before the test begins.

When the test begins, start by going over the instructions carefully, even if you already know what to expect. Make sure you avoid any careless mistakes by following the directions.

Then begin working through the questions, pacing yourself as you've practiced. If you're not sure on an answer, don't spend too much time on it, and don't let it shake your confidence. Either skip it and come back later, or eliminate as many wrong answers as possible and guess among the remaining ones. Don't dwell on these questions as you continue—put them out of your mind and focus on what lies ahead.

Be sure to read all of the answer choices, even if you're sure the first one is the right answer. Sometimes you'll find a better one if you keep reading. But don't second-guess yourself if you do immediately know the answer. Your gut instinct is usually right. Don't let test anxiety rob you of the information you know.

If you have time at the end of the test (and if the test format allows), go back and review your answers. Be cautious about changing any, since your first instinct tends to be correct, but make sure you didn't misread any of the questions or accidentally mark the wrong answer choice. Look over any you skipped and make an educated guess.

At the end, leave the test feeling confident. You've done your best, so don't waste time worrying about your performance or wishing you could change anything. Instead, celebrate the successful completion of this test. And finally, use this test to learn how to deal with anxiety even better next time.

> **Review Video: <u>Test Anxiety</u>**
> Visit mometrix.com/academy and enter code: 100340

Important Qualification

Not all anxiety is created equal. If your test anxiety is causing major issues in your life beyond the classroom or testing center, or if you are experiencing troubling physical symptoms related to your anxiety, it may be a sign of a serious physiological or psychological condition. If this sounds like your situation, we strongly encourage you to seek professional help.

Additional Bonus Material

Due to our efforts to try to keep this book to a manageable length, we've created a link that will give you access to all of your additional bonus material:

mometrix.com/bonus948/crrn